Prentice Hall Health
review manual
for the EMT-Basic
Self-Assessment Exam Prep

Joseph J. Mistovich, M.Ed., NREMT-P
Chair and Associate Professor
Department of Health Professions
Youngstown State University
Youngstown, Ohio

Edward B. Kuvlesky, AAS, NREMT-P
Battalion Chief
Indian River County EMS
Indian River County, Florida

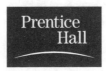

Prentice
Hall

Upper Saddle River, New Jersey 07458

Library of Congress Cataloging-in-Publication Data

Mistovich, Joseph J.
  Prentice Hall Health's Q & A review EMT-basic self assessment exam prep /
Joseph J. Mistovich, Edward B. Kuvleskey.
     p. cm. — (Prentice Hall Health review series)
  Includes index.
  ISBN 0-8359-5134-0 (alk. paper)
    1. Emergency medicine—Examinations, questions, etc. 2. Emergency medical
technicians—Examinations, questions, etc. I. Title: Q & A review EMT-basic self
assessment review manual. II. Title: Prentice-Hall Health's questions & answer review
EMT-basic self assessment review manual. III. Title: EMT-basic self-assessment exam
prep. IV. Kuvleskey, Edward B. V. Title. VI. Series.

RC86.9 .M563 2003
616.02'5'076—dc21   2002038112

Publisher: Julie Levin Alexander
Publisher's Assistant: Regina Bruno
Executive Editor: Marlene Pratt
Editorial Assistant: Monica Silva
Senior Managing Editor: Lois Berlowitz
Director of Production and Manufacturing: Bruce Johnson
Managing Production Editor: Patrick Walsh
Manufacturing Manager: Ilene Sanford
Manufacturing Buyer: Pat Brown
Production Liaison: Jeanne Molenaar
Production Editor: Emily Bush, Carlisle Communications, Inc.
Design Director: Cheryl Asherman
Design Coordinator: Maria Guglielmo-Walsh
Cover and Interior Design: Janice Bielawa
Senior Marketing Manager: Katrin Beacom
Product Information Manager: Rachele Strober
Composition: Carlisle Communications, Inc.
Printing and Binding: Banta Harrisonburg
Cover Printer: Phoenix Color

Pearson Education LTD.
Pearson Education Australia PTY, Limited
Pearson Education Singapore, Pte. Ltd
Pearson Education North Asia Ltd
Pearson Education Canada, Ltd
Pearson Educación de Mexico, S.A. de C.V.
Pearson Education—Japan
Pearson Education Malaysia, Pte. Ltd

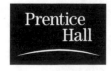

10 9 8 7
ISBN 0-8359-5134-0

Contents

Preface

The purpose of this review manual is to help prepare you for examinations in your EMT-Basic course and your certification examination. The manual consists of a series of self-assessment sections that can identify your strengths and weaknesses in relation to the information you are studying. If you are a currently certified EMT-Basic, this manual can serve as a refresher tool itself or as a method to determine where your knowledge has deteriorated and the need for specific review.

The *EMT-Basic Self-Assessment Exam Prep* consists of multiple-choice type items that are organized according to the U.S. Department of Transportation's National Standard EMT-Basic Curriculum. Enhancement sections are included on stroke, seizures, and abdominal pain that are beyond the D.O.T. curriculum. Every item has a corresponding answer and rationale. In addition, every item, with the exception of those that are considered "enhancement items," is referenced to a specific D.O.T. objective. This can be found in the Answers and Rationales section. Therefore, it is possible for you to refer back to any one of the EMT-Basic textbooks for more specific information on that item or overall concept.

The authors, contributing item writer, and manuscript reviewers all have extensive knowledge and experience as EMS educators. The items they contributed were developed in a "teacher-made test format" to allow you to test your knowledge and understanding of the material. When compiled into a series of sections, the items serve as a self-assessment tool to identify particular strengths and weaknesses in your knowledge and understanding of the information. This allows you to concentrate on specific sections that have been identified as a weakness. A comprehensive examination has also been provided to allow you to test your knowledge at the EMT-Basic level.

This manual should be used as a tool to better prepare you for your examinations. However, there is no better preparation than studying and understanding the information that has been presented to you in your course. To best ensure your success on the examination, we encourage you to study first until you feel confident that you know the information and then use this manual as a self-assessment to determine how well you know the information. When you have identified areas of weakness, do not simply study the manual or review items. Go back and study the information presented to you, study the textbook, and use other sources to better understand the information. Once you again feel confident you know the material, retest yourself using the review manual to determine if you are better prepared for that section.

We hope this manual assists you in preparing for your examination. However, when it comes time to manage a patient in the prehospital environment, there is no time for preparation. You must draw on your existing knowledge and skills to successfully and efficiently treat the patient. Thus, it is imperative to good patient care that you are truly prepared not only to pass that examination but to take care of each and every patient you encounter to the best of your ability. Good luck in your EMS endeavors!

Joseph J. Mistovich
Edward B. Kuvlesky

SPECIAL ACKNOWLEDGMENT

We would like to thank Helen Verdream for her assistance in putting the material together in this book. Her skill, patience, and constant words of encouragement were invaluable in moving this project to completion. Thank you!

CONTRIBUTORS

Craig N. Story, BS, EMT-P
Former EMS Program Director
Polk Community College
Winter Haven, Florida

Matthew S. Zavarella, BSAS, NREMT-P
Program Director
Paramedic Education
Medical College of Ohio
Toledo, Ohio

REVIEWERS

Rhonda J. Beck, NREMT-P
Houston County EMS
Central Georgia Technical College

Stephen J. Rahm, NREMT-P
Dept. of Combat Medical Training
Fort Sam Houston, Texas

Eric Stokley, AAS, EMT-P
Global Education
Lilburn, Georgia

Dedication

This book is dedicated in memory of my father, who provided me with the love and encouragement that allowed me to pursue my dreams. He will always be my inspiration to continue living life to its fullest, no matter what obstacles I encounter. To my beautiful wife Andrea, who continues to be my greatest supporter and best friend. To my wonderful children, Katie, Kristyn, Chelsea, Morgan, and Kara for helping me get through another project. Your energy, hugs, kisses, and smiles make every day so much brighter! I love you all dearly!

Joseph J. Mistovich

To my best friends, Ed my father and Linda my wife, for their unreserved love, constant support, and unfailing encouragement to pursue my dreams of writing and inventing. To my beautiful loving children Ashley, Joshua, Matthew and Kyle for their unconditional love, unending inspiration and childlike spiritual support, I am so proud of you all. To my dear friend Ernie McCloud for taking a step of faith, my family and I are eternally grateful. I love you all.

Edward B. Kuvlesky

Introduction

 SUCCESS ACROSS THE BOARDS:
THE PRENTICE HALL HEALTH REVIEW SERIES

Prentice Hall Health is pleased to present *EMT-Basic Self-Assessment Exam Prep* as part of a review series on the various EMS education levels. The authoritative text gives you expert help in preparing for certifying examinations.

COMPONENTS OF THE SERIES

The series is made up of a book and CD combination.

ABOUT THE BOOK:

- **EMT-Basic Self-Assessment Exam Prep:** This manual has been designed to help students prepare for the written course and certification exams. It can also be used as a review for currently certified EMT-Basics. More than one thousand multiple-choice items are organized by the sections covered in the 1994 U.S. Department of Transportation's National Standard EMT-Basic Curriculum. The multiple-choice items are similar to those found on teacher-made exams and certifying exams. Working through these items will help you assess your strengths and weaknesses in each section.

- **D.O.T. Objectives:** A D.O.T objective reference number located in the answer and rationale section allows you to refer back to the specific D.O.T. Curriculum objective that the item was written from. This will allow you to seek more information for each item from popular textbooks written to the D.O.T. objectives. For the enhancement material that is beyond the D.O.T. objectives, respective answers and rationales do not have objective reference numbers. The D.O.T. objectives are presented in full in the Appendix.

- **Answers and Rationales:** Correct answers and comprehensive rationales are provided and assist you in better understanding each item. Rationales for incorrect answers are typically presented so that you may also learn why that answer is incorrect.
- **EMT-Basic Self-Assessment Practice Test:** An EMT-Basic comprehensive self-assessment test is provided as a practice exam to test your overall knowledge of the information.

ABOUT THE CD-ROM:

A CD-ROM is included in the back of this book. The accompanying CD includes 120 multiple-choice questions for extra practice. A glossary of words and definitions is included to help you review the necessary terminology. In addition the D.O.T. objectives are presented in full.

STUDY TIPS

So, you're getting ready for an exam. Congratulations for making it to this point; now let's help you make the next step—doing your best on this exam. Some people find test taking unsettling, while many consider tests unnerving and even scary! Use this book as an opportunity to practice preparation, information review, and exam techniques.

PHYSICAL PREPARATION

The key to maximizing your potential on a test is to be at your personal best. Along with mental preparation, physical preparation should be included in a good study strategy. Physical preparation includes getting adequate rest and exercising. It also includes eating a balanced meal the night before and the morning of the exam. Your brain works best when it has access to a supply of glucose. So fruits, grains, vegetables, and pasta are important foods. Try to avoid caffeine and foods with high sugar content on the morning of the exam. These foods provide a short burst of energy but when they are used up the slump will significantly reduce your ability to function.

Try some physical exercise the days before the exam but not to the point of exhaustion. Increasing cardiovascular perfusion will also increase perfusion to the brain. More oxygen circulating in the brain can only be good, right?! Exercise is also an outlet for stress, making it easier to get a good night's sleep.

INFORMATION REVIEW

Against popular belief, preparing for the exam should not include extensive studying. You've been studying for months, you know the material, and cramming now will probably cause an intellectual shut down. Review the material for short periods of time, and take frequent breaks. Try study groups of 3 to 5 people for review; the active discussion will be an excellent way to reinforce the material and retain the information.

While knowing the material is essential, physical preparation is equally important. Remember, review only in brief intervals, use a study group, and don't cram.

TAKING THE EXAMINATION

An exam is not written by happenstance; it's an art and a science. Each time you take an exam it's a chance to evaluate your knowledge, as well as to master the test-taking process. It might seem hard, but exams are generally built to measure *minimum* competency. Certification or recertification exams are usually not designed to test total knowledge, ability to expertly function in the field, or even your level of professionalism. They are an attempt to evaluate your reading comprehension and judgment.

There are two basic kinds of questions found on most certification exams; multiple choice and true/false. Each of these question types is built in a specific way to test your ability and your knowledge. Knowing how the questions are constructed may help you during the exam.

Multiple-choice questions consist of two parts: stems and answers. A stem is the actual question part, and the list of answers that follow are called distracters. Distracters are designed to, what else, distract you from the correct response. Multiple-choice questions require you to use knowledge, judgment, and expertise in order to answer the question. *Hint*: Use the process of elimination.

When answering a multiple-choice question, read the question and all of the answers first. Then begin the process of elimination, starting with the most incorrect and sorting your way through until you're left with one or two possible answers. Got a problem picking from those? Then re-read the stem. If it would make it easier, then re-phrase the question, looking for key words that give you a hint about the answer. Don't forget to look at the grammar; is the stem in plural form or singular? Whatever process you use, try not to spend more than two minutes on any one question.

You may find a topic is covered in several consecutive questions. In this case, be sure all your answers are similar and seem to fit together. It might be helpful to use the previous answers to validate each new set of choices. Another option is to check the next question because sometimes the answer, or a strong hint to one question, is the stem of the following questions. Remember, when reading multiple-choice responses the correct answer may be the most comprehensive choice—the one that combines several of the other answers or includes more details.

If the exam contains true/false questions, remember that statements containing absolute terms like *never, always,* and *only* will usually be false. Very little of medicine, or life itself, is absolute. Statements that contain words like *maybe* or *sometimes* tend to be true. These are some hints that may help you when reading true/false questions.

The scientific part of test building is putting all the information into questions, and it is an art form the way the questions are put together to evaluate you. The key is to read each question carefully—try not to scan because you miss important key words like *incorrect* or *not* that would cause you to waste time or, more important, miss the answer. Be prudent, pace yourself, and use patience, your all important three "P's."

WRAPPING UP

You know how people say to go with your first hunch; well, they're right. Your brain makes immediate connections based on stored information and your experience. Don't be afraid that the answer is wrong just because you didn't go through all the usual steps of logic. Research shows that first impressions tend to be correct.

It's okay to choose the same letter answer two or three times in a row. The answers are put into a question at random so it could be that the same letter shows up as being correct up to five times. Don't change your answer if you have chosen the same letter more than once.

Well, you have done the most you can by participating in class, practicing your skills, and reading your material. You know it all by now so trying to teach yourself the curriculum just won't work and ultimately your patients will suffer. Trust yourself and your abilities. Practice some of the tips in this section as you proceed through this book. In the days before the exam remember to eat well, exercise, and get sleep. Good luck.

1 Preparatory

module objectives

Questions in this module relate to D.O.T. objectives 1-1.1 to 1-6.15.

DIRECTIONS Each of the questions or incomplete statements below is followed by suggested answers or completions. Select the **one answer** that is best in each case.

1. Which of the following is not one of the components of an EMS system identified by the "Technical Assistance Program Assessment Standards" provided by the National Highway Traffic Safety Administration?
   A. regulation and policy
   B. equipment
   C. communications
   D. resource management

2. The assurance of a safe rescue operation begins with the:
   A. incident commander.
   B. individual EMT-B.
   C. ranking fire officer.
   D. scene safety officer.

3. You arrive on the scene of a shooting in a housing project and find a patient lying on the sidewalk in a pool of blood. An obvious large gaping open wound to the upper thigh is spurting blood. The patient is still clutching a pistol while thrashing around and screaming. Your first action should be to:
   A. immediately apply direct pressure to the open thigh wound.
   B. restrain the patient and attempt to control the weapon.
   C. retreat and clear the bystanders from around the patient.
   D. attempt to knock the gun from the patient's hand.

4. Medical direction in an EMS system is:
   A. provided by a supervising nurse in the emergency department.
   B. provided by the employing agency's training or education staff.
   C. the ultimate responsibility of a physician medical director.
   D. provided by the use of well-defined treatment protocols.

5. When dealing with a patient diagnosed as having terminal lung cancer, you notice the patient is silent, distant, and despairing. The emotional stage the patient most likely is exhibiting is:
   A. denial.
   B. bargaining.
   C. acceptance.
   D. depression.

6. A terminally ill patient who is coping with his disease and is prepared to die is likely to be exhibiting:
   A. denial.
   B. bargaining.
   C. acceptance.
   D. depression.

7. If your family and friends lack an understanding of emergency medical services and your responsibilities as an EMT-Basic it will most likely:
   A. lead to a stressful relationship.
   B. relieve them of undue worry while you are working.
   C. lessen their frustrations with the requirements of your job.
   D. reduce their fear of separation.

8. A version of Critical Incident Stress Debriefing that is held within 1 to 4 hours following a critical incident is called a(n):
   A. review.
   B. defusing.
   C. follow-up.
   D. incident recap.

9. You are treating a trauma patient with a large laceration to his upper extremity that is spurting blood. You should use all of the following body substance isolation equipment **except:**
   A. eyewear with side shields.
   B. latex gloves.

C. vinyl gloves.

D. a HEPA respirator.

10. Your legal right to function as an EMT-Basic is contingent upon:

A. acquiring medical direction.

B. maintaining malpractice insurance.

C. mastery of the necessary skills.

D. acting in an ethical manner.

11. Permission must be obtained prior to rendering care to a patient. This is termed:

A. consent.

B. an "acknowledgment of care."

C. EMS treatment recognition.

D. a pre-care protocol.

12. You arrive on the scene and find a 45-year-old patient lying on the street corner who responds to your questions with inappropriate words and phrases. You should:

A. immediately assess your patient and initiate emergency care.

B. attempt to determine the patient's name, address, and phone number.

C. contact the police and wait for their consent to initiate care.

D. assume that the words indicate expressed consent and begin treatment.

13. Which patient is most likely capable of refusing treatment?

A. a patient who grabs your arm when obtaining consent

B. a patient who is under the influence of alcohol

C. a patient who gestures you away when obtaining consent

D. a patient who speaks with inappropriate words

14. You are assessing a 62-year-old female patient who complains of chest pain and refuses transport. Her husband requests that you transport her. You initiated treatment prior to her refusing transport. Given these circumstances you should:

A. continue treatment and begin transport.

B. cease additional treatment and gain written permission from her husband.

C. immediately reevaluate her level of competency.

D. transport her and then contact medical control for additional assistance.

15. A patient refuses treatment. She is alert and oriented and answers questions appropriately. She refuses to sign a "Release from Liability Form." Your best action would be to:

A. have both you and your partner sign for the patient.

B. leave the scene and have your partner sign as a witness to the refusal.

C. leave the scene quickly and advise the husband to call back if needed.

D. have the husband sign the form as a witness to the wife's refusal.

16. A patient continues to refuse treatment or transport after assessment and explanation of the consequences of refusing care and transport. Prior to departing the scene you should:

A. say nothing and avoid any eye contact with the family and patient.

B. try again to persuade the patient to accept treatment and transport.

C. prepare to transport the patient in spite of her repeated refusals.

D. describe complications of refusal to the patient, using the appropriate medical terminology.

17. You transport a patient to an emergency department that is extremely busy. The ward clerk yells out to move the patient to any of the rooms that are empty. While you and your partner move the patient to a hospital bed, you are toned out for another emergency. On

your way out of the emergency department, you can only find the ward clerk to tell her that the patient is in room 2A. You then respond to your next call. This action could result in:

A. a continuous quality improvement investigation for improper consent.

B. a charge of abandonment by the patient you just transported.

C. a charge of negligence by the patient that you are responding to.

D. better continuation of care delivered by the emergency department.

18. A woman contacts you who states she is the grandmother of a minor patient you transported. She requests information related to the assessment findings and care of the patient. She states she is the patient's legal guardian. The best action for you to take is to:

A. provide the information requested and document the conversation.

B. provide the information, there is no need to document the conversation.

C. provide the information and then contact your supervisor.

D. not release the information until a release form is obtained.

19. Your patient has a deformity to the midshaft of the forearm. You choose to check the radial pulse. In relation to the deformity, this pulse would be considered:

A. proximal.

B. transverse.

C. lateral.

D. distal.

20. The term dorsal refers to which part of the body?

A. front

B. side

C. back

D. top

21. In order to place the patient in a Fowler's position, you would position him:

A. lying face up with the upper body elevated at a 45 to 60 degree angle.

B. lying on his left or right side with his legs elevated 45 to 60 degrees.

C. lying face up with his lower body elevated 12 inches.

D. lying face up with the upper body elevated 15 degrees.

22. Away from or being the farthest from a point of origin is referred to as:

A. distal.

B. proximal.

C. deep.

D. superficial.

23. The midaxillary line is located at the center of:

A. the sole of the foot.

B. each collarbone.

C. the armpit.

D. the anterior chest.

24. The term bilateral refers to:

A. both lungs.

B. one side.

C. frontal skull.

D. both sides.

25. Which of the following is not considered a baseline vital sign?

A. breathing

B. breath sounds

C. capillary refill

D. skin, color, temperature, and condition

26. Upon assessment of a patient, you find minimal movement of the chest during inhalation and exhalation. You would best describe this characteristic as:

A. labored.

B. shallow.

C. retractive.

D. noisy.

27. Unequal pupils would most likely indicate that the patient is possibly suffering from:

A. hypoperfusion.

B. a head injury.

C. inadequate breathing.

D. a chest injury.

28. Pupils should be assessed for:

A. location, constriction, and equality.

B. size, equality, and constriction.

C. equality and reactivity.

D. size, equality, and reactivity.

29. Unequal pupils may be an indication of:

A. drug use.

B. cardiac arrest.

C. stroke.

D. hypoxia.

30. Which of the following is NOT considered a sign?

A. abdominal pain

B. retractions

C. bleeding from the forehead

D. hot skin temperature

31. While lifting a patient from the ground, your back should be:

A. curved slightly outward and not locked.

B. curved slightly inward in a locked-in position.

C. in a relaxed position of comfort.

D. parallel to the ground and in a locked-in position.

32. Which technique best protects your back from injury when carrying a heavy object?

A. When lifting, lift with a twisting motion.

B. Hyperextend your back by leaning backwards.

C. Keep the weight as close to your body as possible.

D. Keep your back in a relaxed unlocked position.

33. Your patient, who is alert and oriented and has no critical illness or injury, is on the second floor of his house in the back bedroom. The best possible method to move the patient down the steps to the ground floor is by:

A. securing the patient in a seated position in a stair chair.

B. using the stretcher with the carriage in the up position.

C. securing the patient to a long backboard with immobilization straps.

D. carrying the patient using a two-person extremity lift.

34. To help prevent injury when performing a one-handed carrying technique you should refrain from:

A. keeping your abdominal muscles tight.

B. bending at the hips, try to bend at the waist.

C. positioning your back in a locked-in position.

D. leaning to the opposite side excessively.

35. The preferred method to move a responsive, non-injured patient down steps is by the use of a:

A. long spine board.

B. ambulance stretcher.

C. stair chair.

D. vest type immobilization device.

36. Which of the following is correct and should be used to aid against injury when performing a logroll?

A. Use your shoulder muscles whenever possible.

B. Lean towards the patient from your waist, not your hips.

C. Use your lower back muscles to support your weight.

D. Keep your back in a relaxed position by leaning back.

37. Whenever possible when moving an object it should be:

A. pushed rather than pulled.

B. lifted from the waist.

C. pulled as low as possible to the ground.

D. lifted as far from the body as possible.

38. In which of the following situations would an emergency move be appropriate to move a patient?

A. to shield him or her from curious onlookers (protect modesty)

B. to gain access to another patient that is critically injured

C. so law enforcement officers can direct traffic through the scene

D. to provide adequate space for the traffic investigation team

39. You arrive on the scene and find a 34-year-old male patient lying in a hospital bed in his home. The dispatcher notifies you that the patient is HIV positive and has AIDS. When you arrive at the scene you are greeted at the door by his sister. She informs you that the patient is coughing up blood-tinged sputum, has been sweating at night profusely, and has lost weight recently. Your next immediate action should be to:

A. refuse to enter the scene because of your risk of contracting HIV.

B. put on gloves, eye protection, and a HEPA respirator before entering.

C. apply a surgical mask to the patient to reduce the risk of droplet spread.

D. contact medical direction to determine if you should enter the scene.

40. You arrive on the scene and find a 20-year-old male patient who was involved in an auto crash. Upon your assessment, you note the patient can not tell you what date it is, where he is, or whom he is with. The patient refuses to let you examine him further and refuses any emergency care. You should:

A. have the patient sign a refusal form and then leave the scene.

B. turn the patient over to the police on the scene and then leave.

C. begin to administer emergency care to the patient and then transport, using restraints if necessary.

D. have the police place the patient under protective custody so that you can administer emergency care.

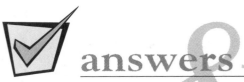

answers & rationales

1.

B. Equipment is not one of the recommended standards identified by the "Technical Assistance Program Assessment Standards." The ten standards are regulation and policy, resource management, human resources and training, transportation, facilities, communications, public information and education, medical direction, trauma systems, and evaluation. (1-1.1) (EC 6-8 PEC 2-5)

2.

B. Each individual is responsible for his or her own personal safety. Other rescuers have specific responsibilities for assuring a safe rescue operation by observing for unsafe activities. This does not relieve the EMT-B from the responsibility of assuring personal safety at all times. (1-1.3) (EC 10 PEC 6-7)

3.

C. Personal safety is your primary role and responsibility, while safety of the crew, patient, and bystander is your second priority. Once safety is assured, the patient's needs become your first priority. (1-1.4) (EC 10 PEC 6-7)

4.

C. The physician medical director of an EMS system is responsible for all patient care and clinical aspects of system management. The other individuals listed in the question do play roles in medical direction, although they do not assume ultimate responsibility. (1-1.6) (EC 15-16 PEC 9-10)

5.

D. The patient may display five various emotional stages associated with death and dying. Depression is associated with silent, distant, sad, and despairing behavior. (1-2.1) (EC 30-33 PEC 15)

6.

C. Acceptance is when the patient appears to accept death. He or she typically is no longer afraid to die. (1-2.3) (EC 35 PEC 14-15)

7.

A. A lack of understanding of your role and responsibility as an EMT-Basic will likely lead to a stressful relationship with family and friends. Other stress responses by family and friends may include fear of separation or of being ignored, worry about on-call situations, frustration with the inability to plan, and frustration with your desire to share your experiences. (1-2.4) (EC 33 PEC 17)

8.

B. A formal CISD is held within 24 to 72 hours after a critical incident. A team of peer counselors guide rescuers through varied phases of discussion. Defusing is a version of CISD that is held within 1 to 4 hours following a critical incident. The defusion is attended by those directly involved in the incident. (1-2.6) (EC 33-34 PEC 16-19)

9.

D. A high efficiency particulate air (HEPA) respirator or N-95 mask is used to filter out the organism responsible for transmitting tuberculosis. Unless your patient is exhibiting signs and symptoms of tuberculosis, there is no need to wear a HEPA respirator. Vinyl or latex gloves, eye wear with side shields, and gowns are appropriate to wear when contact with spurting blood or splashes are suspected. (1-2.10) (EC 23-30, 35-40 PEC 19-26)

10.

A. Your legal right to function as an EMT-Basic is contingent upon acquiring medical direction through protocols and standing orders. Without medical direction, you can not function. It is an ethical responsibility to strive to achieve mastery of your skills. (1-3.1) (EC 45 PEC 30-31)

11.

A. Consent is the permission to care for a patient. Consent must be obtained from all patients prior to treatment. There are three primary forms of consent: expressed, implied, and consent to treat a minor or mentally incompetent adult. (1-3.3) (EC 45-46 PEC 32, 34)

12.

A. Based on the concept of implied consent, you should immediately assess your patient and initiate emergency care. (1-3.4) (EC 46 PEC 34)

13.

C. A competent adult has the right to refuse treatment. A patient with an altered mental status or under the influence of alcohol or drugs may be considered incompetent. Incompetency would depend upon the extent to which the drugs or alcohol are clouding the patient's judgment. Orally refusing or other actions (such as gestures) that imply refusal are considered valid forms of patient refusal. (1-3.6) (EC 46-48 PEC 34)

14.

C. When dealing with refusal issues it is important to determine the patient's competency or lack of competency. A competent adult has the right to refuse treatment or to withdraw from treatment once it has started. (1-3.6) (EC 46-48 PEC 34)

15.

D. The best answer is to have the patient's husband sign as a witness to the refusal. The witnessed refusal form becomes a part of the legal documentation of the patient's refusal. You must document all aspects of the patient encounter to include history obtained and physical exam findings. Also, document your attempts at treatment and transport. (1-3.6) (EC 46-48 PEC 34)

16.

B. Before leaving any patient who has refused treatment or transport, always try one last time to persuade the patient to accept emergency care and transport. (1-3.6) (EC 46-48 PEC 34)

17.

B. Termination of care without assuring the proper continuation of care by a competent practitioner can result in a charge of abandonment. If in the hospital, proper transfer of care to an equally or higher qualified health care practitioner must occur. Failure to properly transfer that care can result in a charge of abandonment. (1-3.7) (EC 47, 50-51 PEC 34, 35-36)

18.

D. Releasing confidential information requires a written release form signed by the patient or a legal guardian. Do not release confidential information about the patient to someone claiming to be a legal guardian. Guardianship must be established. (1-3.9) (EC 51-52 PEC 36)

19.

D. Distal is best described as distant from the point of reference. In most cases, the point furthest from the heart could be referred to as distal. In this case, the radial pulse is away from the heart and from the midshaft deformity, the point of reference. (1-4.1) (EC 61-63 PEC 43, 45)

20.

C. Dorsal refers to the back of the body. Posterior and dorsal have the same meaning; however, posterior is a more commonly used descriptive anatomical term. (1-4.1) (EC 61-63 PEC 43-45)

21.

A. The Fowler's position is when the patient is placed supine, on his back, with his upper body elevated at a 45 to 60 degree angle. The Trendelenburg position is where the patient is placed supine with his legs elevated 12 inches. (1-4.1) (EC 61-63 PEC 43-45)

22.

A. Distal is distant or away from the point of reference. (1-4.1) (EC 61-63 PEC 43-45)

23.

C. The midaxillary line extends from the middle of the armpit to the ankle. It is used as an anatomical point of reference. (1-4.1) (EC 61-63 PEC 43-45)

24.

D. *Bilateral* refers to the patient's right and left or both sides. (1-4.1) (EC 61-63 PEC 43-45)

25.

B. Breath sounds are assessed as part of the focused history and physical exam and are not considered a component of the baseline vital signs. Capillary refill, usually more accurate in infants and young children, is considered a vital sign. (1-5.1) (EC 212 PEC 74)

26.

B. Shallow breathing is characterized by slight movement of the chest or abdomen during breathing. It is an indication that very little volume of air is moving in and out of the lungs. It is considered to be a sign of inadequate breathing. Positive pressure ventilation must be initiated when the breathing is shallow. (1-5.4) (EC 216 PEC 75)

27.

B. Unequal pupils may indicate a head injury, stroke, or artificial eye. Usually, one pupil is also fixed or not reacting to light. Hypoxia and hypoperfusion may cause the pupils to become sluggish, but not unequal. Chest injury would most likely cause hypoxia resulting in sluggish pupils. (1-5.16) (EC 218, 219 PEC 79)

28.

D. Pupils should be assessed for three factors. Size, equality, and reactivity to light. (1-5.15) (EC 218, 219 PEC 79-80)

29.

C. Unequal pupils may indicate a stroke or head injury. Don't overlook the possibility that the patient has an artificial eye. (1-5.18) (EC 218, 219 PEC 79-80)

30.

A. A sign is something you can observe. You can see retractions, you can see bleeding, and you can feel skin temperature. Abdominal pain is a condition that cannot be observed and it must be described by the patient. This is known as a symptom. (1-5.24) (EC 224 PEC 83)

31.

B. When lifting a patient, the back should be kept in a locked-in position that naturally forces an inward curve. (1-6.1) (EC 101 PEC 87)

32.

C. Try to carry objects as close to your body as possible to prevent injury. Refrain from lifting and twisting at the same time. Keep your back locked in a natural position, not hyperextended. (1-6.2) (EC 101-103 PEC 87-90)

33.

A. When possible and if medically appropriate, use a stair chair to move the patient down stairs. Typically, it is too difficult to maneuver the stretcher up and down steps. An extremity lift is used only to place the patient onto a device to move the patient. (1-6.4) (EC 101-103 PEC 90-93)

34.

D. When carrying an object with one hand you should avoid leaning too far to the opposite side. Keeping your back in a locked-in position by keeping your abdominal muscles tight will help to prevent this unnatural position. When bending, you should bend at the hips, not at the waist. (1-6.5) (EC 101 PEC 90-91)

35.

C. The preferred method is to use a stair chair. A stair chair is used for the responsive patient who does not have a spinal injury. Using a stair chair will reduce the potential for EMT-B lifting injuries. (1-6.6) (EC 109 PEC 91)

36.

A. When performing the logroll technique try to use your stronger shoulder muscles rather than your weaker back muscles. Support your body with your free hand, not your back muscles. When leaning toward the patient try to lean at the hip, not the waist. (1-6.8) (EC 106-107 PEC 92)

37.

A. Always push the object if possible. You are less apt to sustain an injury. (1-6.9) (EC 102-103 PEC 92-93)

38.

B. You should use an emergency move only if there is an immediate danger to the patient or rescuer or to gain access to a more critically injured patient. Moving the first patient to gain access to a second patient that needs immediate life saving treatment is correct. (1-6.11) (EC 103 PEC 865)

39.

B. The patient is displaying signs of possible tuberculosis infection, such as blood-tinged sputum, night sweats, and weight loss. Also, he is at higher risk for TB infection due to his HIV status. You should put on gloves and eye protection as a normal routine of body substance isolation protection and also put on a HEPA respirator or a N-95 mask. The HEPA respirator or N-95 mask will block out the very small TB bacteria and prevent transmission of the disease to you. If you are using a HEPA respirator that does not have an exhalation valve, you can place one on the patient also to reduce the incidence of a respiratory droplet transmission. (EC 23-30, 35-40 PEC 19-26)

40.

C. The patient has an altered mental status and is disoriented to time, place, and person. At this point, the patient is unable to make a rational decision and should be treated based on implied consent. If necessary, restrain the patient and provide emergency care. (EC 46 PEC 34)

2 | Airway

module objectives

Questions in this module relate to D.O.T.
objectives 2-1.1 to 2-1.41.

DIRECTIONS Each of the questions or incomplete statements below is followed by suggested answers or completions. Select the **one answer** that is best in each case.

1. The epiglottis:
   A. closes shut over the trachea during inhalation.
   B. opens the esophagus during exhalation.
   C. blocks the opening of the trachea during swallowing.
   D. keeps air from entering the esophagus during ventilation.

2. The cricoid cartilage is located:
   A. in the superior portion of the larynx.
   B. lateral to the larynx.
   C. at the bifurcation of the trachea.
   D. in the inferior portion of the larynx.

3. Which range of respiratory rates indicates adequate breathing for a 6-year-old?
   A. 8 to 12 times a minute
   B. 12 to 20 times a minute
   C. 15 to 30 times a minute
   D. 25 to 50 times a minute

4. Which patient is breathing adequately?
   A. 8-year-old breathing 12 times a minute with a shallow tidal volume
   B. 3-month-old breathing 40 times a minute with abdominal movement
   C. 22-year-old breathing 26 times a minute with excessive accessory muscle use
   D. 61-year-old breathing 42 times a minute with a history of smoking

5. A sign of inadequate breathing in an infant is:
   A. a respiratory rate of 25 to 50 per minute.
   B. a "seesaw" breathing motion.
   C. a regular respiratory pattern.
   D. an equal and full chest expansion.

6. If you are uncertain if a patient is breathing adequately after your assessment, you should:
   A. begin positive pressure ventilation.
   B. reevaluate the patient's respiratory status.
   C. administer oxygen by non-rebreathing mask.
   D. count the patient's respirations carefully over 1 minute.

7. A patient with retractions above the clavicles, between the ribs and below the rib cage, is most likely showing signs of:
   A. adequate breathing with tachypnea.
   B. bradypnea and hyperpnea.
   C. apnea and asystole.
   D. inadequate breathing.

8. You note a snoring sound upon assessment of the airway in an unresponsive patient who is found lying in bed. You should:
   A. place the patient on a non-rebreather mask at 15 lpm.
   B. tilt the head back and lift the chin forward.
   C. begin positive pressure ventilation with a pocket mask.
   D. assess to determine if a carotid pulse is present.

9. When performing a maneuver on an infant to open the airway, the head should be:
   A. hyperextended.
   B. kept in a neutral position or slightly extended.
   C. flexed forward.
   D. maximally extended with the shoulders elevated.

10. You are on the scene and find a 20-year-old female who has fallen from a second story window. The patient is breathing inadequately. You should open the airway by:
    A. head-tilt chin-lift maneuver.
    B. head hypertension maneuver.
    C. lateral head lift maneuver.
    D. jaw-thrust maneuver.

11. When manually opening the airway of an infant without a suspected spinal injury, the preferred method is:
    A. head-tilt, chin-lift with the head in a hyperextended position.
    B. jaw-thrust maneuver with the head and neck in a neutral position.
    C. head-tilt, chin-lift with the neck and head in a neutral position.
    D. jaw-thrust maneuver with the neck in a hyperextended position.

12. You are treating a 6-year-old who was struck by a car. The patient is unresponsive and has no gag reflex. You should open and maintain the airway by:
    A. jaw-thrust maneuver with head hyperextended.
    B. head-tilt, chin-lift and oropharyngeal airway.
    C. head-tilt, chin-lift and a nasopharyngeal airway.
    D. jaw-thrust maneuver and an oropharyngeal airway.

13. When performing the jaw-thrust maneuver, the EMT-B's elbows should:
    A. remain at least 2 inches above the surface upon which the patient is lying.
    B. remain at least 6 inches above the surface upon which the patient is lying.
    C. remain on the surface upon which the patient is lying.
    D. be cradled securely on the rescuer's abdomen.

14. The jaw-thrust maneuver opens the airway by:
    A. displacing the mandible forward.
    B. tilting the head back.
    C. tilting the head back and moving the jaw forward.
    D. retracting the lower lips.

15. What type of catheter is preferred for suctioning the oropharynx?
    A. soft
    B. rigid
    C. French
    D. bulb

16. After opening the mouth to assess the airway of a trauma patient during your initial assessment, you note a large amount of blood in the oropharynx. Your next immediate action should be to:
    A. suction the blood from the mouth.
    B. apply a non-rebreather mask and administer oxygen at 15 lpm.
    C. begin ventilating the patient with a pocket mask.
    D. assess the carotid or radial pulse.

17. Which of the following is the appropriate catheter and pressure for suctioning the nasal passage of an infant?
    A. soft catheter at 130 to 150 mmHg
    B. rigid catheter at 80 to 120 mmHg
    C. tonsil tip catheter at 130 to 150 mmHg
    D. French catheter at 80 to 120 mmHg

18. Select the correct statement pertaining to suction equipment or the technique:
    A. French or soft catheters are inserted beyond the base of the tongue in the infant.
    B. Suction should be limited to 15 seconds in the adult and 5 seconds in the infant.
    C. Suction should be applied before the catheter is inserted into the mouth.
    D. The convex side of the rigid catheter is placed against the tongue.

19. You are preparing to use a French catheter to suction the oropharynx of a 20-year-old male. To determine the length of the catheter needed you would measure:
    A. from the corner of the patient's mouth to the tip of the ear.
    B. from the corner of the patient's mouth to the Adam's apple.

C. from the tip of the patient's nose to the tip of the patient's ear.

D. from the tip of the patient's nose to the patient's cricoid cartilage.

20. When using a pocket face mask to ventilate a non-breathing patient, the oxygen flow should be set at _____ lpm.

   A. 4
   B. 6
   C. 10
   D. 15

21. When ventilating an adult with a pocket mask, the breaths should be delivered over _____ to _____ seconds.

   A. 0.5, 1.0
   B. 1.0, 2.0
   C. 2.5, 3.0
   D. 3.0, 3.5

22. You arrive on the scene and find a patient who fell off a scaffolding from about 30 feet. Upon assessment, you find sonorous (snoring) sounds, respirations are approximately 30 per minute and shallow, a radial pulse is absent, the carotid pulse is weak and rapid at about 130/minute, and the skin is pale, cool, and clammy. You should immediately:

   A. immobilize the patient on a spine board.
   B. apply a cervical spinal immobilization collar.
   C. stabilize the head and neck and apply a non-rebreather at 15 lpm and transport the patient.
   D. perform a jaw-thrust with in-line stabilization and begin bag-valve-mask ventilation.

23. When ventilating a patient while performing the jaw-thrust maneuver, it is necessary to:

   A. maintain a mask seal with one hand while tilting the forehead backwards.
   B. keep the mandible immobilized in a neutral position.

C. hold a mask seal while lifting the mandible forward.

D. flex the neck forward and push the mandible backwards.

24. The bag-valve-mask device without an oxygen source will deliver _____ percentage of oxygen to the patient?

   A. 21%
   B. 44%
   C. 61%
   D. 100%

25. Which statement is true pertaining to the bag-valve-mask device?

   A. The BVM generates a higher tidal volume than mouth to mask.
   B. The BVM is difficult to use and fatiguing to the operator.
   C. A non-disabling pop off valve is a preferred feature on the BVM.
   D. Oropharyngeal airways are contraindicated when using the BVM.

26. You are preparing to ventilate a patient with the bag-valve-mask. Choose the correct sequence for mask placement procedure:

   A. Place the narrow part of the mask over the bridge of the nose and the wider part over the cleft of the chin at the same time.
   B. Place the wider part of the mask over the cleft of the chin; then place the narrow part over the bridge of the nose.
   C. Place the narrow part of the mask over the cleft of the chin and then the wider part over the bridge of the nose.
   D. Place the narrow part of the mask over the bridge of the nose and then the wider part over the cleft of the chin.

27. When ventilating an adult with a bag mask device connected to supplemental oxygen the breaths should be delivered over _____ to _____ seconds.

   A. 0.5, 1.0

B. 1.0, 2.0

C. 2.5, 3.0

D. 3.0, 3.5

28. Ventilation of a patient with a bag-valve-mask device is best performed by a minimum of _____ rescuers.

A. one

B. two

C. three

D. four

29. All of the following are indications that you are ventilating your patient adequately **except:**

A. the chest rises and falls with each ventilation.

B. the heart rate slows from 130/minute to 80/minute in an adult patient.

C. the movement of the abdomen increases with each ventilation.

D. the skin color begins to return to normal.

30. You arrive on the scene and find a 7-year-old patient who was pulled from a pond after being submerged for 10 minutes. The first response crew is on the scene when you arrive. The patient is being ventilated by mouth-to-mask with supplemental oxygen at a rate of 15 ventilations per minute. The patient remains cyanotic. You should immediately:

A. increase the ventilation rate to a minimum of 20 per minute.

B. increase the oxygen liter flow from 10 lpm to 15 lpm.

C. compress the stomach in case there is gastric distention.

D. apply cricoid pressure to the cricoid cartilage.

31. A technique to determine if you are ventilating the patient effectively is by:

A. observing the chest rise while squeezing the bag.

B. listening for air sounds while squeezing the bag.

C. feeling the bag deflate when applying pressure.

D. watching the patient's cheeks flare when ventilating.

32. Which of the following is likely to cause the abdomen to become distended while ventilating with the bag-valve-mask?

A. setting the oxygen supply regulator at 15 liters per minute

B. allowing for passive exhalation after each ventilation

C. using a nasopharyngeal airway

D. ventilating once every second with a high tidal volume

33. The first step in ventilating a patient with a flow-restricted, oxygen-powered ventilation device is to ensure:

A. an adequate, constant oxygen supply is available.

B. the relief valve is open at 30 cm of water pressure.

C. 60 lpm oxygen peak flow rate is delivered by the device.

D. 100 lpm oxygen flow is delivered by the device.

34. You are attempting to ventilate a patient with a flow-restricted, oxygen-powered ventilation device. The patient's chest does not rise. You should:

A. increase the oxygen flow from 40 lpm to 100 lpm.

B. cover the pressure relief valve with your thumb.

C. reevaluate the head position and the mask seal.

D. increase the ventilation time from 1.5 to 3.0 seconds.

35. When ventilating a patient with a flow-restricted, oxygen-powered ventilation device the valve should be depressed until:
   A. the pressure relief valve opens.
   B. resistance is felt on the trigger.
   C. the chest begins to rise.
   D. the audible alarm sounds.

36. When performing mouth-to-mouth ventilation, you should:
   A. not break the seal of your mouth on the patient's face between ventilations.
   B. deliver the ventilation forcefully over less than one second.
   C. allow for adequate exhalation by removing your mouth between ventilations.
   D. increase your rate of ventilation since supplemental oxygen is not used.

37. While performing bag-valve-mask-to-stoma ventilation, you note minimal chest rise and fall and air escaping from the mouth and nose with each ventilation. You should:
   A. pinch the nose and close the mouth and continue ventilation through the stoma.
   B. secure a mask seal over the nose and mouth, occlude the stoma, and continue ventilating the patient.
   C. apply a non-rebreather over the nose and mouth and administer 15 lpm of oxygen.
   D. insert a nasopharyngeal airway in the stoma and ventilate with a pediatric pocket mask.

38. During insertion of the nasopharyngeal airway, resistance is felt. This:
   A. is normal. Use force to ensure rapid placement of the device.
   B. should alert the EMT-B to quickly remove the device.
   C. is not normal and would require deep nasal suctioning.

   D. frequently occurs. Twist and turn the device as you untwine to insert. If additional resistance occurs, remove the device and try the other nostril.

39. You determine the proper size of an oropharyngeal airway by:
   A. measuring from the tip of the nose to the tip of the earlobe.
   B. measuring from the corner of the mouth to the tip of the earlobe.
   C. choosing the same length airway as the length of the index finger.
   D. using the size formula (16 + the patient's age in years) ÷ 4.

40. Which of the following statements is **false** pertaining to the oropharyngeal airway?
   A. The OPA protects the airway from aspiration of secretions and vomitus.
   B. The mental status of the patient will determine if the OPA can be used.
   C. Using an OPA that is too long can cause a complete obstructed airway.
   D. Measure from the center of the mouth to the angle of the jaw for correct size.

41. The oropharyngeal airway is contraindicated in which of the following patients?
   A. trauma patient who responds to verbal stimuli
   B. cancer patient in cardiac arrest
   C. unresponsive diabetic patient
   D. stroke patient without a gag reflex

42. Prior to insertion, a nasopharyngeal airway should be lubricated with:
   A. a water-soluble lubricant.
   B. the patient's oral secretions.
   C. a petroleum based lubricant.
   D. sterile saline or sterile water.

43. To determine the proper length of a nasopharyngeal airway, measure from the patient's:
   A. corner of the edge of the mouth to the tip of the nose.

B. corner of the edge of the mouth to the tip of the earlobe.

C. bridge of the nose to the tip of the chin.

D. tip of the nose to the tip of the earlobe.

44. A properly sized nasopharyngeal airway should:

A. fit snugly in the nostril and extend 2 inches beyond the tip of the nose.

B. fit loosely in the nostril and extend 2 inches beyond the base of the tongue.

C. be seated firmly with the flange against the nostril.

D. blanch the skin of the nostril, insuring proper diameter.

45. When applying a non-rebreather mask or nasal cannula to the patient:

A. apply the device to the patient, attach the oxygen tubing to the flowmeter, and open the flowmeter to the desired lpm.

B. attach the oxygen tubing to the flowmeter, open the flowmeter to the desired lpm, and apply the device to the patient.

C. open the flowmeter and set the desired lpm, apply the device to the patient, attach the oxygen tubing to the flowmeter.

D. attach the oxygen tubing to the flowmeter, apply the device to the patient, open the flowmeter and set the desired lpm.

46. An oxygen tank is full when the pressure gauge reads:

A. 500 psi.

B. 2000 psi.

C. 3000 psi.

D. 5000 psi.

47. When using a non-rebreather mask, the oxygen flow regulator should be set at:

A. 15 liters per minute

B. 10 liters per minute

C. 8 liters per minute

D. 6 liters per minute

48. You are treating a 62-year-old with a history of chronic obstructive pulmonary disease (COPD). The patient states, "I can't breathe and presents with signs of hypoxia." The preferred method for delivering oxygen to this patient is:

A. non-rebreather mask with the oxygen set at 10 liters per minute.

B. non-rebreather mask with the oxygen set at 15 liters per minute.

C. nasal cannula device with the oxygen set at 8 liters per minute.

D. nasal cannula device with the oxygen set at 6 liters per minute.

49. The preferred prehospital device for oxygen delivery to a patient who has adequate ventilation is the:

A. nasal cannula.

B. simple face mask.

C. non-rebreathing mask.

D. Venturi mask.

50. The non-rebreathing mask provides high concentrations of oxygen to a patient by:

A. utilizing high oxygen liter flow rates.

B. its rebreather mask design.

C. connecting the oxygen supply tubing directly to the mask.

D. allowing the patient to inhale the oxygen from an oxygen reservoir bag.

51. Your patient refuses to keep a non-rebreather mask on her face, even with extensive coaching. You should next:

A. remove the non-rebreather mask.

B. remove the non-rebreather mask and apply a nasal cannula.

C. continue to coach the patient and hold the mask to her face.

D. blow oxygen by her face with oxygen supply tubing.

SCENARIO

Questions 52–54 refer to the following scenario:

You and your partner Wilson are enjoying a well-deserved break when you are dispatched to 8356 64th Avenue for a patient complaining of shortness of breath. While en route, you both take body substance isolation precautions. Upon your arrival, you find the scene is safe. You both enter the house to find a 35-year-old female walking around the house complaining, "I can't breathe." You have the patient sit down, and you perform an initial assessment. The patient is breathing 20 times per minute, there is good chest rise, and you feel adequate air during exhalation. Her heart rate is 102 beats per minute and her skin is pale, cool, and clammy. Auscultation of the lungs during formal medical exams reveals lower lobe wheezes. You ask the patient if she has been prescribed a metered dose inhaler (MDI). She states, "My puffer is on the night stand."

52. You determine the patient is breathing _____ and _____.
   A. inadequately, perform the Heimlich maneuver
   B. inadequately, provide positive pressure ventilation
   C. adequately, place the patient on non-rebreather mask
   D. adequately, place the patient on nasal cannula at 6 lpm

53. You and Wilson have obtained orders to administer the metered dose inhaler (MDI).

Prior to administering the MDI, you explain the common side effects of a beta agonist drug, which include:
   A. bradycardia and blurred vision.
   B. hypertension and salivation.
   C. tachycardia and nervousness.
   D. hypotension and sweating.

54. Wilson notices that the patient is breathing faster and with increased effort. The patient's mental status has deteriorated. She is also using her accessory muscle. You quickly auscultate the lungs and hear no air exchange in the lower lungs and slight wheezes in the upper lungs. You should immediately:
   A. provide positive pressure ventilation with the bag-valve-mask and oxygen.
   B. administer high flow oxygen by non-rebreather mask at 15 liters per minute.
   C. apply a nasal cannula at 6 lpm.
   D. prepare to suction the lower airway with a French catheter and low suction.

55. When ventilating a patient with a bag-valve-mask device with a reservoir that is connected to an oxygen source flowing at 15 lpm, you should deliver a tidal volume of:
   A. 10 to 15 ml/kg over 2 seconds.
   B. 8 to 10 ml/kg over 1 to 2 seconds.
   C. 6 to 7 ml/kg over 1 to 2 seconds.
   D. 3 to 4 ml/kg over 1 to 2 seconds.

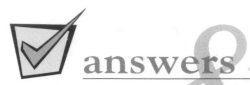

answers & rationales

1.

C. The epiglottis is a cartilaginous flap of tissue that is responsible for closing shut over the opening of the trachea during swallowing. This prevents aspiration of food or other substances into the trachea and lungs. (2-1.1) (EC 128-129 PEC 97-100)

2.

D. The cricoid cartilage, the only completely circumferential cartilaginous ring, is located in the inferior portion of the larynx. The cricoid ring is the landmark to perform the Sellick maneuver, also known as cricoid pressure. (2-1.1) (EC 128-129 PEC 97-100)

3.

C. The typical breathing rate range for children is 15 to 30 times each minute. The typical respiratory rate for the adult is 12 to 20 times each minute. The breathing rate of an infant is typically 25 to 50 times each minute. (2-1.2a) (EC 130-133 PEC 113)

4.

B. A 3-month-old breathing 40 times a minute with use of the abdomen is considered normal. An 8-year-old breathing 12 times a minute is slightly slow (average range is 15 to 30 times a minute). Low tidal volume means the depth of breathing is low (low air volume entering the lungs). A 42-year-old breathing 26 times a minute is fast (average range is 12 to 20 times a minute). Use of accessory muscles indicates increased effort to inflate the lungs. A 61-year-old breathing 42 times a minute is too fast, whether he or she is a smoker or not. (2-1.2b) (EC 130-133 PREC 113)

5.

B. A sign of inadequate breathing in an infant is a "seesaw" breathing motion. This results from the abdomen and chest moving in opposite directions during breathing. A respiratory rate of 25 to 50 in an infant is the average range. You should expect a regular respiration with equal and full chest expansion. (2-1.3) (EC 129-133 PEC 114-115)

6.

A. You should begin positive pressure ventilation immediately. It is best to err on the side of safety and provide ventilation. (2-1.3) (EC 129-133 PEC 114-115)

7.

D. A patient with retractions above the clavicles, between the ribs and above the sternum, is most likely showing signs of inadequate breathing. Tachypnea is a rapid respiratory rate, bradypnea is a slow respiratory rate. Apnea is the absence of respiration. (2-1.3) (EC 129-133 PEC 114-115)

8.

B. Snoring is an indication that the tongue is partially occluding the upper airway. Perform a head-tilt, chin-lift maneuver as a priority in establishing an airway. If the patient is suspected of having a possible spine injury, a jaw-thrust maneuver should be performed. (2-1.4) (EC 135 PEC 104-105)

9.

B. Due to the underdeveloped structures of the upper airway in the infant, the head should be kept in a neutral position or slightly extended when performing a head-tilt, chin-lift maneuver. Hyperextending the head may actually cause the trachea to become occluded causing an airway obstruction. (2-1.4) (EC 135 PEC 104-105)

10.

D. The jaw-thrust maneuver does not require movement of the head or neck. This technique should be used when you suspect the patient may have a spine injury. The head-tilt chin-lift requires the head to be moved, thus compromising the spine. (2-1.5a) (EC 133-136 PEC 105)

11.

C. The preferred method for opening the airway of an infant without a suspected spinal injury is the head-tilt, chin-lift. It is important to remember in the infant the head should be placed in a neutral position or slight sniffing position. If the head is overextended in the infant or child, the trachea may become obstructed. (2-1.5b) (EC 133-136 PEC 105)

12.

D. This patient may have a spinal injury; thus, you should open the airway by using the jaw-thrust maneuver. An oropharyngeal airway will aid in keeping the tongue away from the oropharynx, helping to maintain an open airway. (2-1.5c) (EC 133-136 PEC 105)

13.

C. When performing the jaw-thrust maneuver the rescuer's elbows should be placed on the surface upon which the patient is lying. This provides a solid surface to maintain spinal stabilization. (2-1.6) (EC 136 PEC 105)

14.

A. The jaw thrust maneuver opens the airway by displacing the mandible forward while maintaining the head in a neutral position. (2-1.6) (EC 136 PEC 105)

15.

B. A hard or rigid suction catheter—also known as a tonsil tip, tonsil sucker, or Yankauer—is the preferred catheter for performing oropharyngeal suctioning. The soft or French catheter is usually used to suction the nose, nasopharynx, or oropharynx. (2-1.7) (EC 151 PEC 106)

16.

A. Blood, vomitus, or other substances in the airway must be cleared immediately with suction. Failure to do so may lead to aspiration and severe hypoxia. It is necessary to always have your suction equipment ready for use. (2-1.7) (EC 151 PEC 106)

17.

D. The French or soft catheter is correct when suctioning the nasal passage of an infant. When suctioning the nasal passage of an infant you should use low to medium suction (-80 to -120 mmHg). A rigid (tonsil tip) catheter will cause injury to the soft tissue of the nasal passage. Suctioning at too high of suction (over 120 mmHg) may cause injury to the soft tissue of the nasal passage. (2-1.8a) (EC 153, 155 PEC 106-108)

18.

B. Suctioning longer than 15 seconds in the adult and 5 seconds in the infant can cause hypoxia. The patient should be oxygenated before and immediately after suctioning. Inserting the catheter beyond the base of

the tongue may injure soft tissue or stimulate nerves and cause a decrease in the heart rate. Suction should only be applied after the catheter is in place. The convex side of the rigid catheter is placed against the roof of the mouth, not the tongue. (2-1.8b) (EC 153, 155 PEC 106-108)

19.

A. The correct length of a French or soft catheter is determined by measuring from the patient's corner of the mouth to the tip of the ear when preparing to suction the oropharynx. If you are preparing to suction the nose or nasopharynx, you should measure from the tip of the patient's nose to the tip of the earlobe. (2-1.8c) (EC 153, 155 PEC 106-108)

20.

D. When using a pocket face mask to ventilate a non-breathing patient, the oxygen flow should be set at 15 lpm. (2-l.9) (EC 138-140 PEC 117-119)

21.

B. When ventilating an adult with the pocket mask, the breaths should be delivered over 1.0 to 2.0 seconds. This slow ventilation helps to prevent gastric distention and subsequent aspiration. (2-1.9) (EC 138-140 PEC 117-119)

22.

D. The sonorous (snoring) sounds indicate a partially occluded airway. Thus, a manual maneuver must be performed to immediately open the airway. A jaw-thrust is the most appropriate due to the risk of possible spinal injury. Also, the patient's breathing is inadequate due to the poor tidal volume and excessively high rate. Therefore, it is necessary to immediately begin ventilation. Manual in-line stabilization should be performed at this point until the immediate life threats to the airway and breathing have been managed effectively. A cervical spinal immobilization collar should be applied during the focused history and physical exam. (2-1.10) (EC 141, 142-143 PEC 122-123)

23.

C. When performing the jaw-thrust maneuver, it is necessary to displace the mandible forward while keeping the head and neck in a neutral in-line position. This procedure is most commonly used for patients with suspected spinal injuries. (2-1.10) (EC 141, 142-143 PEC 122-123)

24.

A. Using the bag-valve-mask without an oxygen source will result in delivering only 21% oxygen, the amount found in the air we breath. When used with an oxygen source at 15 lpm and with an oxygen reservoir, you can achieve nearly 95% oxygen concentration delivered to the patient. (2-1.11a) (EC 140 PEC 119)

25.

B. The BVM is difficult to use and fatiguing to the operator. If available, two EMT-Bs should be used to ventilate a patient. One EMT-B should hold the mask on the patient's face, while the other squeezes the bag. The BVM rarely is able to generate higher tidal volumes than the rescuer providing mouth to mask. A non-disabling pop off valve is not preferred. A pop off valve that is not disabled may lead to ineffective ventilation in some patients. The oropharyngeal airway will help to maintain an open airway in the unresponsive patient and is an appropriate adjunct to use when ventilating with the BVM. (2-1.11b) (EC 140 PEC 119)

26.

D. The proper sequence to place a BVM mask on a patient's face is to first place the narrow part of the mask over the bridge of the nose, then lower the mask over the nose and mouth until the wider part meets the cleft of the chin. This sequence will aid in a better seal on the patient's face. If the mask does not cover the bridge of the nose and the cleft of the chin you need to select a more appropriate size mask. (2-1.11c) (EC 140 PEC 119)

27.

B. When ventilating an adult with the bag-valve-mask that is attached to oxygen the breath should be delivered over 1.0 to 2.0 seconds. This slow ventilation prevents gastric distention and subsequent aspiration. Observe for adequate chest rise and fall. (2-1.12) (EC 141-143 PEC 119-121)

28.

B. Ventilation of a patient with a bag-valve-mask device is best performed by a minimum of two rescuers. One rescuer bag-valve-mask ventilation is discouraged. It is difficult for one rescuer to maintain an effective seal and adequate volume of ventilation. (2-1.12) (EC 141-143 PEC 119-121)

29.

C. An increase in abdominal movement or distention with each ventilation is an indication that air is being forced into the esophagus and stomach. This could potentially result in severe gastric distention that impedes ventilation and leads to aspiration. (2-1.13) (EC 137 PEC 120-121)

30.

A. The patient is not being adequately ventilated at a rate of 15 ventilations per minute. Infants and children must be ventilated at a minimum of 20 ventilations per minute. Increasing the oxygen liter flow will not necessarily increase the delivered amount of oxygen to the patient. Never decompress the stomach unless the gastric distention impedes ventilation. (2-1.13) (EC 137 PEC 120-121)

31.

A. When ventilating a patient, watch for the chest to rise and fall when squeezing the bag. Often you will hear air sounds, however, this could be air escaping around the mask. The bag should deflate with little resistance while ventilating. If the bag progressively becomes more difficult to squeeze, consider repositioning the head, using an airway adjunct, or suspecting a tension pneumothorax. Often the cheeks will flare out with ventilations due to their flexibility; however, this is not a sign that the lungs are being ventilated. (2-1.14a) (EC 137 PEC 121-122)

32.

D. Ventilating too fast with too high of a tidal volume will force air into the esophagus and into the stomach, lessening the effectiveness of ventilation. To prevent air from entering the stomach you should ventilate over 2 seconds and allow for passive exhalation. (2-1.14b)(EC 137 PEC 121-122))

33.

A. The first step in ventilating a patient with a flow-restricted, oxygen-powered ventilation device is to ensure an adequate oxygen supply. The pressure relief valve opens at 60 cm of water pressure, not 40. The device should deliver a peak flow rate of 40 lpm, not 60 or 100 lpm. (2-1.15) (EC 144, 145 PEC 123-124)

34.

C. The oxygen flow is delivered at a constant 40 lpm and can not be altered. The inspiratory pressure control valve opens at 60 centimeters of water pressure. Increasing the ventilation time will not correct the problem if due to improper head position or mask seal. If after checking the head position and mask seal, the chest still does not rise, an airway obstruction must be considered. (2-1.15) (EC 144, 145 PEC 123-124)

35.

C. When ventilating a patient with a flow-restricted, oxygen-powered ventilation device the valve should be depressed until the chest begins to rise. Dependence on a pressure relief valve and an audible alarm is inappropriate. (2-1.15) (EC 144, 145 PEC 123-124)

36.

C. When performing mouth-to-mouth ventilation, you should break the seal of your mouth between ventilations to allow for adequate exhalation by the patient. This also allows you to breathe an adequate volume to deliver to the patient on the next ventilation. Ventilations should not be forceful and should be delivered over a 2 second period to reduce the incidence of gastric distention. (2-1.16) (EC 137, 145 PEC 117, 136)

37.

A. Air escaping from the nose and mouth while ventilating a patient through his stoma is an indication that the patient has a partial laryngectomy. You should pinch the nose and close the mouth and continue ventilation through the stoma. (2-1.16) (EC 137, 145 PEC 117, 136)

38.

D. A certain amount of resistance is expected when inserting a nasopharyngeal airway. If excessive resistance is encountered, remove the device and try the opposite nostril. Ensure that the airway is properly lubricated and try gently rotating the airway from side to side. (2-1.17) (EC 146-147 PEC 109-111)

39.

B. The proper size oropharyngeal airway is determined by measuring from the corner of the mouth to the tip of the earlobe. You can also measure from the center of the mouth to the bottom of the angle of the jaw. The sizing formula (16 + the patient's age in years) ÷ 4 is used to determine the proper size endotracheal tube in patients over 1 year of age. (2-1.17a) (EC 146-147 PEC 109-111)

40.

A. The OPA does not protect the airway from aspiration of vomitus or secretions. Suction should always be available. You should only use the OPA on completely unresponsive patients. Failure to do so may result in the patient gagging and vomiting. Using an OPA that is too long may force the epiglottis to close over the trachea, blocking the airway. (2-1.17b) (EC 146-147 PEC 109-111)

41.

A. The oropharyngeal airway must only be used on completely unresponsive patients without a gag reflex. If the patient is semiresponsive it is likely the patient will gag or possibly vomit causing further complications. (2-1.17c) (EC 146-147 PEC 109-111)

42.

A. Prior to insertion, a nasopharyngeal airway should be lubricated with a water-soluble lubricant. Never use a petroleum based lubricant. (2-1.18) (EC 147-148 PEC 111-112)

43.

D. To determine the proper length of a nasopharyngeal airway, measure from the tip of the nose to the tip of the earlobe. (2-1.18) (EC 147-148 PEC 111-112)

44.

C. The presence of blanching at the nasal opening indicates that the nasopharyngeal airway is too large. Use a smaller diameter airway. Blanching occurs when the nasal opening becomes white. This is a result of blood being forced from the area from excessive pressure. The airway should be inserted until the flange is seated firmly on the nostril. (2-1.18) (EC 147-148 PEC 111-112)

45.

B. When administering oxygen to the patient, you should first set up the oxygen delivery system. Second, prepare and attach the oxygen delivery device to the flowmeter, set the desired lpm flow, then apply the device to the patient. Applying a non-rebreather to the patient without oxygen flow can reduce the patient's tidal volume and cause or increase hypoxia. (2-1.19) (EC 156-160 PEC 125-132)

46.

B. The best way to measure the volume in the oxygen tank, regardless of the size of tank, is the pressure gauge. A full tank has 2000 pounds per square inch (psi) of pressure. As the tank volume decreases, so does the pressure in the tank. (2-1.19) (EC 156-160 PEC 125-132)

47.

A. When using a non-rebreather oxygen mask the oxygen regulator must be set so that the reservoir on the mask remains inflated. Typically the oxygen flow required to keep the reservoir inflated is 15 liters per minute. (2-1.20a) (EC 167-168 PEC 129)

48.

B. In the prehospital setting, always provide high flow oxygen to the COPD patient who is complaining of shortness of breath. The nasal cannula may not deliver enough oxygen to this patient; thus, the non-rebreather mask should be used. A nasal cannula set at 6 liters per minute will deliver only 44% oxygen. (2-1.20b) (EC 167-168 PEC 129)

49.

C. The preferred prehospital device for oxygen delivery is the non-rebreathing face mask. It delivers about a 90% to 95-1 oxygen concentration to the patient with adequate ventilation. Adjust the flow meter to prevent the non-rebreathing oxygen reservoir bag from completely collapsing when the patient inhales. This is usually 15 lpm. The nasal cannula is used only when a patient is not able to tolerate a non-rebreathing mask. (2-1.21) (EC 167, 168 PEC 130)

50.

D. The non-rebreathing mask provides high concentrations of oxygen primarily because the device contains an oxygen reservoir bag that collects 100% oxygen. The reservoir, in conjunction with high oxygen liter flow rates, allows the patient to inhale high concentrations of oxygen with each breath. (2-1.21) (EC 167, 168 PEC 130)

51.

B. If a patient is unable to tolerate a non-rebreather mask, you should first attempt to coach the patient. If that is not effective, a nasal cannula should be applied. If the patient can not tolerate the nasal cannula, oxygen should be administered by the blow-by technique. (2-1.22) (EC 167, 168 PEC 130-131)

52.

C. This patient's breathing status is adequate because the respiratory rate is normal, there is good chest rise, and there is good air volume being exchanged in the lungs. The patient was found walking around the house. Many patients with inadequate ventilation will assume a tripod position. You should administer high flow oxygen by non-rebreather mask. During your reassessment of the patient's breathing, if the breathing becomes inadequate you should provide positive pressure ventilation. (2-2.2) (EC 128-170 PEC 97-138)

53.

C. The common side effects of a beta agonist drug are tachycardia, tremors, shakiness, nervousness, dry mouth, nausea and vomiting. It is important to explain these common side effects to your patient prior to administering the drug. Explaining the common side effects will help to reduce the patient's stress and apprehension. (2-2.8) (EC 128-170 PEC 97-138)

54.

A. The patient's breathing has changed from adequate to inadequate. You should immediately provide positive pressure ventilation with the BVM and supplemental oxygen. Administering high flow oxygen will not help this patient. You must facilitate delivery of oxygen to the lungs by using the BVM and positive pressure ventilation. This patient does not need deep suctioning. The wheezes in the upper lungs and the absent lung sounds in the lower lungs are caused by bronchoconstriction. (2-2.5) (EC 128-170 PEC 97-138)

55.

C. A tidal volume of 10 ml/kg over a two second period should be delivered when providing ventilation by bag-valve-mask device or mouth-to-mask with an oxygen concentration less than 40%. If an oxygen concentration of equal to or greater than 40% is delivered by either device, the tidal volume delivered is reduced to 6 to 7 ml/kg and is delivered over a 1 to 2 second period. The smaller tidal volumes will reduce the risk of gastric inflation. If using a pocket mask, a minimum liter flow of 10 lpm is necessary to achieve an oxygen concentration of 40% or greater. However, the recommended liter flow to be used with the bag-valve-mask device and pocket mask is 15 lpm. (EC 128-170 PEC 97-138)

3 Patient Assessment

module objectives

Questions in this module relate to D.O.T. objectives 3-1.1 to 3-8.11.

DIRECTIONS Each of the questions or incomplete statements below is followed by suggested answers or completions. Select the **one answer** that is best in each case.

1. Scene safety begins:
   A. when you have reached the patient's side.
   B. just prior to reaching the patient's side, so the patient will not be distracted when performing the initial assessment.
   C. as you are arriving at the scene and before even exiting the ambulance.
   D. as you approach the scene once you have exited the ambulance.

2. Scenes that are potentially hazardous are:
   A. crash sites.
   B. incidents involving rescuing of the victim.
   C. crime scenes.
   D. all of the above.

3. While on the scene of an automobile crash, you find a small diameter power line lying across the vehicle. Which of the following is correct regarding power lines?
   A. Power lines can safely be removed by using rubber gloves and a long pipe or pole.
   B. Consider all power lines to be energized until a power company representative tells you they are not.
   C. Power lines that are knocked down on the ground are grounded and pose no threat to the EMT-B.
   D. Small diameter power lines are low energy and can be safely removed without injury to you.

4. If during the scene size-up, you identify a potentially hostile environment, you should:
   A. approach the scene cautiously to further assess the scene.
   B. make brief contact with the patient to explain you will return.
   C. drive past the scene and wait for the police to arrive.

   D. make patient contact and quickly transport.

5. You are called, on a winter morning, to the house of an elderly couple who are complaining of flulike symptoms with a rapid onset. You should suspect:
   A. toxic environment.
   B. influenza virus.
   C. hypothermia.
   D. poor nutrition.

6. Which of the following scenes would MOST likely pose a threat to the EMT-B?
   A. a known crime scene
   B. a large crowd
   C. a hypoxic patient
   D. a bar with intoxicated patrons

7. Your major responsibility at a crime scene is to:
   A. provide emergency medical care.
   B. prevent unnecessary people from entering the scene.
   C. identify potential weapons and preserve evidence.
   D. console the family.

8. Immediately upon arriving at a crash scene, you should:
   A. determine the total number of patients.
   B. determine if downed wires are present.
   C. survey and assess the entire scene and its surrounding area.
   D. determine if any patients are ambulatory.

9. A patient who opens his eyes when spoken to is:
   A. disoriented and responsive to verbal stimuli.
   B. responsive to verbal stimuli.

C. alert and disoriented.

D. alert and oriented.

10. All calls are typically categorized during the scene size-up and initial assessment as being:

    A. medical or obstetric.

    B. either medical or trauma.

    C. trauma or cardiac.

    D. cardiac or respiratory.

11. Mechanism of injury includes all the following **except:**

    A. falls.

    B. myocardial infarction.

    C. motor vehicle crash.

    D. shootings.

12. You arrive on a scene and determine that there are more patients than you and your partner can manage. When should you call for additional assistance?

    A. before making patient contact

    B. after making patient contact

    C. after the police have arrived

    D. after a fire official has arrived

13. Determining the total number of patients at a scene is a part of the:

    A. initial assessment.

    B. focused history.

    C. patient assessment.

    D. scene size-up.

14. You arrive on the scene of a two car motor vehicle crash and find four injured patients who appear to have significant injuries on scene size-up. You should immediately:

    A. triage the patients.

    B. transport the most critical patient.

    C. contact the hospital to notify it of the number of patients.

    D. call for additional ambulances.

15. Categorization of the patient as trauma is based on what two factors?

    A. scene size-up and the patient's vital signs

    B. immediate assessment of the scene and the initial assessment

    C. assessment of the scene and the mechanism of injury

    D. immediate assessment of the scene and the patient's mental status

16. While performing painful (tactile) stimulation to assess mental status, the patient responds with non-purposeful movement. Which of the following is an example of non-purposeful movement?

    A. The patient arches his or her back and flexes the arms towards the chest.

    B. The patient reaches up and grabs your hand in an attempt to remove pain.

    C. The patient makes attempts to move away from the painful stimulation.

    D. The patient moves his or her arm upwards and outwards in a sweeping motion toward the pain.

17. Which of the following would be a sign of a partially occluded airway?

    A. a patient who is able to give you his or her chief complaint with garbled speech

    B. an alert patient who has stridor on inhalation and is unable to speak

    C. a child who is crying vigorously and swallowing air

    D. an infant who is alert, sitting still, and drooling

18. You find a diabetic patient lying supine on the floor at the bottom of the stairs. Your first priority should be to:

    A. determine the mental status.

    B. provide manual in-line spinal stabilization.

C. assess the patient's airway.

D. assess the patient's breathing and pulse.

19. The most effective method to determine breathing status during the initial assessment is to:

    A. auscultate for breath sounds.

    B. inspect for retractions.

    C. apply a pulse oximeter.

    D. look, listen, and feel for air exchange.

20. During your assessment of an elderly patient found lying supine in bed you determine the patient is apneic. Your initial management should be to:

    A. immediately provide positive pressure ventilation.

    B. manually stabilize the cervical and lumbar spine.

    C. assess the circulation by checking a radial pulse.

    D. assess perfusion by checking the skin temperature.

21. You have been dispatched to the scene of a shooting. The local police have secured the scene. They direct you to the patient who is a male about 16 years of age. There is a large bloodstain on the patient's left lateral chest region. The patient's eyes are closed and he does not move as you approach. Your partner takes manual in-line stabilization and opens the airway using the jaw-thrust maneuver. Your next immediate action should be to:

    A. apply a gauze dressing to the chest wound.

    B. assess the breathing status.

    C. size and place a cervical collar on the patient.

    D. palpate the chest for signs of chest injury.

22. You are providing positive pressure ventilation by bag valve mask with an oropharyngeal airway in place. Your partner has sealed a sucking chest wound and controlled bleeding from the chest. You find that it is becoming increasingly difficult to squeeze the bag valve mask device to ventilate the patient. You should immediately:

    A. auscultate the chest for wheezing.

    B. recheck the patient's blood pressure.

    C. assess the breath sounds and neck.

    D. recheck the liter flow of oxygen to the BVM.

23. During your detailed physical exam you find a second bullet wound in the occipital region of the patient's head. The patient's pupils are unequal and a straw-colored fluid is draining from his right ear. You should:

    A. quickly remove the oropharyngeal airway.

    B. decrease the oxygen concentration provided.

    C. ventilate the patient between 8 to 12 ventilations per minute.

    D. hyperventilate the patient at 20 ventilations per minute.

24. During the initial assessment you determined the unresponsive infant has an obstructed airway from a foreign body. Your initial action should be to perform:

    A. five quick chest thrusts.

    B. five abdominal thrusts.

    C. a blind finger sweep.

    D. five rapid back blows.

25. The presence of a palpable radial pulse:

    A. indicates an estimated BP at 100 mmHg diastolic.

    B. is not an accurate way to determine blood pressure.

    C. estimates the systolic blood pressure at 80 mmHg.

D. provides an estimate of a diastolic blood pressure.

26. When initially assessing the pulse in an adult the _____ artery is palpated, whereas in an infant you will be palpating the _____ artery. (3-2.13)
    A. carotid, brachial
    B. radial, brachial
    C. radial, femoral
    D. brachial, radial

27. You arrive on the scene and find a patient that fell from a tree. His pants are soaked with blood. You expose the injured area and find a large laceration with a steady flow of blood. You should immediately:
    A. press your gloved hand firmly over the wound.
    B. apply a tourniquet directly below the wound.
    C. place a pressure dressing over the wound site.
    D. apply digital pressure to the nearest proximal pressure point.

28. Which of the following are abnormal skin temperature findings?
    A. hot
    B. cool
    C. cold
    D. all of the above

29. Capillary refill is most reliable sign in:
    A. adults.
    B. children over 8 years of age.
    C. children less than 6 years of age.
    D. newborns only.

30. When reconsidering the mechanism of injury in the focused history and physical exam, you should determine if:

A. the further evaluation of the mechanism of injury met criteria to be considered significant.
B. any hazards or potential hazards that could harm you or the patient were missed.
C. specific injury to organs can be identified.
D. the airway or breathing is compromised.

31. Significant mechanism of injury in the infant and child includes all the following **except**:
    A. falls greater than 10 feet.
    B. motor vehicle collisions of low speed.
    C. bicycle collisions.
    D. motor vehicle collision with the death of a passenger in the same compartment as the patient.

32. In what order would you conduct an assessment of a patient with a significant mechanism of injury?
    A. rapid trauma assessment, baseline vitals, SAMPLE history
    B. baseline vitals, rapid trauma assessment, SAMPLE history
    C. baseline vitals, SAMPLE history, rapid trauma assessment
    D. SAMPLE history, rapid trauma assessment, baseline vitals

33. You arrive at the scene of a motor vehicle crash with significant vehicle damage. You find the patient unrestrained in the front seat. Following the scene size-up, you should immediately:
    A. perform an initial assessment.
    B. perform a focused physical exam to the head, chest, and abdomen.
    C. obtain a set of baseline vital signs.
    D. perform a rapid trauma assessment.

34. The rapid trauma assessment:
    A. focuses on a specific injury site.
    B. is a quick head-to-toe exam.

C. begins with obtaining a SAMPLE history.

D. does not include reassessment of vital signs.

35. The decision to perform a rapid trauma or focused physical exam is based on the:

A. baseline vital signs.

B. SAMPLE history.

C. mechanism of injury and initial assessment findings.

D. findings in the ongoing assessment.

36. You performed a focused trauma exam on a patient who suffered a leg injury from a fall. En route, the patient suddenly becomes disoriented and repeatedly asks you what happened. You should:

A. contact medical control for orders for further emergency care.

B. conduct a focused exam to the patient's head.

C. obtain a SAMPLE history.

D. perform a rapid trauma assessment.

37. A physical exam that is conducted to identify life-threatening injuries to the head, chest, abdomen, pelvis, or extremities is:

A. a focused trauma exam.

B. an ongoing assessment.

C. an initial assessment.

D. rapid trauma assessment.

38. Upon initial assessment you find the patient complaining of severe pain to his ankle following a fall while playing basketball. When questioned, he cannot identify where he is. This patient requires:

A. a rapid medical assessment.

B. a focused physical exam.

C. a rapid trauma assessment.

D. an initial assessment and rapid transport.

39. The mnemonic DCAP-BTLS stands for:

A. deformities, contusions, avulsions, pooling blood, breaks, trauma, lacerations, and swelling.

B. deformities, contusions, avulsions, penetrations, breaks, tenderness, lacerations, swelling.

C. deformities, contusions, abrasions, punctures, burns, tenderness, lacerations, swelling.

D. distention, contusions, abrasions, punctures, burns, tenderness, lacerations, swelling.

40. The rapid trauma assessment is performed using a systematic approach, starting at the _____ and ending at the _____?

A. lower extremities, head

B. head, upper extremities

C. head, posterior body

D. upper extremities, lower extremities

41. When assessing the head and face of a trauma patient during the detailed physical exam, you should:

A. remove the head immobilization device to allow for better examination of the head.

B. firmly press on the skull, using the tips of your fingers to feel for depressions.

C. note any areas of tenderness or swelling to the maxilla and mandible.

D. apply pressure to each eye, assessing for injury to the globe.

42. While assessing the chest during the rapid trauma assessment, you find very minimal chest rise during inhalation. You should:

A. complete the assessment followed by application of oxygen by non-rebreather mask.

B. complete the assessment and then provide positive pressure ventilation.

C. immediately administer oxygen by non-rebreather mask and then continue the assessment.

D. immediately begin positive pressure ventilation and continue with the assessment.

43. When performing a rapid trauma assessment, which of the following represents a critical finding that must be managed immediately?
    A. paradoxical chest wall movement
    B. a closed fibia fracture
    C. flat jugular veins with patient sitting at a 45°
    D. an open humerus fracture with the bone protruding from the skin

44. The rapid trauma assessment is performed to:
    A. prevent patient complaints.
    B. identify life-threatening injuries or conditions.
    C. recognize life threats to the airway and breathing.
    D. identify detailed information about the injury.

45. When assessing a medical patient it is important to ask questions concerning the chief complaint to:
    A. further assess the history of the present illness.
    B. base all treatment of the patient on.
    C. determine if ALS assistance is needed.
    D. determine the mechanism of injury.

46. Which of the following should be used to collect information about the chief complaint?
    A. detailed physical exam
    B. DCAP-BTLS mnemonic
    C. AVPU mnemonic
    D. OPQRST mnemonic

47. The OPQRST is a mnemonic for:
    A. onset, pain, quantity, radiation, sensation, time.
    B. onset, provocation/palliation, quality, radiation, severity, time.
    C. onset, pain, quality, radiation, sensation, time.
    D. onset, provocation, quantity, radiation, sensation, time.

48. When asking the patient about provocation/palliation, you are trying to determine:
    A. what makes the pain better or worse.
    B. what started the pain.
    C. the approximate time the pain started.
    D. what the patient was doing when the symptoms were first noticed.

49. While assessing a patient's complaint you ask, "Does the pain move to the jaw or down the arms?" This question is assessing the:
    A. quality.
    B. radiation.
    C. provocation.
    D. severity.

50. When assessing the quality of a patient's chest pain, you would ask which of the following questions?
    A. What does the pain feel like?
    B. Where is the pain?
    C. What makes the pain worse?
    D. When and how did the pain begin?

51. The focused history and physical exam for the responsive medical patient is performed in what sequence?
    A. history, focused exam, vital signs
    B. history, vital signs, focused exam
    C. focused exam, vital signs, history
    D. vital signs, history, focused exam

52. The focused history and physical exam for the unresponsive medical patient is performed in which sequence?
    A. history, rapid medical assessment, vital signs
    B. history, vital signs, rapid medical assessment
    C. rapid medical assessment, vital signs, history
    D. vital signs, history, rapid medical assessment

53. An unresponsive medical patient is a:
    A. low priority.
    B. medium priority.
    C. high priority.
    D. not a priority patient.

54. When assessing the unresponsive medical patient:
    A. perform a complete detailed physical exam prior to transport.
    B. inspect the scene for information about the nature of the illness.
    C. do not ask bystanders and family members questions regarding the incident.
    D. perform the initial assessment after the rapid medical assessment.

55. Unequal pupils may indicate:
    A. carbon monoxide poisoning.
    B. head injury.
    C. severe hypoxia.
    D. heat emergency.

56. Your medical patient responds to painful (tactile) stimulation with non-purposeful movement during the initial assessment. After the initial assessment, you should next perform a:
    A. focused physical exam.
    B. SAMPLE history interview.
    C. detailed physical assessment.
    D. rapid medical assessment.

57. The unresponsive medical patient should be placed in which position?
    A. Trendelenburg position
    B. semi-Fowler position
    C. prone position, legs extended
    D. left lateral recumbent position

58. You have just completed the initial assessment on a medical patient complaining of shortness of breath. You would next:
    A. perform a rapid medical assessment.

B. evaluate the chief complaint using the OPQRST mnemonic.
    C. perform certain components of a detailed physical exam.
    D. assess the patient by performing a focused medical exam.

59. The purpose of a detailed physical exam is to:
    A. identify all non-life-threatening injuries/conditions and provide appropriate emergency medical care.
    B. identify all life-threatening injuries and manage those injuries.
    C. evaluate the initial assessment.
    D. determine if the mechanism of injury correlates with the patient's injuries.

60. When performing the detailed physical exam, you should use information collected from:
    A. the scene size-up.
    B. the initial assessment.
    C. focused history and physical exam.
    D. all of the above.

61. Which of the following components of the assessment would not occur during the detailed physical exam?
    A. initial assessment of vital signs
    B. evaluation of breath sounds
    C. palpation of the abdomen
    D. reassessment of pupillary function

62. While inspecting the eyes during the detailed physical assessment, you find the sclera are yellow. You would likely suspect possible:
    A. heart failure.
    B. liver failure.
    C. drug overdose.
    D. head injury.

63. During your assessment, the neck appears to be swollen, and crepitation is felt directly under the skin. You would most likely suspect trauma to the:
    A. head.

B. trachea.

C. abdomen.

D. spine.

64. You are performing an assessment on a patient involved in a fall. You find a portion of the chest wall moves inward during inspiration, and then moves outward during exhalation. The condition the patient is suffering from is a:

A. flail chest.

B. tension pneumothorax.

C. simple pneumothorax.

D. collapsed lung.

65. Injuries found during the detailed physical exam are managed:

A. after completion of the exam.

B. when found during the exam.

C. after the patient is transported.

D. just prior to patient transport.

66. A trauma patient is unable to close his mouth. Your major concern is:

A. maintenance of spinal immobilization.

B. potential damage to teeth.

C. immobilizing a fracture of the maxilla.

D. maintaining a patent airway.

67. When examining the eyes of a patient during the detailed physical exam:

A. it is necessary to remove any foreign bodies embedded in the eye to further examine it.

B. the eyelid should be forced open if injuries to the eyelid are observed.

C. both eyes should react simultaneously to a light shone in one eye.

D. pressure should be applied to the globe of the eye to control bleeding.

68. A pupil that is large in size and not responding to light is referred to as:

A. profiled.

B. fixed and dilated.

C. pytosis.

D. a false dilation.

69. The eyes moving together in one direction is referred to as:

A. visual acuity.

B. consensual movement.

C. conjugate movement.

D. conjugate gaze.

70. A patient who has unequal pupils but is alert and oriented requires:

A. rapid treatment and transportation.

B. positive pressure ventilation at 24 breaths per minute.

C. insertion of a nasopharyngeal airway.

D. assessment for a possible direct injury to the eye.

71. During palpation of a trauma patient's neck you feel an unusual sensation of air under the skin. This is referred to as:

A. a tension pneumothorax.

B. a pericardial tamponade.

C. hematoma infiltration.

D. subcutaneous emphysema.

72. A pale tongue in a trauma patient may be an indication of:

A. hypoxia.

B. head injury.

C. laryngeal trauma.

D. poor perfusion.

73. When auscultating a patient's chest, the presence of wheezing may indicate:

A. fluid in the smaller airways.

B. dilation of the airway.

C. constriction of the trachea.

D. constriction of the bronchiole.

74. During your ongoing assessment of a head injured patient, you would repeat the initial assessment for all the following reasons **except:**
    A. to determine if the patient's injuries have begun to worsen.
    B. to make sure you did not miss any injuries in the rapid trauma exam.
    C. to determine if treatment provided is beneficial.
    D. to determine if you need to provide a different treatment.

75. Your patient was struck on the head with a hammer and lost consciousness. How often should you repeat the ongoing assessment?
    A. every 3 minutes
    B. every 5 minutes
    C. every 10 minutes
    D. every 15 minutes

76. Your patient tells you that he has a history of an abdominal aortic aneurysm. The patient begins to experience a sharp tearing pain that radiates to his lower back. You should conduct the ongoing assessment because:
    A. the patient's aneurysm may be leaking.
    B. the patient's circulatory system may be compromised.
    C. the patient's condition now may require a different destination hospital.
    D. all of the above.

77. Your patient has an altered mental status of an unknown etiology. You have inserted an oropharyngeal airway to maintain an open airway. While you continue with the initial assessment, you should assess all the following **except:**
    A. positioning of the airway.
    B. for vomitus in the airway.
    C. the vital signs.
    D. the respiratory effort.

78. While performing repeated ongoing assessments, the information gathered should:
    A. be compared with the initial examination.
    B. provide you with a current patient status.
    C. allow for quicker identification of patient deterioration.
    D. all of the above.

79. When performing an ongoing assessment on an unstable patient, you should repeat and record vital signs and assessment findings every:
    A. 5 minutes.
    B. 10 minutes.
    C. 15 minutes.
    D. 20 minutes.

80. While performing an ongoing assessment your patient—who was initially alert and talking—is no longer talking and has his eyes closed. You should reassess the mental status using which mnemonic?
    A. OPQRST
    B. AVPU
    C. GLASGOW
    D. SAMPLE

81. During the ongoing assessment you note the patient's pulse rate has decreased and is a poor quality. You should suspect:
    A. a low blood sugar level (hypoglycemia).
    B. a head injury or severe hypoxia.
    C. a heat related emergency.
    D. an allergic reaction (anaphylaxis).

82. Which of the following is not a basic reason for performing an ongoing assessment?
    A. to determine a diagnosis of the patient's condition
    B. to detect any changes in the patient's condition
    C. to change the emergency care as needed
    D. to locate and identify missed injuries and conditions

83. Why should you wait at least one second after you push the transmit button before you begin speaking into the radio?
   A. to eliminate static in the background
   B. so your battery will last longer
   C. to allow the radio to broadcast farther
   D. to allow the repeater time to open the channel and prevent cutting off the first part of the communication

84. After you are finished with your transmission you should:
   A. turn the radio off to save power.
   B. say "Over" and wait for confirmation from the other participant.
   C. say "Over" and turn your radio off to free the airwaves.
   D. none of the above.

85. Identify the correct sequence for communicating patient information to medical direction.
   1. patient age and sex
   2. history of present illness
   3. chief complaint
   4. past illness
   5. vitals
   6. mental status

   A. 1, 2, 3, 5, 6, 4
   B. 1, 3, 2, 6, 5, 4
   C. 1, 3, 2, 4, 6, 5
   D. 1, 3, 5, 6, 2, 4

86. Once you have received a correct order from medical direction, you should:
   A. repeat the order back word for word.
   B. ask medical direction to repeat the order.
   C. repeat the order to dispatch.
   D. ask your partner to repeat the order to you.

87. Clear communication with medical control is most important because:
   A. patient confidentiality statutes must be followed.
   B. the FCC requires accurate transmission of information.
   C. of your department's concern about medical legal liability.
   D. receiving accurate orders is necessary for good patient care.

88. Essential information that needs to be summarized in the oral report includes:
   A. patient's chief complaint, vital signs at the scene, treatment given en route, response to the treatment, and pertinent history not given earlier.
   B. patient's chief complaint, vital signs en route, and treatment en route.
   C. patient's chief complaint, vital signs taken en route, treatment given en route, response to the treatment, and pertinent history not given earlier.
   D. patient's chief complaint, vital signs en route, and treatment given.

89. To improve communication with your patient, especially children and infants, you should:
   A. immediately establish that you are in charge and allow the patient to speak only to you.
   B. position yourself at the same level or lower than that of the patient.
   C. address all patients by their first name.
   D. remove any other family, toys, or distracters from the area directly around the patient.

90. When dealing with an older patient, it is important to remember:
   A. not all older patients have auditory deficits.
   B. some older adults need more time to rationalize what you are saying.
   C. allow enough time for the patient to respond to you.
   D. all of the above.

91. Information given in the oral report:
    A. is not important because a written report is always provided.
    B. is important information that helps the hospital ensure continuity of care.
    C. generally requires only your unit identification and the patient's chief complaint.
    D. is of little importance because a written report is always provided.

92. Which of the following is an appropriate procedure when using the radio to communicate with other members of the EMS team?
    A. Push the press to talk (PTT) button and immediately begin speaking.
    B. Speak with your mouth at least 12 to 18 inches from the microphone.
    C. Give objective or relevant subjective information, and avoid offering a diagnosis.
    D. After receiving medical control orders, stop the transmission and initiate treatment.

93. All of the following are responsibilities of the Federal Communications Commission **except:**
    A. training response personnel.
    B. approving equipment for use.
    C. monitoring field operations.
    D. assigning call signs.

94. A major disadvantage of cellular telephones for EMS use is that they:
    A. require a special FCC EMS license.
    B. do not work well in urban areas.
    C. may be overwhelmed in a disaster.
    D. are expensive to maintain and operate.

95. A device that receives a transmission from a relatively low-powered source such as a mobile radio and rebroadcasts the signal on another frequency and a higher power is called a(n):
    A. encoder.
    B. duplexer.
    C. repeater.
    D. decoder.

96. CAD, when used in Emergency Medical Service dispatching, stands for:
    A. computer-aided dispatch.
    B. critical-area dispatch.
    C. common-area dispatch.
    D. constant-action dispatch.

97. Recording of response times:
    A. should be accurately transcribed by the EMT-B.
    B. does not need to be precisely recorded by the EMT-B.
    C. is not required in EMS systems.
    D. is generally only handled by the Emergency Medical Dispatcher.

98. The agency that has jurisdiction over all EMS radio operations in the United States is the:
    A. APCO.
    B. NTSHA.
    C. D.O.T.
    D. FCC.

99. You have received what appears to be an inappropriate order from medical control. In this circumstance you should:
    A. perform the request.
    B. question the order.
    C. perform the request and document the order.
    D. contact your supervisor for instructions.

100. Medical direction insists that you perform a procedure outside of your scope of practice. You should:
    A. question the order.
    B. follow the order.
    C. call your supervisor.
    D. disregard the order.

101. When speaking to an elderly patient who has been in an automobile crash, you should:
    A. speak loudly and assertively with authority.
    B. use medical terms to convey intelligence.
    C. speak slowly, calmly, and distinctly.
    D. use codes to protect the patient from stress.

102. The patient care report must include:
    A. chief complaint, level of responsiveness, and systolic blood pressure.
    B. skin perfusion, color, and temperature.
    C. pulse rate, respiratory rate, and effort.
    D. all of the above.

103. The D.O.T. requires all the following administrative information be placed on the prehospital care report **except:**
    A. time the incident was reported and the time the unit was notified.
    B. time the unit spent in the hospital and the time it was placed back into service.
    C. time the unit arrived at the hospital and the time of transfer of patient care.
    D. time of arrival at the scene and the time the unit left the scene.

104. The Department of Transportation requires minimum data to be collected on the prehospital care report (PCR). Which is an element of the Department of Transportation's minimum data set?
    A. patient's legal name
    B. level of responsiveness
    C. age and sex of the patient
    D. diastolic blood pressure

105. The narrative section of the patient care report (PCR) should include all of the following **except:**
    A. patient's chief complaint.
    B. SAMPLE history.
    C. mechanism of injury.

    D. patient's name, age, and sex.

106. What is an acceptable abbreviation for "four times a day"?
    A. QID
    B. SOB
    C. TID
    D. NTG

107. Information that the Department of Transportation requires on all patient care reports is called the:
    A. transport care information.
    B. D.O.T PCR data.
    C. minimum data set.
    D. D.O.T patient care information.

108. All of the following are important considerations related to the collection of information for patient care reports **except:**
    A. clocks should be accurate and synchronous.
    B. only one set of vital signs should be obtained.
    C. the patient narrative contains objective information.
    D. the patient narrative contains subjective information.

109. Noting information and signs that were not found during the physical assessment would be referred to as:
    A. pertinent negative.
    B. negative complaint.
    C. reverse symptom.
    D. compound complaint.

110. Knowingly providing false information on the patient care report:
    A. is acceptable if limited to only the vital signs.
    B. is acceptable if an act of omission occurs.

C. is acceptable if an act of commission occurs.

D. is never acceptable in any circumstances.

111. Patient refusals of treatment require:

A. less documentation than if a patient is transported.

B. about the same amount of information as a transported patient.

C. complete documentation of your efforts to provide care.

D. more documentation than if a patient is transported.

112. Confidentiality of information contained in the patient care report is

A. not important and requires little vigilance.

B. required only if covered by local or state law.

C. required only if the patient makes a formal request.

D. important and should be maintained at all times.

113. If a patient refuses to sign your refusal document you should:

A. leave the scene before the patient changes his mind.

B. place an X in the refusal box.

C. tell the patient he will have to sign or go to the hospital.

D. have a family member, police officer, or bystander sign the report verifying that the patient refused to sign.

114. When a patient signs a refusal, the EMT-B must be completely assured that the patient:

A. is not under the influence of alcohol or other drugs.

B. is able to make a rational informed decision about his or her care.

C. does not have an altered mental status from an injury or illness.

D. all of the above.

115. In the refusal report, the EMT-B should include all the following information **except:**

A. complete patient assessment or documentation explaining why it was not completed.

B. statement that the EMT-B advised the patient of the consequences of refusing transport, including the potential of death.

C. statement advising the patient not to call EMS if the patient will not allow the EMT-B to perform his or her job.

D. documentation of any and all communication with medical control or other authorities.

116. To correct an error in the patient care report (PCR), you should:

A. erase the error completely, then write over the area with the correction.

B. draw a single horizontal line through the error; then initial the correction.

C. write directly over the error with a different color ink; then initial the correction.

D. cover the error completely with correction fluid; then write directly over the area.

SCENARIO

Questions 117–119 refer to the following scenario.

You and your partner Emil are dispatched to a call for a fight at 69 Over Street. Dispatch advises that the scene is secured by police, and they are requesting you to expedite your response. Upon your arrival, you are met by a police officer who states an elderly man named Carl Luis has been shot in the chest. As you approach the patient you quickly gain the impression that he is severely injured. You see blood escaping freely from a penetrating wound to the upper right chest. The patient is breathing approximately 20 times a minute.

117. As you proceed with the initial assessment, your first action should be to:

A. assess mental status using AVPU.

B. assess airway, breathing, and circulation.

C. perform a focused history and physical.

D. place your gloved hand over the chest wound.

118. The next action performed as part of the initial assessment of this patient is to:

A. open the airway using the head-tilt chin-lift.

B. assess mental status using the mnemonic AVPU.

C. obtain a SAMPLE history and a detailed exam.

D. establish manual in-line stabilization of the spine.

119. Relating to the mechanism of injury of this patient, which physical exam should you perform?

A. focused trauma assessment

B. rapid trauma assessment

C. detailed physical assessment

D. concentrated trauma assessment

120. You have responded to a call for a patient who fell. You arrive on scene and find a patient with a deformity to the toe. The patient requests care and transport. The hospital is located close by. Your departmental policy requires at least two sets of vital signs to be taken on all patients. Due to your close proximity to the hospital, you only obtain one set. How should you handle this situation?

A. Report the same vital signs as recorded earlier.

B. Use a standard set of vitals based upon the age.

C. Document that you failed to obtain the vital signs.

D. Use the same vital signs but change them slightly.

121. While completing your patient care report, you note that the patient complained of intense pain in his toe. This is an example of _____ information.

A. subjective

B. orthopedic

C. minor

D. objective

122. You are returning to quarters and stop by a convenience store to purchase a soft drink. A gentleman approaches and asks what was going on across the street from his house a few minutes ago. He identifies himself as the neighbor of the patient you just transported. How should you respond to his request?

A. Tell him exactly what happened, but don't use any names.

B. Tell him only if he promises not to tell where he got the information.

C. Tell him this is "Off the record" and then relay the information.

D. Tell him you are not allowed to divulge such information.

123. You arrive on the scene and find a 27-year-old man in the bathroom of his home. During your initial assessment, you determine he is not alert. The next immediate action you should take is to:

A. open the airway by using a jaw-thrust maneuver.

B. ask him to open his eyes or talk to you.

C. insert an oropharyngeal airway.

D. check for a radial pulse and skin color, temperature, and condition.

124. You arrive on the scene and find a young male construction worker who was crushed under a wall that collapsed on top of him. You determine the scene is safe and approach the patient. He is severely cyanotic and appears not to be breathing. Blood is spurting out of his cut pant leg. Your next immediate action should be to:

A. begin positive pressure ventilation with supplemental oxygen.

B. expose and apply direct pressure to the bleeding leg wound.

C. assess the radial pulse and skin for perfusion status.

D. take manual in-line stabilization and apply a non-rebreather mask.

125. You arrive on the scene and find a 30-year-old male patient with a gunshot wound to the chest. During your general impression you note blood in the mouth, severe cyanosis to the face and neck, and no chest wall movement. You should immediately:

A. suction the airway and occlude the gunshot wound to the chest.

B. expose the patient and check for other serious gunshot wounds.

C. begin BVM ventilation with supplemental oxygen and place your gloved hand over the wound.

D. occlude the open wound, apply a non-rebreather mask at 15 lpm and begin your initial assessment.

126. You are assessing a 40-year-old male patient who crashed his motorcycle. He complains of pain to his right leg. You suspect the tibia and fibula are fractured. Which of the following would be the best indicator of a suspected fracture?

A. crepitation

B. pain

C. ecchymosis

D. edema

127. Which of the following provides the least accurate information when assessing circulation in the adult patient?

A. capillary refill

B. skin color

C. skin condition

D. peripheral pulse

128. While conducting your general impression, which of the following would cause you to believe the patient is dyspneic?

A. The patient is gasping for air while crying loudly.

B. The patient is lying supine on the couch while explaining how he feels.

C. The patient says a few words and takes a breath.

D. The patient is on home oxygen at 2 lpm.

129. You arrive on the scene of an auto crash and find a 23-year-old woman who was the driver of the vehicle. During the initial assessment you find cyanosis to the face and neck, a large depression with moderate bleeding to the left temporal region, a respiratory rate of 12/minute with shallow breathing, and weak peripheral pulses. You should immediately:

A. apply direct pressure to the head injury and apply a non-rebreather at 15 lpm.

B. perform a jaw-thrust and begin positive pressure ventilation with supplemental oxygen.

C. take a blood pressure and apply a pulse oximeter to determine the blood oxygen concentration.

D. dress the wound to the head and then begin BVM ventilation with supplemental oxygen.

130. A 25-year-old female patient was thrown off her horse. She is responsive and complains of pain to her head. Following the initial assessment you should:

A. conduct a focused physical exam of the head.

B. begin transport.

C. conduct a detailed exam of the head.

D. conduct a rapid trauma assessment.

131. You arrive on the scene and find a 28-year-old female who fell 20 feet while roofing a house. As you exit the ambulance, she appears to be unresponsive. You notice a large pool of blood around her left thigh. There is blood draining from the mouth and nose. Your first priority is to:

A. suction the airway and begin BVM ventilation.

B. look for safety hazards before approaching the patient.

C. expose the left thigh and find any possible major bleeding.

D. open her airway using a jaw-thrust and apply a non-rebreather mask at 15 lpm.

132. You arrive on the scene and find a 10-year-old male patient who was struck by a car while riding his bike. He is unresponsive to painful stimuli. You have opened the airway with a jaw-thrust and find the respirations to be 20/minute and shallow. His radial pulse is barely palpable. You should immediately:

A. apply a non-rebreather at 15 lpm.

B. begin chest compressions.

C. begin bag-valve-mask ventilation.

D. apply a cervical spinal immobilization collar.

133. A 62-year-old female patient whom you find sitting in her recliner at home is complaining of severe abdominal pain as you walk in the door. As you approach the patient, she states that her "belly is real sore and aching bad." Your next action in assessing the patient is to:

A. assess the circulation and gather a SAMPLE history.

B. open the airway and assess the breathing status.

C. begin BVM ventilation and connect supplemental oxygen.

D. conduct a rapid medical assessment and assess vital signs.

134. You arrive on the scene and find an 8-year-old boy at the local gym who was knocked out while playing basketball. Following your assessment you suspect he has a head injury. You should immediately:

A. transport without treatment due to the lack of parental consent.

B. initiate emergency care and transport.

C. wait for the police to arrive before initiating treatment.

D. contact the parents for consent to begin treatment.

135. You arrive on the scene and find a 23-year-old female patient who stepped on a piece of glass and lacerated her foot while walking through the front yard. She is sitting on the ground holding her foot as you approach her. She complains that her foot "hurts like hell" and is bleeding. Your next immediate action is to:

A. assess the amount of bleeding to determine if it is uncontrolled and major.

B. apply a non-rebreather mask at 15 lpm.

C. immediately begin a rapid trauma assessment to assess for life-threatening injuries.

D. perform a jaw-thrust maneuver and assess the breathing status.

136. Following the initial assessment of a medical patient complaining of chest pain, you determine that the patient is not oriented and is speaking inappropriately. The next step in your assessment is to:

A. repeat the initial assessment.

B. perform an ongoing assessment.

C. conduct a focused history and physical exam.

D. perform a rapid medical assessment.

137. You arrive on the scene of an auto crash involving a frontal collision and find the patient seated in the front seat of the driver's side of the vehicle. You determine that the scene is safe and approach the patient. You should immediately:

A. determine the mental status.

B. open the airway using the jaw-thrust.

C. establish manual in-line stabilization of the head and neck.

D. assess the radial pulse and carotid pulses and the skin.

138. Tracheal deviation is:
    A. an early sign of a pneumothorax.
    B. a late sign of a tension pneumothorax.
    C. a sign of pericardial tamponade.
    D. a late sign of hypovolemic shock.

139. You arrive on the scene and find a 20-year-old male patient who was involved in an auto crash. Upon your assessment, you note the patient can not tell you what date it is, where he is, or whom he is with. The patient refuses to let you examine him further and refuses any emergency care. You should:
    A. have the patient sign a refusal form and leave the scene.
    B. turn the patient over to the police on the scene and leave.
    C. begin to administer emergency care to the patient and then transport him, using restraints if necessary.
    D. have the police place the patient under protective custody so that you can administer emergency care.

140. Capillary refill would be most reliable and provide the most information on which of the following patients?
    A. a 3-year-old trauma patient who is trapped in a vehicle in 10° temperature
    B. an 8-year-old who is having an asthma attack
    C. a 30-year-old who was shot in the chest three times
    D. a 5-year-old who lacerated his femoral artery on broken glass and is bleeding profusely

141. Blood mixed with clear fluid coming from the ears in a patient who was struck in the head would most likely indicate:
    A. a fractured skull.
    B. a concussion.
    C. an injury to the ear canal.
    D. a lacerated meningeal artery.

142. You arrive on the scene and find a 65-year-old male patient sitting on the couch at home complaining that he "can't breathe." The patient is alert and oriented and his radial pulse is rapid and strong. His skin is slightly pale, cool, and clammy. You should immediately:
    A. apply a non-rebreather mask at 15 lpm.
    B. assess his baseline vital signs.
    C. perform a rapid medical exam.
    D. place the patient in a supine position.

143. You arrive on the scene and find a 74-year-old male patient who collapsed at home. As you approach the patient you note his eyes are not open, you hear a loud gurgling noise, and it appears he is breathing at about 6 times per minute. You should immediately:
    A. assess the radial and then the carotid pulse.
    B. begin bag-valve-mask ventilation with supplemental oxygen and assess his mental status.
    C. apply a non-rebreather mask and assess the blood pressure.
    D. suction the mouth until clear and then begin positive pressure ventilation.

144. The respiratory rate of an infant:
    A. is approximately the same rate as that of an adult.
    B. is usually slightly slower than that of an adult.
    C. is higher at birth and progressively decreases with age.
    D. is irregularly irregular.

145. Which of the following would be the best indicator of hypoxia in a patient complaining of dyspnea?
    A. The patient states his difficulty of breathing is a 10 on the severity scale.
    B. The pulse oximeter reads 93% while the patient is on a non-rebreather mask at 15 lpm.

C. The skin is slightly pale, cool, and clammy.

D. The patient is using his sternocleido-mastoid muscles to breathe and you see intercostal retractions.

146. You arrive on the scene and find a patient who is complaining of dizziness and nausea. You find the radial pulse is present and the skin is warm, moist, and flushed. You should next:

A. determine the level of responsiveness.

B. begin a rapid medical assessment.

C. gather a SAMPLE history.

D. assess the patient's abdomen for tenderness and rigidity.

147. The skin is assessed during the initial assessment to determine the:

A. level of hypoxia.

B. number of circulating red blood cells.

C. the perfusion status of the patient.

D. need for oxygen therapy.

148. Which of the following is **not** considered a life-threatening injury?

A. fractured ribs

B. bilateral femur fractures

C. open wound to the posterior thorax

D. unstable pelvis

SCENARIO

Questions 149 and 150 refer to the following scenario.

You arrive on the scene and find a 77-year-old male patient lying in bed. He does not respond to verbal stimuli. He is breathing at 22 times per minute with good tidal volume and his radial pulse is 78 per minute. The skin is warm, dry, and normal in color.

149. Your next immediate action in this patient is to:

A. apply a non-rebreather mask and begin a rapid medical assessment.

B. establish manual in-line spinal stabilization and insert an oropharyngeal airway.

C. obtain a set of baseline vital signs and begin transport.

D. begin bag-valve-mask ventilation with supplemental oxygen.

150. The skin of the patient most likely indicates:

A. hypovolemic shock.

B. inadequate delivery of hemoglobin to the cells.

C. good tissue perfusion.

D. hypoxia and hypercarbia.

151. The unresponsive medical patient should be placed in what position?

A. supine with head slightly elevated

B. Fowler's

C. left lateral recumbent

D. Trendelenburg

152. Which of the following is considered subjective patient information?

A. "The patient has a swollen, deformed extremity."

B. "The patient's pulse is 110 beats per minute."

C. "The patient's blood pressure was 110/80."

D. "The patient is in pain."

SCENARIO

Questions 153 and 154 refer to the following scenario.

As you are pulling up to the scene of a construction accident you spot a patient lying prone on the ground next to a pile of rubble. It appears a building has collapsed.

153. Your immediate action is to:

A. take in-line spinal stabilization and logroll the patient onto his back.

B. assess the mental status and determine if he is responsive.

C. search for more than one patient and call for additional resources.

D. wait by the ambulance until the engineer has indicated that the structure is safe to enter.

154. The next step in managing the patient is to:
   A. roll the patient onto his side to check for responsiveness and for an open airway.
   B. insert an oropharyngeal airway and begin positive pressure ventilation.
   C. establish manual in-line spinal stabilization and logroll the patient into a supine position.
   D. gather a SAMPLE history from someone at the scene while your partner gets a set of baseline vital signs.

155. A detailed physical exam is performed:
   A. to identify and manage life-threatening injuries.
   B. to identify and manage other non-life-threatening injuries.
   C. to determine trends in the patient's condition.
   D. before any emergency care can be done.

156. Which of the following breath sounds would be expected in a patient with alveoli that collapse after exhalation and re-expand with each inhalation?
   A. crackles (rales)
   B. wheezing
   C. pleural friction rub
   D. rhonchi

157. You arrive on the scene and find a 16-year-old male patient lying on the living room floor in a fetal position (curled up with his knees drawn to his chest). His positioning would cause you to most likely suspect he is suffering from:
   A. an asthma attack.
   B. congestive heart failure.

C. appendicitis.
D. a migraine.

158. When assessing the pupils during the detailed physical exam, you shine the light in the right eye while inspecting the left pupil reaction. This is testing the:
   A. consensual reflex.
   B. extra ocular eye movements.
   C. muscle palsies.
   D. sclera.

159. You arrive on the scene of a bar fight and find a male patient who is approximately 26 years of age who was struck several times in the face. The patient is hostile and not cooperating. He can not remember his address or his last name and does not know where he is. He refuses to allow you to assess him or provide any emergency care. You should?
   A. have him sign a refusal form and leave the scene.
   B. explain the consequences of not allowing you to assess and treat him, document it on the PCR, and have the patient and a witness sign the refusal form.
   C. call for the police, restrain the patient, and conduct a rapid trauma assessment to identify any life-threatening injuries.
   D. have his friend who is at the bar with him drive him to the hospital as you follow close behind.

160. You arrive on the scene and find a 23-year-old pregnant patient trapped in her car that is on its roof following a broadside collision. Upon arrival at the scene you should:
   A. gain access to the vehicle and take manual in-line spinal stabilization.
   B. immediately apply a non-rebreather mask at 15 lpm to the patient to try to protect the fetus.
   C. contact a second ambulance in case she would go into labor and deliver at the scene.

D. wait until the fire department has stabilized the vehicle before gaining access to the patient.

161. A 40-year-old male patient was struck in the face by a softball. During your detailed exam, you note that his eyes both deviate upward with a conjugate gaze. You would suspect he is possibly suffering from:
    A. an infraorbital fracture.
    B. a nasal fracture.
    C. a zygomatic contusion.
    D. a third cranial nerve injury.

162. During your rapid trauma assessment of a patient who fell down the steps, you note that the unresponsive patient's left pupil is fixed and dilated. You would suspect the patient most likely:
    A. has suffered a brain injury.
    B. injured the eighth cranial nerve.
    C. has injured the eyeball during the fall.
    D. fractured the maxilla and mandible.

163. If the left pupil is fixed and dilated in the brain injured patient, you would suspect the impact and injury most likely occurred to which side of the head?
    A. frontal region
    B. left region
    C. right region
    D. occipital region

164. A positive Babinski sign is when the:
    A. toes fan up and out.
    B. patient withdraws his foot.
    C. large toe moves laterally.
    D. toes curl downward toward the sole.

SCENARIO

Questions 165 and 166 refer to the following scenario.

You arrive on the scene and find a 34-year-old female patient who crashed her motorcycle. During your assessment, you note that the skin is pale, cool, and clammy, abdomen is rigid and tender, and the radial pulse is weak and rapid.

165. Based on this information, you would suspect the patient is most likely suffering from which of the following?
    A. intra-abdominal bleeding
    B. a pelvic fracture
    C. a pneumothorax
    D. bilateral femur fractures

166. The abdominal pain and tenderness in the patient is most likely due to:
    A. blood collecting around the femur.
    B. blood irritating the peritoneal lining.
    C. fecal material causing diaphragmatic irritation.
    D. the pleural lining collapse.

167. While you are collecting the SAMPLE history during the focused history and physical exam on a medical patient complaining of dyspnea, the patient states that he feels his breathing is much better when he sits straight up. This would be reported as an item addressing what component of the mnemonic OPQRST?
    A. severity
    B. provocation/palliation (alleviation)
    C. radiation
    D. quality

168. Pain upon palpation of the symphysis pubis most likely indicates:
    A. a bladder infection.
    B. a ruptured ovary.
    C. a pelvic fracture.
    D. intra-abdominal bleeding.

169. You are transporting a 46-year-old male patient from the scene of an auto crash. He is complaining of pelvic pain and abdominal discomfort. An ongoing assessment should be conducted every:
    A. 30 minutes.

B. 15 minutes.

C. 5 minutes.

D. 2 minutes.

170. A patient with right-sided heart failure would likely have:

A. a distended abdomen.

B. jugular vein distention.

C. tracheal deviation.

D. pain to the lower extremities.

171. You are conducting a focused physical exam on a patient complaining of chest pain. Which of the following assessments would **not** be included in your examination?

A. oral mucosa

B. breath sounds

C. ears and nose

D. pedal pulses

172. You have just transported a patient suspected of having a heart attack to the emergency department. Upon your arrival you are greeted at the door by the ward clerk who instructs you to place the patient in room B. As you are transferring the patient over to the hospital bed, you receive a tone from your dispatcher for another emergency call. You should:

A. immediately leave the emergency department and respond to the call.

B. wait to notify the nurse or physician of the patient's condition prior to leaving.

C. refuse to take the call until your prehospital report is completely done.

D. instruct the ward clerk to pass the information about the patient to the physician.

173. Which of the following **would not** be considered a significant mechanism of injury?

A. an auto crash with frontal impact

B. a gunshot wound to the neck

C. a deformed steering wheel in a rear-end collision

D. a fall of less than two times the height of the patient

SCENARIO

Questions 174–176 refer to the following scenario.

You arrive on the scene and find a patient who fell off a balcony at a hard rock concert. He struck several people when he fell before being impaled on a broken piece of plastic. Upon your arrival at the scene, you note three people lying on the ground next to the patient.

174. As you enter the scene, what would be your immediate action?

A. Perform an initial assessment on each patient to determine who is the most severely injured.

B. Ask that the police remove all of the people at the concert before approaching the patient.

C. Call for at least two additional ambulances to respond to the scene.

D. Go right to the patient impaled on the plastic and begin your assessment.

175. You are now treating the patient impaled on the plastic. You take in-line spinal stabilization and note a large pool of blood around the left thigh where the clothing is soaked in blood. The patient is moaning and groaning in pain. You should immediately:

A. apply a tourniquet to the leg to stop the bleeding.

B. expose the extremity to assess for major bleeding.

C. check the radial pulse to determine if the patient is in shock.

D. assess the airway and breathing and apply a non-rebreather mask at 15 lpm.

176. Which of the following would **not** be an indicator of a patient priority status?

A. absent radial pulses with a weak and thready carotid pulse

B. pale, cool, clammy skin in a trauma patient

C. dizziness and weakness in a diabetic patient

D. open wound to the lateral chest at the fourth intercostal space

177. A 30-year-old female patient fell off of her bicycle. She was not wearing a helmet. During your detailed physical exam you notice discoloration to the mastoid process behind her left ear. This is most likely a sign of a(n):

A. infraorbital fracture.

B. basilar skull fracture.

C. fractured nose.

D. zygomatic arch injury.

178. You are treating a 2-year-old girl who has been vomiting and suffering diarrhea for the past 3 days. The best method to assess whether she has lost a significant amount of volume is by:

A. taking a systolic and diastolic blood pressure.

B. assessing the radial pulses and skin color, temperature, and condition.

C. determining the mental status and if she is oriented × 3.

D. inspecting the sclera for redness.

179. When conducting the initial assessment, you should always assume that the patient with an altered mental status:

A. has a head injury.

B. can not maintain his or her own airway.

C. needs bag-valve-mask ventilation with supplemental oxygen.

D. will not have radial pulses.

180. You arrive at the scene of a bar fight and find a 25-year-old man who has been stabbed several times and is bleeding severely from a wound to the neck, which is spurting bright red blood. The assailant is still on the scene in the bathroom, cleaning blood off of his hands. You can hear the sirens of the police who are not yet on the scene. How would you proceed?

A. Try to keep the assailant calm and in the bathroom while you quickly apply direct pressure to the knife wound in the patient's neck.

B. Both you and your partner ask the assailant to put the knife down so that you can enter the house and take care of the patient.

C. Remain in the ambulance until the police arrive on the scene and indicate it is safe to enter.

D. As soon as you see the police cars, quickly enter the scene and apply direct pressure to the wound, and drag the patient to safety.

181. An example of paradoxical motion of the chest is when:

A. a segment moves inward on exhalation.

B. a segment moves outward on exhalation.

C. a segment moves outward on inhalation.

D. a segment does not move with respiration.

182. Stridor is an indication of:

A. fluid or vomitus obstructing the upper airway.

B. bronchoconstriction and mucus obstructing the lower airway.

C. the tongue blocking the upper airway.

D. laryngeal edema partially occluding the upper airway.

183. You arrive at the scene of a fall and find a 42-year-old woman sitting on the ground next to a ladder. She says she only fell a couple of feet and twisted her ankle. She is complaining of a sharp stabbing pain in her ankle. Which component of the initial assessment must be assessed next in this patient?

A. mental status

B. airway

C. breathing

D. circulation

184. A 62-year-old female patient who has been working in her garden has hot, dry skin. This patient may be suffering from:

A. a heart attack.

B. heat exposure.

C. shock.

D. stroke.

185. The decision to perform a rapid medical assessment or SAMPLE history first in the medical patient is determined by:

A. the mechanism of injury.

B. the nature of the illness.

C. the signs of medical illness.

D. the mental status of the patient.

186. You are assessing a 23-year-old female patient who is complaining of abdominal pain. While you are gathering your history, it is important to ask her which of the following questions?

A. When was the last time you had intercourse?

B. Have you ever smoked crack cocaine?

C. Are you a drug user?

D. When was your last period?

187. You are assessing a patient complaining of chest pain. You obtain a set of vital signs and find the following: BP 112/64, HR 112/minute, and RR 16/minute. You should report that the patient has:

A. a narrow pulse pressure.

B. tachypnea

C. tachycardia.

D. hypertension.

188. While assessing the trauma patient, you logroll the patient and find an open wound to the posterior thorax. You should immediately:

A. increase the liter flow of oxygen to 15.

B. begin bag-valve-mask ventilation.

C. assess the lower extremities for other wounds.

D. apply an occlusive dressing.

189. The medical term for swelling is:

A. erythema.

B. edema.

C. ecchymosis.

D. contusion.

190. Once you have inspected and palpated the neck in the rapid trauma assessment, the next step is to:

A. move on to inspecting the chest.

B. apply a cervical spinal immobilization collar.

C. relieve your partner of holding in-line stabilization if there is no pain or obvious injury.

D. auscultate the chest for decreased breath sounds.

191. You arrive on the scene and find a patient who aspirated a large amount of vomitus. You would expect to find which of the following in the assessment?

A. pale, cool, clammy skin

B. cyanosis

C. constricted pupils

D. absent breath sounds

192. You arrive on the scene and find a patient who has fallen down the steps. As you approach the patient she states, "I am fine, but embarrassed. Just leave me alone and I'll be fine." You should immediately:

A. take in-line spinal immobilization.

B. open the airway and check inside the mouth.

C. have her sign a refusal form.

D. ask if it is okay to assess her to determine if she is injured.

193. A patient suffering an allergic reaction would most likely have:

A. crackles.

B. decreased breath sounds on one side.

C. wheezing.

D. gurgling sounds in the upper airway.

194. You arrive on the scene and find a patient who claims that his abdominal pain was less intense following ingestion of an antacid. In your history, this would be reported as:

A. provocation or aggravation.

B. premedication.

C. palliation or alleviation.

D. past medical history.

195. Which of the following may be a sign in an unresponsive patient that he may have suffered a seizure?

A. a rapid radial pulse

B. an increased systolic blood pressure

C. poor capillary refill in the nail beds

D. a lacerated tongue

196. Subcutaneous emphysema would most likely indicate which of the following conditions?

A. a myocardial infarction

B. pericardial tamponade

C. ruptured aorta

D. lacerated bronchiole

197. Which of the following assessment components may be skipped due to the patient's condition or estimated time of arrival to the hospital?

A. initial assessment

B. focused history and physical exam

C. ongoing assessment

D. detailed physical exam

198. A patient with a tension pneumothorax will also have:

A. a widened pulse pressure with a low diastolic blood pressure.

B. a decreased heart rate and weak peripheral pulses.

C. warm, dry skin that is moist to touch.

D. a decreased systolic blood pressure.

199. An initial assessment must be conducted on:

A. patients who present with an altered mental status only.

B. all patients with either an illness or injury.

C. those patients who would require an immediate intervention.

D. patients when time and patient condition permits.

200. A 26-year-old female patient is found responsive and alert at the scene of a car rollover. She complains of upper abdominal pain. Following an appropriate patient assessment, you decide to transport. En route she becomes less responsive. Her breathing rate increases. As a part of your ongoing assessment you should immediately:

A. repeat the focused history and physical exam.

B. repeat the detailed physical exam.

C. repeat the initial assessment.

D. contact medical control.

201. The purpose of the rapid trauma assessment is to:

A. identify and manage life threats to the patient.

B. locate all injuries to the patient.

C. assess the airway, breathing, and circulatory status.

D. identify injuries that will require surgical interventions.

202. Which of the following signs would indicate that the patient is having trouble breathing?

A. The patient talks in a normal speech pattern.

B. The patient is crying vigorously.

C. The patient says a few words and gasps for a breath.

D. The patient complains his throat feels as though it is closing.

203. You are treating a 28-year-old female who fell 20 feet while roofing a house. After determining she is unresponsive, you would immediately:
    A. open her airway using a head-tilt chin-lift maneuver.
    B. apply in-line stabilization and open her airway.
    C. start high concentration oxygen using a non-rebreather mask.
    D. open her airway and start high concentration oxygen.

204. You are treating a 78-year-old female patient who was found at home on the living room floor by her daughter. She is unresponsive to painful stimuli. Her respirations are 15 per minute with very minimal chest wall movement. What should you do first?
    A. Apply a non-rebreather mask at 15 lpm and assess the pulse.
    B. Provide two ventilations and reassess the mental status.
    C. Immediately move the patient to the ambulance and begin transport.
    D. Insert an oropharyngeal airway and begin bag-valve-mask ventilation.

205. During palpation of the abdomen in the rapid trauma assessment, the patient makes a facial grimace and draws his knees upward. You would note this as abdominal:
    A. rigidity.
    B. tenderness.
    C. guarding.
    D. pain.

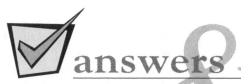

answers & rationales

1.

C. The scene survey should begin as you are pulling up to the scene. You should be identifying potential hazards (fire, downed power lines, gas leaks) and also looking for clues to identify an unsafe scene (all the lights off in the house, general atmosphere of the scene, listening for arguing or fighting) before leaving the confines of the ambulance. (3-1.1) (EC 178-181 PEC 143-152)

2.

D. All the scenes listed could potentially present a hazard or rapidly deteriorate to a hazardous scene. Do not become a victim due to carelessness and complacency. (3-1.1) (EC 178-181 PEC 143-152)

3.

B. All power lines are considered energized until a power company representative arrives on the scene and advises you they are not. Downed power lines pose a serious threat to rescuers and the public. You should advise the patients to remain inside the vehicle until you can safely remove them. Never try to move power lines. Power lines that are on the ground can energize the area around them. Keep a safe distance away. (3-1.2a) (EC 178-181 PEC 143-152)

4.

C. If at any time you feel the scene is not safe, you and your partner should make it safe or leave the scene. There is no reason to assess this scene further. You have already determined it is unsafe. Do not make contact with bystanders or the patient until the scene is secured by the police. (3-1.2b)(EC 178-181 PEC 143-152)

5.

A. In a closed environment like a house, when more than one patient complains of the same symptoms, you should suspect a toxic environment such as carbon monoxide poisoning. Clues that lead you to suspect a toxic environment in this situation include winter morning (furnace use), inside the house (enclosed space), more than one patient with same symptoms (husband and wife). (3-1.2c) (EC 178-181 PEC 143-152)

6.

D. Of the scenes listed the barroom is the most likely place for the EMT-B to be injured. Calls to barrooms may or may not involve a police response. The EMT-B should not enter the known crime scene unless accompanied by law enforcement. A large crowd is not necessarily a threat. (3-1.3) (EC 183-184 PEC 143-152)

7.

A. Your first and foremost responsibility at the crime scene is to provide emergency medical care. If possible, prevent destruction of evidence by not touching weapons and preventing unnecessary personnel from entering the crime scene. Your own personal safety is the ultimate priority. (3-1.3) (EC 183-184 PEC 143-152)

8.

C. Upon arriving at a crash scene, assess and observe the entire scene. Don't become focused on the vehicles or patients involved. Look to the right, left, above, and below the vehicle to ensure a safe scene. Remember that the area encompassing an accident scene can extend hundreds of feet in high speed crashes. (3-1.3) (EC 183-184 PEC 143-152)

9.

B. You can't determine if a patient is oriented by simple eye openings in response to verbal stimuli. The patient is reported to respond to verbal stimuli. (3-2.3) (EC 200, 202, 205, 207 PEC 170)

10.

B. All calls can be categorized as trauma or medical. If the EMT rules out injury or potential for injury, the call can typically be classified as a medical emergency. (3-1.4) (EC 184-191 PEC 153-155)

11.

B. Falls, motor vehicle crashes, and shootings all involve injury or the potential for physical injury due to the mechanism of injury. A myocardial infarction is a true medical emergency that does not involve physical injury from a blunt or penetrating force. (3-1.4) (EC 184-191 PEC 153-155)

12.

A. When you arrive at a scene and you determine there are more patients than you can effectively manage, immediately call for additional assistance before making patient contact. If you make patient contact prior to calling for additional assistance, you may become focused on that one patient and not the whole scene. (3-1.5a) (EC 191 PEC 147-148, 155-156, 157)

13.

D. Determining the total number of patients is a major element of the scene size-up. Try to determine the total number of patients before making patient contact. The total number of patients will determine how many additional resources are needed. (3-1.5b) (EC 191 PEC 147-148, 155-156, 157)

14.

D. Any requests for additional help and assistance should be made prior to patient contact. If you wait until patient contact you are likely to become focused on the patient's needs and not call for additional help. (3-1.6) (EC 191 PEC 145-151, 155-156)

15.

C. The general overall impression is based on the scene findings and the mechanism of injury. These two assessments will allow you to categorize your patient into medical or trauma categories and determine priority of care. (3-2.1) (EC 196-200 PEC 166-170)

16.

A. Non-purposeful movement has no purpose relative to the painful (tactile) stimulation. A purposeful movement is one in which the patient makes an active attempt to remove the source of painful stimulation. There are two types of non-purposeful movement.

Decorticate (flexion) posturing is when the patient arches the back and flexes the arms towards the chest. Decerebrate (extension) posturing is when the patient arches the back and extends the arms parallel to the body. (3-2.2) (EC 200-202 PEC 170-171)

17.

B. An alert adult who is gasping for air, is unable to speak, or has stridor indicates some type of partial airway obstruction. The process of talking in complete sentences and crying or drooling may indicate simply a sore throat. (3-2.4) (EC 200, 202, 205, 207 PEC 171-173)

18.

B. If you suspect the patient may have an injured spine, you must provide in-line spinal stabilization prior to continuing with the assessment. The patient may have fallen down the stairs. If you were to ask the patient questions before stabilizing the spine, the patient will likely look towards the person speaking to him or her, thus compromising the spine. (3-2.5) (EC 196-200 PEC 169)

19.

D. The most effective way to determine if a patient is breathing is by looking at the patient's chest for chest rise and fall and listening and feeling for air exchange over the patient's mouth and nose. (3-2.6) (EC 200-201, 202, 207 PEC 173-175)

20.

A. Your initial action for an apneic patient is to provide immediate positive pressure ventilation. Delaying positive pressure ventilation will likely result in brain damage or cardiac arrest. This patient was found lying in bed and spinal injury is not suspected. (3-2.8) (EC 198, 200-201, 202, 207 PEC 175)

21.

B. After ensuring an adequate airway, assess the patient's breathing status. If in doubt as to the adequacy of the breathing, provide positive pressure ventilation. Applying a gauze pad is not appropriate for an open chest wound. (3-2.9) (EC 200-201, 202 PEC 175)

22.

C. The patient may be presenting with a sign of a tension pneumothorax, a serious chest injury. Immediately auscultate for absent breath sounds and check for additional signs such as jugular venous distention (JVD) and a tracheal deviation. You also should release the occlusive dressing that is covering the sucking chest wound. If absent breath sounds, JVD and/or tracheal shift are not present, you should recheck the airway and ensure proper head position. (3-2.9) (EC 200-201, 202 PEC 175)

23.
D. The patient is potentially suffering from a head injury. The patient requires hyperventilation at 20 ventilations per minute if he is displaying signs of brain herniation such as a fixed and dilated pupil, non-purposeful posturing, and paralysis to one side. Cover the right ear loosely with a sterile dressing. (3-2.9) (EC 200-201, 202 PEC 175)

24.
D. Your initial response to an obstructed airway from a foreign body in the infant is to deliver five rapid back blows. These back blows are delivered to the infant while supporting his or her body over your hand and knee. Chest thrusts are delivered after the back blows. Never administer abdominal thrusts to an infant. Blind finger sweeps are not performed on the infant since this procedure may lodge the foreign body further into the airway. (3-2.11) (EC 198, 200, 202, 205, 207 PEC 173-175)

25.
B. Current research has found the location of perfusing pulses does not accurately estimate systolic blood pressures. (3-2.12) (EC 201, 202, 207 PEC 176-177)

26.
B. In the adult patient you will first palpate the radial pulse, whereas in an infant the brachial artery in the upper arm is assessed. The carotid artery in the adult and femoral artery in the infant are assessed when the peripheral pulses are absent. (3-2.13) (EC 201, 202, 205, 207 PEC 176)

27.
A. Blood flowing from a wound at a steady continuous flow is considered major bleeding. You should immediately apply direct pressure to the wound with a gloved hand. Most bleeding can be controlled by direct pressure. Once the bleeding is controlled, you should apply a pressure dressing. (3-2.14) (EC 201, 202, 207 PEC 177)

28.
D. Hot, cool, and cold skin temperatures are considered abnormal. Hot skin usually indicates hyperthermia (heat emergency) or an infection. Cold skin is found in hypothermia (cold emergency), and cool skin is usually a sign of hypoperfusion (shock). (3-2.16) (EC 201, 202, 207 PEC 178)

29.
C. Capillary refill is most reliable in the infant or child less than 6 years of age. It can be quickly checked in the nail bed, the fleshy part of the palm along the ulnar margin, forehead, or cheeks. Capillary refill is usually less than 2 seconds. (3-2.18) (EC 199, 202, 205, 207 PEC 178)

30.
A. The mechanism of injury may not be very apparent or well understood upon arrival at the scene. You should reconsider the mechanism of injury during the focused history and physical exam to reevaluate whether it was enough to cause critical injuries. (3-3.1) (EC 233, 245 PEC 183-184)

31.
B. Falls, if greater than 10 feet, bicycle collisions, and a motor vehicle collision where a person in the same passenger compartment of the patient has died are all considered significant. Low speed motor vehicle collisions are not considered significant. (3-3.1) (EC 233, 245 PEC 183-184)

32.
A. The patient with a significant mechanism of injury requires a rapid trauma assessment, followed by baseline vitals and then a SAMPLE history. (3-3.3) (EC 246-247 PEC 183)

33.
A. The first step in the assessment of any patient following scene size-up is performing an initial assessment. The initial assessment is followed by the rapid trauma assessment if significant mechanism of injury is suspected. Baseline vital signs and SAMPLE history are the next steps. (3-3.2a) (EC 246-247 PEC 182-183)

34.
B. The rapid trauma assessment is a quick head-to-toe exam performed on patients with a significant mechanism of injury or altered mental status. It is conducted

to identify critical injuries. The focused trauma assessment is performed when you do not have a significant mechanism of injury (MOI) or altered mental status and is focused on a specific injury. The SAMPLE history is performed at the end of the rapid trauma assessment. Reassessment of the vital signs is obtained at the end of the rapid trauma assessment. (3-3.2b) (EC 246-247 PEC 182-183)

35.

C. The type of assessment that is performed on a trauma patient is based on the mechanism of injury (MOI) and initial assessment findings. (3-3.2c) (EC 246-247 PEC 182-183)

36.

D. Immediately perform a rapid trauma assessment to determine if a life threatening injury or condition exists. (3-3.3) (EC 246-247 PEC 183)

37.

D. A rapid head-to-toe assessment that is performed on the injured or ill patient to identify life-threatening injuries is called a rapid trauma or medical assessment. (3-3.3) (EC 246-247 PEC 183)

38.

C. A patient who has a significant mechanism of injury or an altered mental status requires a rapid trauma assessment. Because this patient is not oriented to place, he is considered to have an altered mental status. (3-3.3) (EC 246-247 PEC 183)

39.

C. DCAP-BTLS is the mnemonic for deformities, contusions, abrasions, penetrations/punctures, burns, tenderness, lacerations, and swelling. These are signs of injury that should be identified during your assessment. (3-3.4) (EC 246-253 PEC 186-198)

40.

C. The rapid trauma assessment uses a systematic approach, starting at the head and proceeding down the neck, chest, abdomen, lower extremities, upper extremities, and finally the posterior body. (3-3.4) (EC 246-253 PEC 186-198)

41.

C. Palpate the entire head and face, noting any tenderness or deformities. The immobilization device should not be removed to perform the detailed physical exam. Gently palpate the skull with your hands flattened over the skull. This will prevent you from inadvertently pushing your finger tips into a skull fracture. (3-3.4) (EC 246-253 PEC 186-198)

42.

D. If you find inadequate breathing while performing a rapid trauma assessment, you must immediately stop the assessment and provide positive pressure ventilation. Management of the airway and breathing takes precedence over continued assessment. (3-3.5a) (EC 246-247, 253-254 PEC 188, 203, 205)

43.

A. Paradoxical chest wall movement associated with a flail segment is a critical injury affecting the patient's breathing and must be managed immediately. It is normal to find flat jugular veins with a patient sitting at a 45° angle. Flat jugular veins in the supine patient may indicate a decreased blood volume. An open humerus fracture, unless it is associated with major bleeding, is not considered a life-threatening injury. A tibia fracture is not a life threat. (3-3.5b) (EC 246-247, 253-254 PEC 188, 203, 205)

44.

B. The rapid trauma assessment is performed to determine if additional life-threatening injuries or conditions are present. Subsequent care and treatment will be based upon this examination. (3-3.6) (EC 232 PEC 180-181)

45.

A. In a medical patient there is no mechanism of injury that will tell you about your patient's injuries. Therefore, you must act like a detective and look for any and all clues about the chief complaint. Further assessment of the chief complaint is considered the history of the present illness. (3-4.1) (EC 275 PEC 205-217)

46.

D. The OPQRST mnemonic allows you to rapidly and systematically gather more information about the chief complaint. (3-4.1) (EC 274-275 PEC 205-217)

47.

B. The mnemonic OPQRST stands for onset, provocation, quality, radiation, severity, and finally the length of time the patient has had the symptom. (3-4.1) (EC 274-275 PEC 205-217)

48.

A. Provocation determines what makes the pain worse, whereas palliation determines what makes the pain better. This provides the EMT with the information to help gauge the severity of the illness. A patient that is complaining of severe chest pain while sitting in a chair should concern the EMT more than the patient whose chest pain after shoveling the driveway was relieved with rest. (3-4.1) (EC 274-275 PEC 205-217)

49.

B. The mnemonic OPQRST refers to radiation of pain. This describes if the pain or symptom moves or radiates. (3-4.2a) (EC 274, 275 PEC 215-217)

50.

A. When assessing the quality of a patient's pain you should ask open-ended questions, such as "What does the pain feel like?" Asking leading questions, such as "Is the pain sharp or dull?" may lead to an inaccurate description. Questions regarding what makes the pain worse pertain to provocation and not quality. Asking questions about when and how the pain began, pertains to onset. (3-4.2b) (EC 274, 275 PEC 215-217)

51.

A. Gather the history first in the responsive medical patient. The history will provide valuable information and must be obtained before the patient becomes potentially unresponsive. The history is followed by the focused exam and vital signs. (3-4.3) (EC 274, 277-279 PEC 206-215)

52.

C. In the unresponsive medical patient, you perform a rapid medical assessment to determine the possible nature of the medical illness. This is followed by the vital signs and patient history. (3-4.3) (EC 274, 277-279 PEC 206-215)

53.

C. The unresponsive medical patient is considered a high priority patient. Unresponsiveness is a critical finding. (3-4.3) (EC 274, 277-279 PEC 206-215)

54.

B. Valuable information is commonly obtained when inspecting the area around the unresponsive medical patient. The condition of the patient's environment, presence of home oxygen supply, the patient's position in a hospital bed, and patient's medications are a few examples. (3-4.3) (EC 274, 277-279 PEC 206-215)

55.

B. Unequal pupils are usually an indication of stroke or possible head injury. Changes in pupil size and reactivity are commonly associated with drug overdose, oxygen starvation (hypoxia), or adverse environmental conditions. (3-4.3) (EC 274, 277-279 PEC 206-215)

56.

D. When you have determined that your patient is unresponsive or has an altered mental status during the initial assessment your next assessment step would be to perform a rapid medical assessment. The rapid medical assessment will help to determine the possible nature of the medical illness. The status of the airway, breathing, and circulation is assessed and managed during the initial assessment. (3-4.4a) (EC 274 PEC 206-217)

57.

D. The unresponsive medical patient should be placed in the left lateral recumbent position, also known as the recovery or coma position. This position will help to protect the airway from vomitus, blood, and other secretions. Be prepared to suction the airway if secretions are present. The Trendelenburg (shock) position is used to help increase blood perfusion to the brain and vital organs. The semi-Fowler's position requires the patient to sit at a semireclined position, which may permit secretions and vomitus to enter the airway and lungs. The prone position (face down) will not permit you access to the patient's face and airway. (3-4.4c) (EC 274 PEC 206-217)

58.

B. You will initially assess the responsive medical patient by evaluating the complaint and signs and symptoms by using the mnemonic OPQRST. You should perform a rapid medical assessment on patients you find unresponsive. In the responsive medical patient, perform components of a detailed physical assessment after you make a transport decision. You should perform a focused medical exam in the responsive patient after you obtain a SAMPLE history. (3-4.4c) (EC 274 PEC 206-217)

59.

A. The detailed physical exam is performed after all life-threatening injuries have been managed. During the detailed physical exam the EMT should identify and treat all non-life-threatening wounds or injuries. (3-5.1) (EC 254-255, 258-261 PEC 218-219)

60.

D. The detailed physical exam can be a head-to-toe examination or an exam specific to isolated injuries. You should take into account all information gained in previous assessments. (3-5.1) (EC 254-255, 258-261 PEC 218-219)

61.

A. During the detailed exam the patient is reassessed, other non-life-threatening injuries are identified and treated, the vital signs are reassessed and compared with earlier vital signs to gauge the patient's condition and response to treatment. Initial assessment of vital signs are assessed during the rapid assessment or focused physical exam. (3-5.1) (EC 254-255, 258-261 PEC 218-219)

62.

B. A yellow color to the white portion of the eye (sclera) is called icterus and is an indication of possible liver damage or failure. (3-5.2b) (EC 254-255 PEC 218, 219-229)

63.

B. Trauma to the airway, respiratory tract, lungs or esophagus may cause subcutaneous emphysema. Subcutaneous emphysema is the term that describes trapped air under the skin. Trapped air under the skin can be palpated and feels like crackling or crepitation. This sign should increase your suspicion of further injury. Monitor the patient closely for increased breathing difficulty. (3-5.2c) (EC 254-255 PEC 218, 219-229)

64.

A. Paradoxical movement is the term used to describe the chest wall that moves inward during inhalation and outward during exhalation. This type of movement is indicative of a flail segment. This is a true emergency and must be treated immediately. Often flail segments can be missed during the initial or rapid trauma assessment because the area is stabilized by muscle spasm. The major life-threatening problem associated with a flail segment is the potential for an underlying pulmonary contusion. (3-5.2d) (EC 254-255 PEC 218, 219-229)

65.

B. Any injuries found during the detailed physical exam are managed as discovered. Lacerations are bandaged and fractures immobilized. (3-5.3) (EC 254-255, 258-261 PEC 218,229)

66.

D. A trauma patient who is unable to close his mouth most likely has suffered a fracture or dislocation of the mandible. The most important concern is to closely observe the patient's airway to prevent obstruction and possible aspiration. (3-5.4) (EC 261 PEC 218-229)

67.

C. Do not remove any foreign body embedded in the eye and don't force the eyelids open if eyelid injury is present. Pressure should not be used to control bleeding from the eyeball. Both pupils should respond and react simultaneously to a light source. This is called a consensual reflex. (3-5.4) (EC 261 PEC 218-229)

68.

B. Pupils that are large in size and not responding to light are termed fixed and dilated. (3-5.4) (EC 261 PEC 218-229)

69.

C. Visual acuity is clarity of vision. Conjugate movement describes the eyes moving together. A conjugate gaze is a gaze or stare in one direction. (3-5.4) (EC 261 PEC 218-229)

70.

D. A patient with unequal pupils who is alert and oriented may have sustained a direct injury to the eye. Other possibilities include the presence of a glass eye, localized nerve injury, or use of eye drops such as atropine or pilocarpine that dilate the pupils. (3-5.4) (EC 261 PEC 218-229)

71.

D. Air trapped under the skin may be caused by a tension pneumothorax, but is called subcutaneous emphysema. It may crackle and cause a sound called crepitation. This may be due to trauma to the respiratory tract, airway, lung, or esophagus. (3-5.4) (EC 261 PEC 218-229)

72.

D. The tongue is a very vascular organ and provides a reflection of a patient's perfusion status. A pale tongue may be an indication of poor perfusion and shock. (3-5.4) (EC 261 PEC 218-229)

73.

D. Stridor is a high pitched sound caused by a partial upper airway obstruction. The presence of wheezes during auscultation indicates constriction of the bronchioles in the lower airway. Wheezing produces a high pitched sound heard on exhalation. Ronchi indicate the presence of mucous in the larger airways. Ronchi produce a snoring type sound. (3-5.4) (EC 261 PEC 218-229)

74.

B. The purpose of the ongoing assessment is to monitor the patient and his or her injuries. The ongoing assessment assesses the airway, breathing, and circulation interventions and vital signs. The ongoing assessment is not designed to initially identify life threats. These should have been identified in the rapid trauma assessment (3-6.1) (EC 289 PEC 232)

75.

B. All critically injured patients should be reassessed at least every 5 minutes so that indicators of a worsening situation or an improvement can rapidly be noted. (3-6.1) (EC 289 PEC 232)

76.

D. The patient has telltale signs of a leaking abdominal aortic aneurysm and now becomes a critical patient. This patient can become hemodynamically unstable at any time and should be transported to a hospital where lifesaving surgery could be performed immediately. (3-6.1) (EC 289 PEC 232)

77.

C. The initial assessment does not include taking the time to obtain and record vital signs. This survey rapidly identifies if there are problems with the airway, breathing, and circulation. The vital signs are taken after the initial assessment is completed. (3-6.1) (EC 289 PEC 232)

78.

D. The information gathered from a repeated ongoing assessment should always be compared with previous findings. This will help determine the current patient status, know whether or not the treatment you are providing is helping the patient, and quickly identify a deteriorating patient status. (3-6.1) (EC 289 PEC 232)

79.

A. When reassessing the unstable patient, you should repeat the vital signs and assessment findings at least every 5 minutes. By reassessing and obtaining the vital signs frequently you will assess the effectiveness of your treatment and find other problems that were not found earlier. The stable patient should be reassessed and have the vital signs taken at least every 15 minutes. (3-6.2a) (EC 289-290 EC 231-233)

80.

B. The mnemonic used to assess the mental status of a patient is AVPU. A-alert: Is the patient awake, is the patient able to talk and respond? V-verbal: Does the patient respond to verbal stimulus? P-painful: Does the patient respond to painful stimulus? U-unresponsive: The patient does not respond to pain. (3-6.2b) (EC 289-290 PEC 231-233)

81.

B. A decrease in the pulse rate and pulse quality may indicate a head injury or severe hypoxia. These signs should alert you to other injuries or a need to change your treatment, like providing positive pressure ventilation. A low blood sugar level (hypoglycemia) usually presents with an increased heart rate. A heat related emergency usually presents with an increased heart rate that may be very strong. As the condition continues the heart rate remains high and the quality becomes poor. An allergic reaction (anaphylactic shock) presents with an increased heart rate that can be of a poor quality. (3-6.2c) (EC 289-290 PEC 231-233)

82.

A. An ongoing assessment is done to detect any changes in the patient's condition, to detect any missed injuries or conditions, and to adjust your treatment as needed. The ongoing assessment may reveal that your patient's condition has worsened and that you must change your treatment. As an EMT-Basic, you do not make a diagnosis. (3-6.2d) (EC 289-290 PEC 231-233)

83.

D. By waiting at least one full second you are allowing time for the repeater to "open" the channel, preventing the initial part of your transmission from being cut. (3-7.1) (EC 300-301 PEC 262-264)

84.

B. By saying "Over" you are informing the receiver that you are through with your transmission. By waiting for confirmation you are assured that the other party got your message and has no further questions. (3-7.1) (EC 300-301 PEC 262-264)

85.

C. It is very helpful to keep a standard format when communicating to medical direction. Use the following sequence when communicating with medical direction. 1. Your unit number and level of service. 2. The patient's age and sex. 3. The patient's chief complaint. 4. A brief history of the present illness, including scene assessment and mechanism of injury. 5. Major past history. 6. Patient's mental status. 7. Patient's baseline vital signs. 8. Pertinent findings of your physical exam. 9. Description of the medical care you have administered. 10. The patient's response to the emergency medical care. (3-7.2a) (EC 302 PEC 264-265)

86.

A. After medical direction has given you an order, you should repeat the order back to medical direction word for word. Repeating the order back will help ensure that the order was given and received correctly. This is referred to as the "echo" method. If the person giving you the order has not identified himself or herself, you should ask for his or her name and document it on the run report. (3-7.2b) (EC 302 PEC 264-265)

87.

D. Be sure the information you provide is accurate and that it is reported clearly. A patient's life may depend upon the decisions that are reached. If an order is not understood, ask that it be repeated. Repeat back critical information to medical control. (3-7.3) (EC 303 PEC 265)

88.

C. The oral report should only summarize the information you already gave the staff: any changes that have occurred, current vital signs, and any treatment rendered. The oral report should not be a duplicate of your radio report. (3-7.4) (EC 303 PEC 265)

89.

B. By establishing yourself at the same level of the patient or lower you help decrease the fear and anxiety of the patient. (3-7.4) (EC 303 PEC 265)

90.

D. Do not offend older patients by automatically assuming that you have to raise your voice when speaking to them or by rushing the patients' thoughts or actions. (3-7.4) (EC 303 PEC 265)

91.

B. Effective communication of patient information is important in the oral report. The information is vital and allows hospital personnel to provide for a smooth transition of care. Provide the hospital personnel with your unit's ID number, patient's age/sex, chief complaint, brief pertinent history, major past illness, mental status, vital signs, physical exam findings, care provided and response to this care, and your estimated arrival time at the facility. (3-7.4) (EC 303 PEC 265)

92.

C. Push the press to talk button and wait one second before transmitting. Speak with your mouth 2 to 3 inches from the microphone. After receiving orders from medical control, echo back the orders. Avoid making a diagnosis and provide only objective infor-

mation or important relevant subjective information. (3-7.4) (EC 303 PEC 265)

93.

A. The Federal Communications Commission (FCC) is responsible for licensing base station operations, assignment of call signs, approval of equipment for use, limiting transmitter power output and the monitoring of field operations. The FCC has no responsibility for the training of response personnel. (3-7.6) (EC 299-300 PEC 261-262)

94.

C. Cellular telephone use in EMS is common. The major disadvantage is that they are part of the public telephone system that can easily be overwhelmed in a multiple casualty disaster. (3-7.*) (EC 299 PEC 261)

95.

C. A repeater takes a low-power signal, changes the frequency and increases the power of the signal. Repeaters are common in large areas or where the terrain makes transmission and reception of signals difficult. (3-7.*) (EC 298-299 PEC 261)

96.

A. CAD refers to computer aided dispatch. (3-7.*) (EC 298)

97.

A. Response times must be accurately transcribed and recorded when obtained from the Emergency Medical Dispatcher. These times may become vitally important if the call should lead to a court case. The EMT-B must take the times from dispatch and accurately transcribe these onto the patient care report. (3-7.4) (EC 303 PEC 265)

98.

D. The FCC or the Federal Communications Commission has jurisdiction over all radio operations in the United States. This includes EMS and other public service radios. (3-7.4) (EC 299-303 PEC 265)

99.

B. Anytime you feel an order is inappropriate it is always best to question the order. Medical control may have misunderstood the patient information that you provided. Questioning the order may prevent the administration of a harmful medication or performance of an inappropriate procedure. (3-7.4) (EC 303 PEC 265)

100.

A. If medical direction has given you an order that you feel is inappropriate you should immediately question the order. It is possible that medical direction misunderstood something you said, or medical direction may have misspoken when giving the order. It is best to question the order in a professional manner. (3.75) (EC 303-305 PEC 265-267)

101.

C. Often patients are under a tremendous amount of stress. Speaking calmly and slowly will help to engender confidence in you and reduce stress. You should only raise your voice if the patient is hard of hearing. Avoid medical terms. Speak so the patient can understand you. Do not use codes. This may elevate the stress for the patient. Be truthful to the patient and speak so he or she can understand what is happening. (3-7.8) (EC 303-305 PEC 265-267)

102.

D. The D.O.T. determined that this was the bare minimum to be written on all run reports. Remember accurate documentation will help prevent any questions or problems later. (3-8.1) (EC 314-318 PEC 275-277)

103.

B. The D.O.T. requires times that relate only to the specific call (time to dispatch, response time, time to patient side, on scene time, and transport time). (3-8.1) (EC 314-318 PEC 275-277)

104.

B. The following is the minimum data set that is required by the Department of Transportation: chief complaint, level of responsiveness, systolic blood pressure, skin perfusion, skin color and temperature, pulse rate, respiratory rate and effort. (3-8.2a) (EC 314-318 PEC 276-277)

105.

D. The patient narrative section of the patient care report includes the chief complaint, SAMPLE history, and/or the description of the mechanism of injury. The patient's name, age, and sex are parts of the patient data section, not the narrative section. (3-8.2b) (EC 314-318 PEC 276-277)

106.

A. QID is the acceptable abbreviation for four times a day. For example, the patient is prescribed a bronchodilator treatment QID. SOB is the abbreviation for shortness of breath. This is the only acceptable definition for SOB. TID is the abbreviation for three times a day. NTG is the abbreviation for nitroglycerin. (3-8.2c) (EC 314-318 PEC 276-277)

107.

C. The minimum data set is established by the Department of Transportation to standardize information collected by EMS systems. It will allow for comparisons between systems and improvements in care. (3-8.3) (EC 314-318 PEC 275-277)

108.

B. Clocks should be synchronized to the dispatch clocks so time critical events can be accurately documented. Ideally, at least two sets of vital signs should be obtained. This provides a basis for determining the trend of the vital signs. The patient narrative section of the PCR contains both subjective and objective information. (3-8.3) (EC 314-318 PEC 275-277)

109.

A. A pertinent negative is a complaint that the patient should exhibit but denies having. For example, the patient complains of substernal chest pains but denies the presence of shortness of breath. The patient with AMI type chest pain frequently exhibits shortness of breath. It is pertinent to document this absence of symptom. (3-8.3) (EC 314-318 PEC 275-277)

110.

D. Falsification of the patient care report is NEVER acceptable. This can lead to poor continuity of patient care. Knowingly providing false information can lead to revocation of an EMT-B certification or license. (3-8.3) (EC 314-318 PEC 275-277)

111.

C. Documentation of patient refusals requires careful and complete documentation of your efforts to provide care and transport for the patient. Issues related to the determination of the patient's competency at the time are frequently the areas that are contested. Fully document the patients competency or lack of competency in the patient care report. (3-8.3) (EC 314-318 PEC 275-277)

112.

D. Confidentiality of patient care report information is important and must be maintained. Generally the only individuals who are allowed access to this information are police officers for an investigation, health care workers for continuity of care, legal subpoena, and third party billing information. (3-8.3) (EC 314-318 PEC 275-277)

113.

D. The EMT needs to have proof that the victim did refuse transport. Without a signature it will be the victim's word against yours and your partner's. (3-8.4) (EC 318-319 PEC 277-278)

114.

D. If the EMT suspects that the patient is suffering from any disease, injury, drug, or other substance that can alter the patient's judgment, the EMT may be held liable if he or she does not treat the patient or arrange for the treatment of the patient. (3-8.4) (EC 318-319 PEC 277-278)

115.

C. This EMT should offer suggestions on how to gain care or call EMS back to the scene if the patient wants to go to the hospital. When the EMT offers this help, the patient should not feel stranded and helpless. (3.8.4) (EC 318-319 PEC 277-278)

116.

B. When an error is made on the patient care report, you should draw a single horizontal line through the mistake. The correct information should be written next to the error. Finally, you should initial the area that was corrected. Any other means of correcting an error may be perceived as deception or an attempt to cover up a mistake. Remember the report you write today will be your memory years down the road when called into court. (3-8.5) (EC 310, 313, 318-322 PEC 277-279)

117.

D. While gathering your general impression of the injured patient, any life threats must be managed before proceeding on with the assessment. An open wound to the chest must be immediately managed by placing your gloved hand directly over the wound site. (3-2.1) (EC 196-200 PEC 166-170)

118.

D. Gunshot entrance wounds may be away from the spine; however, after the projectile enters the body it can strike the spine. While forming your general impression of this patient before continuing your assessment, you must provide in-line stabilization of the spine. (3-2.5) (EC 196-200 PEC 169)

119.

B. When the mechanism of injury is significant, as it is with this patient, you should perform a rapid trauma assessment of the patient. The rapid trauma assessment is a complete head-to-toe exam that is performed quickly. The rapid trauma assessment will help to identify other injuries such as additional gunshot wounds or exit wounds. The focused physical exam is completed when you do not suspect a significant mechanism of injury. The focused physical exam is the exam of the specific injury site. (3-3.2) (EC 246-247 PEC 182-183)

120.

C. Although it seems quite innocent when providing care for a patient with a minor injury, falsification of a patient record should never occur. Document the incident accordingly. (EC 321-322 PEC 278-279)

121.

A. This is an example of subjective information: information that is based on the patient's perceptions or expressions of information that you cannot see or feel. Subjective information is described in the patient care report in the patient narrative section. (EC 316-318 PEC 276)

122.

D. This is a rather minor example of maintaining patient confidentiality. Confidentiality is the patient's legal right and it is your ethical responsibility not to divulge such information. (EC 318 PEC 277)

123.

B. The next immediate step in the assessment process is to determine if he responds to verbal stimuli. All you have determined at this point is that he is not alert. He may respond to your voice or command with appropriate communication that would provide information about his airway and breathing status. If he talks to you, there is no need to open the airway manually or to insert an airway adjunct. If he does not respond to verbal stimuli, you would then assess his response to painful stimuli. The pulse and skin check occurs after assessment of the breathing status. (EC 232-265 PEC 143-257)

124.

B. During the general impression of the initial assessment, you inspect for obvious life-threatening injuries that need immediate management. Upon your approach to the patient, if you note a major bleed, such as spurting or steady flowing blood, you or a partner should quickly expose the area and apply direct pressure. Once direct pressure is applied, you should then move on with the remainder of the initial assessment. Positive pressure ventilation is necessary in this patient; however, it will be performed after establishing the airway. Manual spinal stabilization is necessary and should be performed prior to establishing an airway. Oxygen administration is necessary; however, it will be delivered by positive pressure ventilation. A nonrebreather is not appropriate in this patient since it will not provide ventilation. (EC 178-323 PEC 143-257)

125.

A. There are several life threats that must be managed in this patient: the open wound to the chest, the blood in the mouth, the hypoxia, and the poor ventilation status. You must clear the airway immediately—prior to positive pressure ventilation—to prevent aspiration. A non-rebreather is not applied until after assessment of the ventilation status. In this patient, it appears the ventilatory status is poor; therefore, oxygen will be delivered via the ventilation device. The gunshot wound to the chest must be occluded as quickly as possible. (EC 178-323 PEC 143-257)

126.

A. All of the possible choices are signs or symptoms of a possible fracture. However, the most objective is crepitation. Crepitation is a grating sensation found when bone ends rub over each other. Pain, ecchymosis (discoloration), and edema (swelling) could all be found in ligament, tendon, or muscle injuries where there is no actual bone injury. (EC 232-265 PEC 143-257)

127.

A. Capillary refill does not provide as accurate information in the adult patient as in the infant and young child. The adult patient may have preexisting disease conditions that may cause a delay. Research has found that some people have a normally slow capillary refill, some up to 4 seconds. Also, environmental conditions play a role in capillary refill. A cold environment, for example, will cause the refill to be delayed. (EC 218, 289 PEC 178)

128.

C. During the general impression when you are attempting to ascertain the chief complaint, note the patient's speech pattern. A patient who says a few words and then must gasp for a breath is showing objective signs of respiratory distress. It would be normal for a patient who is crying loudly to gasp for a breath. Typically, patients who are dyspneic sit upright or may be propped up in bed with a few pillows. Just because the patient is on 2 lpm of oxygen at home, it does not mean that he or she is dyspneic. (EC 196-293 PEC 143-257)

129.

B. Since the respirations are shallow, indicating an inadequate tidal volume of air being breathed in, the priority of management of this patient is to establish an airway by employing a jaw-thrust maneuver followed by positive pressure ventilation. Application of a non-rebreather will not correct the inadequate tidal volume and will lead to severe hypoxia. A blood pressure will not be taken until after the airway and ventilation are managed and the initial assessment and rapid trauma assessment are completed. It is more important to establish an airway prior to ventilation than to apply a dressing to a moderately bleeding wound. Only severe bleeding is managed during the initial assessment. (EC 196-293 PEC 143-257)

130.

D. Since the patient has the potential for multiple injuries based on the mechanism of injury, a rapid trauma assessment must be conducted. A focused physical exam is used only if there is no possible chance of other injuries. A detailed exam may be conducted after the rapid trauma assessment. The patient should not be transported until after the appropriate assessment is performed and the patient is immobilized to a backboard. (EC 178-323 PEC 143-257)

131.

B. All of the choices must be performed on this patient; however, the first priority is to ensure your own safety. Do not get drawn into dramatic scenes without first conducting a scene size-up to be sure safety hazards have been identified and managed. (EC 196-207 PEC 143-257)

132.

C. The airway has been secured; therefore, the next immediate action is to begin positive pressure ventilation. Even though the rate is adequate, the tidal volume is not. An inadequate rate or tidal volume is an indication of inadequate breathing. Inadequate breathing is treated by providing positive pressure ventilation. Application of a non-rebreather will provide an increased amount of oxygen to the patient; however, most of the oxygen will not reach the alveoli since the volume is inadequate. Chest compressions are not indicated since the patient still has pulses. A cervical spinal immobilization collar will be applied during the rapid trauma assessment, not during the initial assessment. (EC 196-293 PEC 143-257)

133.

A. The patient is complaining orally when you arrive on the scene; therefore, you could assume the airway is open and the breathing is adequate. These are both parts of the initial assessment. In order to complete the initial assessment, you must assess the circulation by checking the pulses and skin. Since the patient is responsive, you would next obtain a SAMPLE history as part of the focused history and physical exam for the medical patient. (EC 196-293 PEC 143-257)

134.

B. Since the patient is a minor, consent becomes an issue of concern. However, because the patient has suffered a critical injury it is necessary to initiate emergency care and transport under implied consent. In the case of a minor injury, it would be prudent to attempt to contact the parents or legal guardian of the child prior to transport. (EC 196-293 PEC 143-257)

135.

A. During the general impression of the initial assessment, it is necessary to manage any obvious major bleeding. Since the bleeding has been identified by the patient, you should quickly assess the foot and determine if the bleeding is spurting or flowing steadily from the wound. If so, you must then control the bleeding. If not, you would proceed with the initial assessment and assess the circulation since the airway is patent and breathing is adequate evidenced by the patient's oral complaints and speech pattern. (EC 196-293 PEC 143-257)

136.

D. Following the initial assessment, you should next perform a rapid medical assessment since the patient has an altered mental status. If the patient was coherent, it would be appropriate to conduct a focused history and physical exam. (EC 196-293 PEC 143-257)

137.

C. You would approach the patient from the front of the vehicle if possible and instruct the patient not to move his head or neck. You or your partner would then gain access to the vehicle and provide manual stabilization of the spine while in the vehicle. Once that is done, you would then proceed with the general impression and the remainder of the initial assessment. (EC 196-293 PEC 143-257)

138.

B. Tracheal deviation, along with jugular venous distension, are late signs of a tension pneumothorax. A tension pneumothorax occurs from an injury to the pleural lining, which allows a large amount of air to enter the pleural space, resulting in a buildup of pressure in the injured side of the chest, causing compression of the mediastinum. This causes the heart and great vessels to be compressed, resulting in a decrease in blood pressure, an increase in heart rate, and a narrow pulse pressure. The patient will complain of severe shortness of breath and will display signs of respiratory distress. The perfusion and respiratory signs, along with severely decreased or absent breath sounds on the injured side, are much earlier signs of a tension pneumothorax. (EC 196-293 PEC 143-257)

139.

C. The patient obviously has an altered mental status; therefore, he could be deemed unable to make a rational decision. Based on implied consent you would assess the patient, begin emergency care, and transport the patient. (EC 196-293 PEC 143-257)

140.

D. Capillary refill is most accurate in younger children. It is used to assess the perfusion status of the patient. Capillary refill is subject to environmental influences such as cold weather that would cause the vessels in the periphery to constrict, thereby reducing the blood flow to that area. This would cause the capillary refill to be reduced. The asthma patient is suffering a ventilation problem, not a perfusion problem. It is appropriate to assess capillary refill in the 30-year-old who was shot in the chest; however, it has been found that the capillary refill test is most accurate in younger children. (EC 218, 289 PEC 143-257)

141.

A. Blood mixed with clear fluid coming from the ears, nose, or mouth is likely blood mixed with cerebrospinal fluid. This is typically an indication of a skull fracture. A "halo test" can be performed to determine if the blood is mixed with cerebrospinal fluid. This is where blood is dropped onto a cotton gauze pad or pillow case. The CSF forms a yellow ring around the blood in the center of cotton cloth. This test has a limited usefulness since research has found that saliva and saline will also cause the same result. (EC 196-293 PEC 143-257)

142.

A. Administration of oxygen is done during the initial assessment. Because the patient is complaining of shortness of breath, it is appropriate to apply oxygen. The baseline vital signs will be assessed during the focused history and physical exam. A patient who is complaining of shortness of breath or one who displays signs of respiratory distress will rarely tolerate being placed in a supine position. These patients typically are more comfortable in an upright position. (EC 196-293 PEC 143-257)

143.

D. The gurgling sound indicates that the patient has blood, vomitus, secretions, or some other substance in the airway. This requires immediate suction. Also, the patient has a respiratory rate of only 6 breaths/minute, which indicates inadequate breathing. After clearing the airway, positive pressure ventilation must be initiated. (EC 196-293 PEC 143-257)

144.

C. The respiratory rate of a newborn may be between 40 to 60 breaths/minute. As the infant grows older, the respiratory rate declines. Once the child reaches adolescence, the respiratory rate is close to that of an adult. (EC 196-293 PEC 143-257)

145.

B. A pulse oximeter is a very useful tool to indicate hypoxia in a patient. A real concern is a low pulse oximeter reading that persists after the application of a non-rebreather mask at 15 lpm. In this case, the patient is on a non-rebreather and his SpO2 is still at 93%. With supplemental oxygen (especially a non-rebreather at 15 lpm), you would expect an SpO2 reading near 100%. If the oxygen were removed from this patient, you would speculate that the SpO2 reading would dip extremely low, indicating hypoxia. The patient complaint of dyspnea does not correlate directly to the level of hypoxia. The skin is a better indicator of perfusion status and not hypoxia, even though you would expect to see cyanosis to the skin. Cyanosis could be a late sign. The retractions and accessory muscle use are great indicators of respiratory distress and respiratory muscle work; however, these do not measure the level of hypoxia. You could assume the patient in respiratory distress is hypoxic; however, other physical signs such as an altered mental status, head bobbing, agitation, and confusion are better indicators of hypoxia. (EC 222-224 PEC 143-257)

146.

C. Since the patient is responsive, the next step is to gather a SAMPLE history and then perform a focused physical exam where you would examine the abdomen and other related body systems. You would have already determined the level of responsiveness during the initial assessment. Also, it appears the patient is continuing to complain, indicating the mental status has not changed. A rapid medical exam would be performed if the patient were unresponsive or had an altered mental status. (EC 212-265 PEC 143-257)

147.

C. The skin is the best indicator of the patient's perfusion status. During the initial assessment you are trying to identify a life threat to the circulation. (EC 216-218 PEC 143-257)

148.

A. All of the injuries, except for the fractured ribs, would be considered possible life threats. If two or more ribs were fractured in two or more places creating a flail segment, it would be considered a life-threatening injury. However, simple rib fractures are not life-threatening unless they lacerate the lung or another underlying organ. Femur fractures and pelvis fractures have a tendency to bleed severely. An open wound to the posterior thorax can lead to a significant amount of air trapped in the pleural space, causing the lung to collapse. This would lead to a compromise in gas exchange and hypoxia. (EC 196-293 PEC 143-257)

149.

A. The patient's airway is open, the breathing is adequate, and his pulse is present. Since he has an altered mental status, you would apply a non-rebreather mask and perform a rapid medical assessment. There is no need for spinal stabilization since there is no mechanism of trauma that would indicate a possible spine injury. The breathing is adequate; therefore, there is no need for bag-valve-mask ventilation. The vital signs will be taken as part of the rapid medical assessment. No transport should be conducted until after the assessment is completed. (EC 196-293 PEC 143-257)

150.

C. The skin is warm and dry and normal in color. This would indicate good tissue perfusion. Hypovolemic shock would result in poor tissue perfusion in which the skin would be pale, cool, and clammy. Hypoxia and inadequate delivery of hemoglobin would cause cyanosis. (EC 216-219 PEC 143-257)

151.

C. The unresponsive medical patient should be placed in a left lateral recumbent position. This is also known as the coma or recovery position. This position is used to allow secretions and vomit to drain from the mouth and airway. (EC 196-293 PEC 143-257)

152.

D. Pain is a subjective complaint. You can not assess and objectively determine if the pain really exists or not. Some signs may tell you the severity of pain, such as a facial grimace. (EC 196-293 PEC 143-257)

153.

D. The first priority is to determine if the scene is safe. The best person at a building collapse to determine the safety hazard of further collapse is the engineer. (EC 196-293 PEC 143-257)

154.

C. Once the scene is cleared of safety hazards, you would approach the patient, apply manual spinal stabilization, quickly assess the posterior thorax, and logroll the patient into a supine position. (EC 196-293 PEC 143-257)

155.

B. The initial assessment and rapid trauma and medical assessments are performed to identify and manage life-threatening injuries or conditions. The detailed physical exam is conducted to identify other non-life-threatening injuries. If you are finding life threats during the detailed physical exam, it is an indication that you did not conduct a proper rapid trauma assessment. The detailed physical exam is time and patient condition dependent. The means, if you do not have the time or if the patient condition does not allow you to perform the detailed physical exam, it would be acceptable not to perform it. (EC 196-293 PEC 143-257)

156.

A. Crackles, also know as rales, will be heard when the terminal bronchiole and alveoli collapse and re-expand with a breath. Wheezing indicates constricted bronchioles. Rhonchi is a snoring type sound that is heard when mucous collects in the larger airways. A pleural friction rub is a leathery creak sound heard on inhalation and exhalation. (EC 196-293 PEC 143-257)

157.

C. A patient who is found in a fetal position is most likely suffering from severe abdominal pain. The fetal position relieves some of the tension of the abdominal wall muscles and places less pressure on the underlying organs. Appendicitis may produce severe abdominal pain. (EC 196-293 PEC 143-257)

158.

A. This technique is assessing the consensual reflex. This reflex causes both pupils to respond simultaneously to light even though it is shone in only one eye. (EC 196-293 PEC 143-257)

159.

C. Because the patient has an altered mental status, you must treat him under implied consent. It would be best to have law enforcement present to assist and witness the restraint process. Do not restrain the patient in prone position. This may interfere with his airway and impede his ventilation. (EC 196-293 PEC 143-257)

160.

D. A car on its roof is considered an unstable vehicle. It is possible that the car may collapse under the weight, thus making it unsafe. The fire department must stabilize the vehicle prior to your entry. (EC 196-293 PEC 143-257)

161.

A. A patient who has suffered a blow to the face, nose, or area around the eye may have suffered a fracture to the bone on the bottom portion of the orbit under the eye (infraorbital). One sign of this type of fracture is the patient may have a gaze upward of both eyes (conjugate gaze). (EC 196-293 PEC 143-257)

162.

A. An unresponsive patient with a fixed and dilated pupil following trauma to his head is most likely suffering from a brain injury with compression and herniation of brain tissue. A patient who is responsive and who has a fixed and dilated pupil is not suffering from herniation of the brain. He is more likely suffering from an injury to the eye itself or an injury to the third cranial nerve. (EC 196-293 PEC 143-257)

163.

B. The brain controls function on the same side of the body above the level of the medulla at around the upper lip and on the opposite side of the body below the upper lip. If the injury occurred to the left side of the brain, the left pupil and right extremities will be affected. (EC 196-293 PEC 143-257)

164.

A. In the adult patient, a positive Babinski sign is when the toes fan up and out when an object such as a pen or your thumb is run up the arch. A positive Babinski sign may be an indication of a brain injury. (EC 196-293 PEC 143-257)

165.

A. A rigid and tender abdomen is a sign of bleeding within the abdominal cavity (intra-abdominal bleeding). Pale, cool, clammy skin and weak rapid radial pulses are indications of poor perfusion. (EC 196-293 PEC 143-257)

166.

B. The abdominal cavity is covered by a peritoneal lining. Blood leaking into the peritoneal cavity will cause irritation of the lining. The irritation will cause abdominal pain, tenderness on palpation, and abdominal wall guarding and rigidity. (EC 196-293 PEC 143-257)

167.

B. Palliation refers to any relief or alleviation of the symptom. Palliation of the breathing difficulty in this patient is achieved by an upright position. (EC 196-293 PEC 143-257)

168.

C. Tenderness and pain on palpation of the symphysis pubis usually indicates a pelvic fracture. When assessing the pelvis, if the patient is already complaining of pain prior to palpation, do not palpate. If not, press down and then inward on the anterior iliac crest, assessing for a pain response, instability, and crepitus. You should then apply pressure to the symphysis pubis. (EC 196-293 PEC 143-257)

169.

C. A patient with abdominal discomfort and pelvic pain may be suffering from a pelvic fracture and intra-abdominal bleeding. This patient is considered unstable; therefore, you should assess the vital signs every 5 minutes. (EC 196-293 PEC 143-257)

170.

B. Because the jugular vein drains into the superior vena cava that empties into the right atrium, a patient suffering from right-sided heart failure would likely be suffering from jugular venous distention. (EC 196-293 PEC 143-257)

171.

C. Assessment of the ears and nose in the chest pain patient would be the least relevant to check. The oral mucosa may provide information about the oxygenation status. The breath sounds are important to assess for abnormal sounds or absence of breath sounds. The pedal pulses will provide information about the perfusion status. (EC 196-293 PEC 143-257)

172.

B. In order to ensure that you have properly transferred the care of the patient to the emergency department, you must provide an oral report to medical personnel who are of equal or higher level of training than yourself. Until that official transfer of care is done, you must remain with the patient, even in the emergency department. (EC 303 PEC 265)

173.

D. A fall of less than two times the height of the patient is not considered to be a significant mechanism of trauma. A fall of **greater than** two times the height of the patient would be considered a significant mechanism of injury. (EC 196-293 PEC 143-257)

174.

D. A component of the scene size-up is to determine the number of patients and call for additional resources. If several patients are found upon entering the scene, you should call for additional resources at that time. (EC 196-293 PEC 143-257)

175.

B. Since the laceration of the leg could be a wound with major bleeding, it is necessary to immediately expose the extremity and inspect the wound. Once the bleeding is controlled, you would continue with the initial assessment. (EC 196-293 PEC 143-257)

176.

C. Dizziness and weakness in a diabetic patient are not indications of an immediate life threat or a priority status. In many diabetic patients, the dizziness and weakness may be related to an episode of hypoglycemia. Administration of glucose will reverse the symptoms. The other selections are all priority indicators. (EC 196-293 PEC 143-257)

177.

B. Discoloration to the mastoid process is also known as Battle's sign. It typically indicates a posterior basilar skull fracture. The discoloration, however, does not occur usually for several hours after the injury. (EC 196-293 PEC 143-257)

178.

B. It is difficult to assess a blood pressure in children less than 3 years of age. It is more important to rely on peripheral and central pulses and the skin signs to determine perfusion status. It would be difficult to assess the orientation in a 2-year-old patient. The reddened sclera does not apply to a dehydrated patient. (EC 196-293 PEC 143-257)

179.

B. A patient with an altered mental status may not be able to control his or her own airway. Therefore, it is important that in any patient with an altered mental status you carefully assess and monitor the airway. (EC 196-293 PEC 143-257)

180.

C. Scene safety is your first concern. Until the scene is determined to be safe, you should remain in the ambulance. (EC 196-293 PEC 143-257)

181.

B. During exhalation, the chest wall is moving inward. A segment that moves opposite or outward when the remainder of the chest is moving inward would be considered to be moving in a paradoxical motion. This is an indication of a flail segment. (EC 196-293 PEC 143-257)

182.

D. Stridor is a high pitched sound that is produced from air rushing past a partial obstruction at the level of the larynx. It is commonly produced by swelling that occurs in the larynx. (EC 196-293 PEC 143-257)

183.

D. Because the patient is talking when you arrive at her side, you have already determined she is alert, her airway is patent, and her breathing is adequate. The next step in the initial assessment is to assess the pulse and skin. (EC 196-293 PEC 143-257)

184.

B. A patient with hot, dry skin may be suffering from a heat related emergency such as heat stroke. This is a dire emergency that requires rapid treatment and transport. Shock and heart attack normally produce cool and diaphoretic skin. A stroke usually presents with no significant skin findings. (EC 196-293 PEC 143-257)

185.

D. The mental status of the patient is the key determinant of whether to perform the rapid medical assessment or SAMPLE history first. If the patient is unable to respond appropriately to your questions, you should proceed with the rapid medical assessment. (EC 196-293 PEC 143-257)

186.

D. Any female patient in child bearing years who is complaining of abdominal pain should be questioned about her menstrual period. You want to determine if she has missed a period, if any abnormal discharge has occurred, bleeding between the period, or if the period was excessively heavy. This may provide you with a clue that the condition may be related to a reproductive organ injury or disorder. (EC 196-293 PEC 143-257)

187.

C. The patient has tachycardia. A heart rate greater than 100 beats/minute in an adult patient is considered to be tachycardia. A narrow pulse pressure is when the difference between the systolic and dia- stolic blood pressure is less than 30 mmHg. Tachypnea is a respiratory rate that is greater than 20 per minute in the adult. Hypertension is defined as a systolic blood pressure greater than 160 mmHg and a diastolic greater than 90 mmHg. (EC 196-293 PEC 143-257)

188.

D. Apply an occlusive dressing to any wound to the thorax. Regardless if the wound is anterior, lateral, or posterior, it may still be a sucking chest wound. This type of wound could easily produce a tension pneumothorax. (EC 196-293 PEC 143-257)

189.

B. The medical term for swelling is edema. Erythema is redness. Ecchymosis means discoloration of a black and blue tint. A contusion is a bruise. (EC 196-293 PEC 143-257)

190.

B. Once the posterior neck or cervical region has been palpated, it is necessary to apply the cervical spinal immobilization collar. Once the collar is applied, manual spinal stabilization must still be maintained until the patient is fully immobilized to the backboard. (EC 196-293 PEC 143-257)

191.

B. Since aspiration would interfere with gas exchange in the alveoli and produce hypoxia, cyanosis may occur. (EC 196-293 PEC 143-257)

192.

D. Even if the patient refuses, attempt to persuade the patient to allow you to assess her. It is important to be sure that you inform the patient of the possible consequences of the possible injuries. (EC 196-293 PEC 143-257)

193.

C. A systemic allergic reaction, also known as anaphylaxis, will cause the bronchioles to constrict and become inflamed on the internal surface. This increase in airway resistance will produce wheezing when air rushes through. (EC 196-293 PEC 143-257)

194.

C. Palliation or alleviation is reported when a medication, position, activity, or lack of activity reduces the symptom's severity or eliminates the symptom. (EC 196-293 PEC 143-257)

195.

D. Approximately 50% of the patients who suffer a tonic-clonic seizure will bite their tongue. If you arrive on the scene of a patient who has a laceration to the tongue, you should suspect a possible seizure. (EC 196-293 PEC 143-257)

196.

D. Subcutaneous emphysema is air trapped under the skin. It is an indication that there is a leak in the respiratory tract lung, or the esophagus. It may be easier to feel the bubble packaging texture than to see the bloated look of the skin when performing your assessment. In the seated patient, the air normally travels upward to the upper chest, neck, and face. (EC 196-293 PEC 143-257)

197.

D. A detailed physical exam is one component of the assessment that may be skipped. It is designed to identify injuries that are not life-threatening; therefore, it is more important to focus on life threats than assess for injuries that are not life-threatening. (EC 196-293 PEC 143-257)

198.

D. Because the heart is compressed in the mediastinum in a tension pneumothorax, the cardiac output will be reduced and the systolic blood pressure decreased. The pulse pressure will become narrowed when the systolic and diastolic blood pressure readings become closer together. (EC 196-293 PEC 143-257)

199.

B. All patients, regardless of how serious or minor the extent of the injury or illness, must have an initial assessment. (EC 196-293 PEC 143-257)

200.

C. You would immediately repeat the initial assessment to determine if her airway is still patent, her breathing is still adequate, and to reassess her pulse and skin. You would then move to repeat the assessment of the abdomen and obtain another set of vital signs. (EC 196-293 PEC 143-257)

201.

A. The purpose of the rapid trauma assessment is to identify and manage life threats to the patient. All other injuries that are not life threats are identified and managed during the detailed physical exam. (EC 196-293 PEC 143-257)

202.

C. When a patient says a few words and then must gasp for a breath, it is a good indication that the patient is having difficulty breathing. A crying patient, or one who talks with a completely normal speech pattern, typically is not having a difficult time breathing. (EC 196-293 PEC 143-257)

203.

B. A fall from the roof of a house would be an indication to suspect a spinal injury. Therefore, it is necessary to take manual spinal stabilization prior to proceeding in the initial assessment. (EC 196-293 PEC 143-257)

204.

D. The patient has inadequate respirations. Because the patient is not responding to painful stimuli, you can insert an oropharyngeal airway to facilitate the ventilation. (EC 196-293 PEC 143-257)

205.

B. Tenderness is pain on palpation. Rigidity is an involuntary abdominal muscle contraction. Guarding is voluntary abdominal muscle contraction. Pain is a patient complaint that occurs without any palpation or manipulation of the area. (EC 196-293 PEC 143-257)

4 Medical/Behavioral/ Obstetrics

module objectives

Questions in this module relate to D.O.T. objectives 4-1.1 to 4-9.29.

DIRECTIONS Each of the questions or incomplete statements below is followed by suggested answers or completions. Select the **one answer** that is best in each case.

GENERAL PHARMACOLOGY 4.1

1. All of the following medications are carried on the EMT-Basic unit **except:**
   A. activated charcoal.
   B. epinephrine.
   C. oxygen.
   D. oral glucose.

2. EMT-Basics can assist with administration of which of the following medications?
   A. epinephrine for allergic reactions
   B. metered-dose inhalers for respiratory emergencies
   C. nitroglycerin for cardiac emergencies
   D. all of the above

3. Which of the following is **not** a medication that the EMT-B can assist the patient in taking during a respiratory emergency?
   A. Decadron
   B. Bronkosol
   C. Ventolin
   D. Alupent

4. Actidose and SuperChar are trade names for a medication that is used:
   A. for patients suffering from hypoglycemia.
   B. to bind with certain poisons to prevent further absorption.
   C. as an antibiotic to prevent wound infection.
   D. to help increase heart rate in cold water drowning.

5. The generic name(s) for Alupent include:
   A. albuterol
   B. isoetharine
   C. metaproterenol
   D. all of the above

6. You are called to the scene for an unknown medical emergency. Upon arrival you find your patient lying on the ground too weak to reach her medication. The medication on the metered-dose inhaler reads salmeterol xinafoate. Is this a medication that you can assist the patient in taking? If so, what type of emergency is it used for?
   A. No. This is not an approved drug for administration by an EMT-B.
   B. Yes. This is an approved drug for administration, and it is used in cardiac emergencies.
   C. Yes. This is an approved drug for administration, and it is used in acute poisoning.
   D. Yes. This is an approved drug for administration, and it is used in respiratory emergencies.

7. If you are unsure about a generic name on a medication, you should:
   A. ask the patient if the generic name is the same as the trade name that you are familiar with.
   B. administer the drug immediately because any delay in the medication administration could harm the patient.
   C. contact medical control and ask the physician.
   D. attempt to find the drug insert information and locate the different names of the medication.

8. The generic name of a medication is:
   A. the name assigned to a drug before it becomes officially listed.
   B. the name listed in the U.S. Pharmacopoeia.
   C. the name that is close to the chemical name.
   D. all of the above.

9. Which of the following is an approved medication to carry on an EMT-Basic ambulance?
   A. LiquiChar
   B. Bronkosol
   C. albuterol
   D. nitrostat

10. The EMT-B may assist with the administration of all the following medications **except:**
    A. metaproterenol.
    B. epinephrine.
    C. albuterol.
    D. Inderal.

11. After a medication has been administered it is important to:
    A. repeat the dose two times.
    B. check the expiration date.
    C. conduct an ongoing assessment.
    D. ask the patient about any allergies.

12. Which of the following drug routes of administration is incorrectly paired?
    A. sublingual - nitroglycerin spray under the tongue
    B. oral - swallowing nitroglycerin
    C. inhalation - topical deposition of beta$_2$ drugs on bronchial smooth muscle
    D. injection - intramuscular administration of epinephrine

RESPIRATORY 4.2

13. Components of the respiratory system include all of the following **except:**
    A. lung.
    B. larynx.
    C. esophagus.
    D. trachea.

14. Which of the following are functions of the nose?
    A. warm inspired air
    B. filter out large dust particles
    C. humidify inspired air
    D. all of the above

15. Which structure is responsible for controlling the movement of food and air between the respiratory and digestive systems?
    A. pharynx
    B. epiglottis
    C. thyroid cartilage
    D. cricoid cartilage

16. The major muscle of respiration is the:
    A. external intercostal muscle.
    B. internal intercostal muscle.
    C. diaphragm.
    D. pectoralis major.

17. When an aduct patient initially becomes hypoxic, the EMT would expect the heart rate to:
    A. increase due to sympathetic discharge.
    B. decrease due to parasympathetic discharge.
    C. increase due to parasympathetic discharge.
    D. decrease due to sympathetic discharge.

18. Signs of hypoxia may include:
    A. tachypnea.
    B. cyanosis.
    C. bradycardia.
    D. all of the above.

19. To determine if the patient has an adequate breathing, the EMT-B should do all the following **except:**
    A. assess the respiratory rate.
    B. auscultate breath sounds bilaterally.
    C. assess the heart rate.
    D. assess the rise and fall of the chest.

20. Signs of adequate ventilation in an adult include all of the following **except:**
    A. respiratory rate of 16 breaths per minute.
    B. breath sounds that are equal and clear bilaterally.
    C. slight cyanosis to the oral mucosa.
    D. equal and full chest rise and fall.

21. The size of the tongue in an infant when compared proportionately with that of an adult is:
    A. smaller.
    B. larger.
    C. equal in size.
    D. extremely small.

22. What is the narrowest portion of the upper airway for infants and children under 10 years of age?
    A. posterior oral pharynx
    B. the epiglottic opening
    C. glottic opening
    D. the cricoid cartilage

23. You arrive on scene to find a frantic mother screaming that her daughter can not breathe. The infant is making high-pitched sounds on inspiration, has good color, is alert, and is gasping for air. You suspect what problem?
    A. acute exacerbation of bronchitis
    B. partial airway obstruction
    C. asthma attack
    D. complete airway obstruction

24. Your treatment for an adult patient with a partial airway obstruction as compared with a complete obstruction varies in that:
    A. in a complete obstruction oxygen is provided by non-rebreather mask, and no oxygen is given in a partial obstruction.
    B. in a partial obstruction you would attempt to view the obstruction, whereas in a complete obstruction no visualization is performed.
    C. in a partial obstruction you would instruct the patient to cough, whereas in a complete obstruction you would deliver abdominal thrusts.
    D. priority is placed on removing the obstruction in the partial obstruction, whereas immediate transport is the key management for a complete obstruction.

25. Signs indicative of a complete airway obstruction include all of the following **except:**
    A. the patient does not cry or talk.
    B. central and or core cyanosis may be present.
    C. the patient will cough forcefully.
    D. there is no chest rise or fall.

26. During the mechanical process of inspiration:
    A. the diaphragm contracts along with the intercostal muscles, causing expansion of the thoracic cavity.
    B. the diaphragm contracts, pulling the ribs inward and causing expansion of the chest.
    C. the diaphragm relaxes, allowing the intercostal muscles to contract and thus causing inspiration.
    D. the intercostal muscles contract, causing the ribs to flare out and pull up on the diaphragm.

27. The process of exchange of oxygen and carbon dioxide at the cell is known as:
    A. oxygenation.
    B. ventilation.
    C. inspiration.
    D. respiration.

28. This structure has a common opening for the respiratory tract and the digestive system:
    A. larynx.
    B. esophagus.
    C. trachea.
    D. pharynx.

29. A common cause of upper airway obstruction in a young child is flexion of the head. The flexion is commonly caused by:
    A. the child's head being proportionately smaller than the rest of the body.
    B. the trachea being underdeveloped.
    C. the child's tongue being so big it forces the forward flexion.
    D. the head being disproportionately larger, causing flexion of the head.

30. Which of the following is adjacent to and covers the outer lung tissue?
    A. parietal pleura
    B. peritoneum
    C. visceral pericardium
    D. visceral pleura

31. The EMT-B can assist the patient with administration of a prescribed inhaler if:
    A. the EMT-B has protocol authorizing the action.
    B. the on-line medical director authorizes the action.
    C. the patient is prescribed the inhaler.
    D. all of the above.

32. The pharynx is divided into two major divisions:
    A. larynx and trachea.
    B. larynx and oropharynx.
    C. larynx and nasopharynx.
    D. oropharynx and nasopharynx.

33. The larynx is commonly referred to as the:
    A. windpipe.
    B. esophagus.
    C. voice box.
    D. master gland.

34. You are called to a residence for a man who is having difficulty breathing. While you are assessing your patient, his wife hands you the telephone stating it's the family doctor. The doctor identifies herself and orders you to administer two puffs of the wife's inhaler because it sounds as if the husband is suffering from the same type of asthma attacks his wife does. You should:
    A. follow the order since it was given by a physician.
    B. advise the physician that you will only follow her orders if she meets you at the emergency room and signs your run report.
    C. explain to the physician that it is against your protocol to help administer the medication since it is not prescribed for your patient.
    D. tell the physician you can perform her order if she writes a prescription for the medication for your patient.

35. Before consulting with medical control for an order to administer a medication, the EMT-B should:
    A. assess the patient and perform any life-saving procedures.
    B. perform a check of the baseline vital signs.
    C. check to make sure the medication is prescribed for the patient and the medication is not expired.
    D. all of the above.

36. You administer oxygen to a patient who is short of breath. Initial auscultation revealed inspiratory and expiratory wheezing in all lung fields. After the oxygen administration, you reassess the patient and find decreased wheezing and diminished breath sounds bilaterally. This is a sign that:
    A. the oxygen therapy is helping since the wheezes are decreasing.
    B. the bronchoconstriction is worsening.
    C. bronchodilation is occurring.
    D. you probably are not listening correctly with your stethoscope.

37. Signs of adequate ventilation when the EMT-B is performing positive pressure ventilation include all of the following **except:**
    A. adequate and equal chest rise and fall.
    B. increased heart rate above 100 bpm.
    C. improving mental status.
    D. equal breath sounds bilaterally.

38. _____ indicates an upper airway obstruction, while _____ indicates a lower airway bronchoconstriction.
    A. Wheezing, stridor
    B. Wheezing, rales
    C. Stridor, wheezing
    D. Stridor, rales

39. Asthma is an example of a(n) _____ airway disease and epiglottitis is a(n) _____ airway disease.
    A. upper, lower
    B. lower, upper
    C. upper, upper
    D. lower, lower

40. A tripod position is a sign of:
    A. severe respiratory distress.
    B. hypoglycemia.
    C. stroke.
    D. heat emergency.

41. The term used to describe a patient in respiratory arrest is:
    A. dyspnea.
    B. bradypnea.
    C. tachypnea.
    D. apnea.

42. Choose the sign or symptom that best indicates severe respiratory distress.
    A. A patient speaks full sentences between breaths.
    B. A patient has a bluish-gray skin color on the neck.
    C. A 10-year-old is breathing 30 times each minute.
    D. A 4-month-old is breathing with abdominal muscles.

43. While assessing a patient who complains of difficulty breathing, you hear stridor when the patient inhales. This is a sign of:
    A. traumatic flail segment.
    B. tension pneumothorax.
    C. sucking chest wound.
    D. partial airway obstruction.

44. All of the following are late signs of respiratory distress in the infant and child **except:**
    A. head bobbing.
    B. bradycardia.
    C. hypertension.
    D. tachpnea.

45. You are treating a patient in respiratory distress. You are unsure if the patient needs positive pressure ventilation. You should immediately:
    A. administer oxygen via non-rebreather mask.
    B. provide positive pressure ventilation.
    C. insert an nasopharyngeal (NPA) airway.
    D. place the patient in the Trendelenburg position.

46. Your patient is complaining of shortness of breath. He has a respiratory rate of 22/minute with an adequate tidal volume. You should:
    A. immediately provide positive pressure ventilation.
    B. provide oxygen by non-rebreather mask at 15 lpm.
    C. provide oxygen by nasal cannula at 6 lpm.
    D. withhold oxygen if he is only complaining of minimal shortness of breath.

47. A late sign of respiratory failure in an infant that indicates the need for positive pressure ventilation is:
    A. loss of muscle tone (limp appearance).
    B. cyanosis of the hands and feet.
    C. increased heart rate (tachycardia).
    D. prolonged exhalation and nasal flaring.

48. You are treating an apprehensive child who is experiencing difficulty breathing. The child will not tolerate the non-rebreather mask and continuously removes it from his face. You should:

   A. do nothing since the child cannot be in distress if he can resist treatment.

   B. have a parent hold the mask near the child's face to deliver the oxygen.

   C. speak to the child calmly while holding the mask over his mouth and nose.

   D. place the child on a nasal cannula at 10 liters per minute and reassure him.

49. You are treating a child who complains of a fever and a sore throat. The child is sitting upright, has his neck jutted out, and is drooling. You should:

   A. inspect inside the child's mouth and oropharynx with a tongue depressor.

   B. perform a finger sweep of the mouth to remove any foreign materials.

   C. provide oxygen by non-rebreather mask and begin immediate transport.

   D. suction the secretions from the oropharynx with the hard suction catheter.

50. Which of the following best describes the actions of aerosolized medication in the metered-dose inhaler (MDI)?

   A. beta agonist that relaxes the bronchiole smooth muscle

   B. beta agonist that contracts the tracheal smooth muscle

   C. alpha agonist that relaxes the bronchiole smooth muscle

   D. alpha agonist that contracts the tracheal smooth muscle

51. A bronchodilator administered by metered-dose inhaler should not be given to the patient in which situation?

   A. The patient has a history of bronchoconstriction.

B. The patient does not respond to verbal stimuli appropriately.

C. The patient takes albuterol, which is prescribed to him or her.

D. The patient complains of shortness of breath with wheezes.

52. Which of the following administration steps is **incorrect** when assisting a patient with a metered-dose inhaler?

   A. Obtain either on-line or off-line orders from medical direction.

   B. Coach the patient to hold his or her breath for 10 seconds.

   C. Depress the canister and then ask the patient to breathe rapidly and deeply.

   D. Instruct the patient to exhale slowly through pursed lips.

53. Which of the following respiratory drugs used by patients with chronic respiratory disease is **not** a beta agonist?

   A. albuterol (Proventil®, Ventolin®)

   B. metaproterenol (Alupent®, Metaprel®)

   C. isoetharine (Bronkosol®, Bronkometer®)

   D. ipratropium bromide (Atrovent®)

54. After assisting your patient with a metered-dose inhaler (MDI), he experiences tachycardia and nervousness. Which of the following is true regarding this finding?

   A. Tachycardia and nervousness are common side effects of the drug.

   B. The patient has overdosed on the medication.

   C. Tachycardia and nervousness occurred because the medication dose was incorrect.

   D. The patient is hypersensitive to the drug.

55. You are treating a 4-year-old patient with a sore throat and fever. When the patient coughs it sounds like a barking seal. You know this as the hallmark sign of:

A. croup, resulting in swelling of the larynx, trachea, and bronchi.

B. croup, resulting in constriction of the bronchioles.

C. epiglottitis, resulting in swelling of the epiglottis in the upper airway.

D. epiglottitis, resulting in upper airway obstruction from a foreign body.

56. Which of the following signs and symptoms are indicative of lower airway disease in a child?

A. audible wheezes and diminished breath sounds

B. cough that produces a sound like a barking seal

C. fever, stridorous airway sounds, drooling patient

D. sudden onset of stridorous airway sounds

57. You are assessing a child who presents with shortness of breath and wheezing with each breath. The patient is prescribed Proventil® by metered-dose inhaler (MDI). You suspect the patient suffers from:

A. an upper airway disease.

B. acute epiglottitis.

C. a lower airway disease.

D. acute croup.

CARDIOVASCULAR 4.3

58. Blood is ejected from the right atrium to the:

A. right ventricle to the lungs to the aorta.

B. left ventricle to the lungs to the left atrium.

C. right ventricle to the lungs to the left atrium to the left ventricle.

D. left ventricle to the lungs to the right ventricle to the left atrium.

59. The site where the exchange of oxygen, carbon dioxide, and other vital nutrients takes place is in the:

A. large arteries.

B. capillaries.

C. arterioles.

D. venules.

60. The heart can be divided into two separate pumps:

A. the low pressure left myocardium and high pressure right myocardium.

B. the high pressure right myocardium and the high pressure left myocardium.

C. the low pressure right myocardium and the high pressure left myocardium.

D. the low pressure right myocardium and the low pressure left myocardium.

61. The AED (automated external defibrillator) should be applied to which patient?

A. a 6-year-old child in cardiac arrest

B. a 17-year-old in traumatic cardiac arrest

C. a 55-year-old patient whose chief complaint is chest pain

D. a 43-year-old patient who is unresponsive, pulseless, and apneic

62. Your patient complains of shortness of breath and has a history of congestive heart failure. What is the most appropriate position to transport the patient?

A. the patient secured to the cot with the head flat, allowing for access to the airway

B. the patient secured to the cot with the feet elevated to reduce the edema of the ankles

C. the patient secured to the cot with the head and chest elevated

D. the patient sitting on the cot unsecured, holding on to the side rails

63. Within the first 8 minutes, what is the most common presenting rhythm in cardiac arrest?

A. asystole

B. ventricular tachycardia

C. ventricular fibrillation

D. pulseless electrical activity

64. The most effective treatment for ventricular fibrillation is:
    A. CPR.
    B. hyperventilation.
    C. defibrillation.
    D. rapid transport.

65. Why should ALS be requested when the EMT-B can defibrillate?
    A. The patient can be transferred to the ALS unit and place the basic unit back into service quicker.
    B. Prehospital ALS is integral in the chain of survival and needs to be activated quickly to allow for earlier definitive care.
    C. The fee for the ALS unit is higher and will generate more revenue.
    D. The ALS unit carries a monitor/defibrillator in case the AED malfunctions.

66. The major difference between a semi-automatic and automatic defibrillator is:
    A. the semi-automatic defibrillator allows a better "picture" of the heart.
    B. the automatic defibrillator requires more involvement by the operator.
    C. the automatic defibrillator requires the operator to push a button to deliver a shock.
    D. the semi-automatic defibrillator requires the operator to push a button to deliver a shock.

67. With a single rescuer, what is the maximum number of shocks to administer before leaving the patient to call for help?
    A. two sets of three shocks totaling six
    B. as many shocks as needed to convert the patient out of ventricular fibrillation
    C. only one shock because the activation of ALS is more important
    D. one set of three shocks

68. When using the AED you should transport your patient when:
    A. the patient regains a pulse.
    B. the AED has given three consecutive "No Shock" messages.
    C. a total of six shocks have been delivered.
    D. all of the above.

69. After the AED is used, a case review would be beneficial for all the following reasons **except:**
    A. determining if steps can be taken to decrease the time to defibrillation.
    B. determining how to work more effectively with ALS backup.
    C. determining if the AED is effective in converting v-fib to a perfusing rhythm.
    D. determining if further training is needed, and in what areas.

70. Once you reach the side of a patient who is pulseless and apneic, the first shock from the AED should be delivered in under:
    A. 3 minutes.
    B. 1 minute.
    C. 4 minutes.
    D. 2 minutes.

71. The speed of delivery of the first shock is dependent on:
    A. provider training.
    B. delaying airway management and oxygen therapy until the shocks are delivered.
    C. delaying the start of CPR until the first shocks are delivered.
    D. all of the above.

72. The most common cause of failure of the AED is due to:
    A. electronic malfunction.
    B. improper placement of the pads.
    C. patient artifact.
    D. a dead battery.

73. By completing the operator checklist, you are assured of all of the following **except:**

    A. the batteries are fully charged.

    B. the cables are in working condition.

    C. the operator is proficient in the use of the AED.

    D. the AED has an adequate amount of ECG paper.

74. To be most effective in converting ventricular fibrillation into a perfusing rhythm, defibrillation should occur within how may minutes of the cardiac arrest:

    A. 10 minutes.

    B. 8 minutes.

    C. 6 minutes.

    D. 4 minutes.

75. If proper CPR is being performed, defibrillation is most successful for up to _____ minutes after the onset of cardiac arrest.

    A. 10 minutes

    B. 8 minutes

    C. 6 minutes

    D. 12 minutes

76. During the first set of three stacked shocks, CPR should be performed:

    A. in between the individual shocks while the machine is assessing the rhythm.

    B. after the second shock.

    C. after the first shock.

    D. only after the third shock is delivered and the pulse is checked.

77. When using a semi-automatic defibrillator, between shocks the operator should:

    A. check pulses before delivering the second and third stacked shocks.

    B. initiate CPR while the machine is analyzing the rhythm.

    C. keep clear of the patient and depress the shock button if advised.

    D. press the shock button as a precaution.

78. Circumstances that may lead to inappropriate defibrillation include all of the following **except:**

    A. placing the AED on a patient who is complaining of chest pain.

    B. placing the AED on a patient in ventricular tachycardia who has a pulse.

    C. placing the AED on a patient who is pulseless and apneic.

    D. mechanical failure caused by poorly maintained or faulty batteries.

79. You arrive on scene and find an unresponsive, apneic, and pulseless patient. While you are preparing the AED, your partner should be:

    A. preparing a backboard and the cot for rapid transport.

    B. performing CPR.

    C. gathering a medical history from family or bystanders.

    D. performing a focused history and exam.

80. What are the initial steps for single rescuer use of the AED?

    A. Take body substance isolation precautions, apply the AED, and press the shock button.

    B. Take body substance isolation precautions, perform the initial survey, start CPR for 1 minute, apply the AED, and press the analyze button.

    C. Take body substance isolation precautions, perform the initial survey, oxygenate the patient with positive pressure ventilation for 1 minute, apply the AED, and press the analyze button.

    D. Take body substance isolation precautions, perform the initial survey, apply the AED, and analyze the rhythm.

81. After successfully defibrillating your patient you are en route to rendezvous with ALS backup. You have applied oxygen and left the AED on the patient. Your patient suddenly becomes pulseless and apneic. Your actions should include:
    A. pulling the ambulance over to the side of the road and turning off the engine.
    B. pressing the analyze button.
    C. delivering three stacked shocks if indicated.
    D. all of the above.

82. While transporting a patient who received a total of six shocks before regaining a pulse, loses his pulse and deteriorates into ventricular fibrillation. You should:
    A. begin CPR and continue transport.
    B. shock the patient only once.
    C. deliver three more stacked shocks.
    D. do nothing and the ventricular fibrillation will degrade into asystole.

83. How often should you reassess the post-resuscitation patient during transport?
    A. when the patient begins to experience chest pain
    B. once during a 20-minute transport
    C. at least every 5 minutes or whenever the patient's condition changes
    D. every 15 minutes if the patient's condition doesn't change

84. The fully automated external defibrillator differs from the semi-automatic external defibrillator in which of the following aspects?
    A. With the fully automated external defibrillator, there is no chance of discharging the machine while a rescuer is still in contact with the patient.
    B. The fully automated external defibrillator analyzes the rhythm and delivers the shock itself.

C. The fully automated external defibrillator delivers the shocks at a higher joule setting.
D. The fully automated external defibrillator delivers the stacked shocks at a slower rate.

85. If your AED is equipped with an event recorder, you should include what information?
    A. unit name or number
    B. location of call/incident
    C. the time and date
    D. all of the above

86. You are working in a rural county as an EMT-B. You answer a call at a physician's office for a patient with chest pain. The physician informs you the patient is experiencing a myocardial infarction. The physician orders you to administer nitroglycerin every 5 minutes for the entire trip to the emergency department (approximately 30 minutes away). You are unable to contact the on-line medical control physician to discuss what to do. As a prudent EMT, you should:
    A. transport the patient following the physician's orders.
    B. transport the patient and administer the nitroglycerin every 5 minutes only if the patient's systolic blood pressure remains above 100 mmHg.
    C. advise the physician that it is against your protocol and you cannot administer the nitroglycerin as he has ordered.
    D. call dispatch to send the ALS unit in the neighboring county to transport the patient and place your unit back in service.

87. To decrease anxiety and the effort of breathing you should place all patients complaining of chest pain in what position?
    A. sitting straight up on the cot
    B. lying flat on the cot

C. lying flat with the feet elevated

D. in a position of comfort

88. The batteries in the AED should be checked:
    A. monthly.
    B. daily.
    C. weekly.
    D. semiannually.

89. Any time the semi-automatic defibrillator advises "No Shock" you should:
    A. stop and turn the machine off.
    B. disconnect the leads from the AED, leaving only the patches in place on the patient's chest.
    C. perform CPR for 1 minute and then check pulse and reanalyze the rhythm.
    D. turn the machine off and then back on to reset the computer.

90. Contraindications for use of the AED include:
    A. a trauma patient.
    B. a child under 8 years of age.
    C. a conscious patient.
    D. all of the above.

91. Place the following steps for use of the AED into order:

    1. Body substance isolation
    2. Deliver shock
    3. Have partner start CPR
    4. Attach device
    5. Determine unresponsiveness
    6. Turn device on
    7. Initiate rhythm analysis
    8. Perform initial assessment
    9. Have partner stop CPR

    A. 1,3,5,8,7,6,2,4,9
    B. 1,5,8,4,3,6,7,9,2
    C. 1,5,8,3,4,9,6,7,2
    D. 1,5,8,4,9,3,6,2,7

92. Before administering a second dose of nitroglycerin, you must:

A. determine the systolic blood pressure.

B. perform a detailed physical examination.

C. call medical control for direction before readministration.

D. all of the above.

93. The right side of the heart:
    A. receives blood from the arteries of the heart and pumps oxygenated blood to the left ventricle.
    B. receives oxygen depleted poor blood from the veins of the body and pumps the blood to the peripheral tissues.
    C. receives oxygen depleted blood from the arteries and pumps oxygenated blood to the left side of the heart.
    D. receives oxygen depleted blood from the veins and pumps oxygenated blood to the lungs.

94. Your patient complains of slight chest discomfort without shortness of breath. The breathing status is adequate with good volume. You should:
    A. administer oxygen by nasal cannula at 6 lpm.
    B. administer oxygen by non-rebreather mask at 15 lpm.
    C. administer oxygen by nasal cannula at 2 lpm.
    D. administer oxygen by non-rebreather mask at 6 lpm.

95. You are preparing to treat a responsive patient who complains of severe chest pain. Your initial treatment should consist of:
    A. assisting with the metered-dose inhaler (MDI).
    B. placing the patient in the Trendelenburg position.
    C. assisting the patient with his or her nitroglycerin.
    D. administering oxygen by non-rebreather mask.

96. You are preparing to assess a 68-year-old patient who was complaining of chest tightness. You should assess the patient in which order?
    A. breathing, circulation, skin, airway, mental status
    B. general impression, airway, circulation, mental status, skin, breathing
    C. breathing, airway, circulation, skin
    D. general impression, mental status, airway, breathing, circulation, skin

97. Approximately 20% of heart attack patients do not experience chest pain. The term used to describe this type of heart attack is known as:
    A. silent heart attack.
    B. muted heart attack.
    C. tranquil heart attack.
    D. quiet heart attack.

98. Nitroglycerin spray is administered by what route?
    A. topical
    B. sublingual
    C. ingestion
    D. injection

99. In which of the following chest pain patients would nitroglycerin be contraindicated?
    A. 62-year-old, lightheaded, heart rate 80/minute, blood pressure 98/52mmHg, respirations 20/minute
    B. 72-year-old who is very anxious, heart rate 102/minute, blood pressure 158/88mmHg, respirations 26/minute
    C. 46-year-old who has taken two doses of nitroglycerin, HR 110/minute, BP 142/68mmHg, R22/minute
    D. 86-year-old with an irregular pulse of 86/minute, difficulty breathing at 38/minute, BP 186/80mmHg

100. All of the following are common side effects of nitroglycerin except:
    A. decrease in systolic blood pressure.
    B. blurred vision.
    C. headache.
    D. tachycardia.

101. You arrive on the scene and find a 42-year-old responsive patient who is experiencing cardiac compromise. Your first assessment concern is:
    A. pulse rate and quality.
    B. SAMPLE history.
    C. airway and breathing status.
    D. skin color and temperature.

102. Which of the following is **not** a link in the American Heart Association's chain of survival?
    A. early access
    B. early CPR
    C. early diagnosis
    D. early defibrillation

103. Which of the following statements is **incorrect** pertaining to ventricular fibrillation and defibrillation?
    A. Ventricular fibrillation is the most common initial rhythm in sudden cardiac arrest.
    B. Early electrical defibrillation is the most successful treatment for ventricular fibrillation.
    C. When CPR is performed, successful defibrillation time may be extended.
    D. Ventricular fibrillation will last long periods of time before deteriorating to asystole.

104. If an advanced life support (paramedic) unit is not available to assist you after three sets of stacked shocks. You should:
    A. continue to defibrillate the patient until the rhythm changes to asystole.
    B. by radio, pronounce the patient dead.
    C. immediately begin transport to the hospital.

D. remain on the scene and provide CPR only.

105. Which of the following represents correct placement of monophasic defibrillator adhesive pads on a cardiac arrest patient?
    A. The (+) is placed below the xiphoid process below the sternum; the (−) is placed over the ribs at the right anterior axillary line.
    B. The (−) is placed below the xiphoid process below the sternum; the (+) is placed over the ribs at the right anterior axillary line.
    C. The (+) is placed on the right upper border of the sternum; the (−) is placed over the ribs at the left anterior axillary line.
    D. The (−) is placed on the right upper border of the sternum; the (+) is placed over the ribs at the left anterior axillary line.

106. You have delivered the second shock in the first set of stacked shocks, using a semi-automated AED. The AED gives a "No Shock" message. Your next action should be:
    A. check the patient's pulse.
    B. deliver the third shock.
    C. reposition the adhesive pads.
    D. begin CPR immediately.

107. The major difference between a semi-automated AED and a fully automated AED is:
    A. the semi-automated AED recognizes asystole and will deliver a shock.
    B. the semi-automated AED is designed to be used on children and adults.
    C. the fully automated AED delivers a shock without operation intervention when appropriate.
    D. The fully automated AED can effectively analyze the rhythm during CPR.

108. Why must CPR be stopped while the AED is analyzing the rhythm?

A. The device emits oral messages that may not be heard during CPR.
B. The device senses the CPR compressions and can not be turned on.
C. The device may automatically deliver a series of three rapid shocks.
D. The device cannot analyze the rhythm while CPR is being performed.

109. The AED is considered safer to use than a manual defibrillator because the AED:
    A. produces less electrical energy.
    B. uses adhesive external pads.
    C. can not shock the rescuers.
    D. can be used safely when wet.

110. While the automated external defibrillator (AED) is performing its analysis between shocks, you should:
    A. perform CPR.
    B. auscultate breath sounds.
    C. check for a carotid pulse.
    D. remain clear of the patient.

111. While transporting a cardiac arrest patient to the hospital, the patient goes back into v-fib. Before analyzing the rhythm with the AED you must:
    A. stop the ambulance and turn the motor off.
    B. stop the ambulance and let the throttle idle.
    C. stop the ambulance and place it in neutral.
    D. stop the ambulance and shut off all lights.

112. All of the following may interfere with the AED's ability to analyze the rhythm, **except:**
    A. vehicle engine vibration.
    B. vehicle interior lighting.
    C. movement of the patient.
    D. two-way radio transmission.

113. You have provided three stacked shocks with the AED. The patient has regained a pulse; your next immediate action should be:
    A. assess the blood pressure.
    B. check the patient's breathing.
    C. perform a focused history.
    D. provide ACLS immediately.

114. Most automated external defibrillator (AED) failures are attributed to:
    A. poor training of personnel.
    B. improper maintenance.
    C. complicated directions.
    D. adhesive pad failure.

SCENARIO

Questions 115–117 refer to the following scenario:

You and your partner Ingrid are exercising at the station when the alerting system sounds, "Medic One respond to 812 Elm Street for a person with chest pain." Upon arrival you introduce yourself and Ingrid. The patient states his name is Wilson, but he would rather be called "Big Joe." Big Joe states, "I was drinking beer and mowing the yard when all of a sudden I became sweaty and my chest began to hurt." Big Joe is a 40-year-old with a prior history of chest pain; he has no other prior medical history and seems in good health. He describes the pain as "sharp" and points to the midsternal area. He describes the pain as an "8" on the 1 to 10 severity scale. He denies any shortness of breath.

115. Oxygen therapy for this patient should be delivered by:
    A. nasal cannula at 6 lpm.
    B. non-rebreather mask at 15 lpm.
    C. positive pressure ventilations with BVM.
    D. blow-by oxygen.

116. To help reduce the anxiety of this patient, you should reassure him and place him in which position?
    A. position the patient is most comfortable
    B. left lateral recumbent (recovery position)
    C. Trendelenburg (shock position)

D. supine with legs bent at the knees

117. After assessing Big Joe, you consult medical direction and are instructed to administer nitroglycerin. A few minutes after administering nitroglycerin, Ingrid advises you that the blood pressure has dropped from 182/78 to 156/62 and the pulse rate has increased from 88 to 100 beats each minute. Your immediate actions should be:
    A. remove the tablet quickly because this patient is too sensitive to this drug.
    B. position the patient appropriately since these are early signs of anaphylaxis.
    C. reassure the patient, explaining these are common side effects of nitroglycerin.
    D. administer another nitroglycerin to stabilize the condition and increase the blood pressure.

118. In which of the following patients would the use of the AED be indicated?
    A. a 60-year-old medical patient who is in respiratory arrest only
    B. a 7-year-old cardiac arrest patient who weighs 15 kg
    C. a 90-year-old medical patient who is pulseless and breathless
    D. a 21-year-old head injured patient who is pulseless and breathless

119. The AED is not indicated for children under age:
    A. 12
    B. 10
    C. 9
    D. 8

120. In general, a patient suffering from a cardiac emergency will fall into one of two broad categories:
    A. unresponsive in cardiac arrest or responsive
    B. dead on scene or cardiac arrest
    C. cardiac arrest or unresponsive

D. immediate cardiac arrest or delayed cardiac arrest

C. agonal

D. pulseless electrical activity

121. Patients who complain of chest pain:
    A. require the application and use of the AED.
    B. require the AED only if in respiratory arrest.
    C. may deteriorate to cardiac arrest.
    D. will go into cardiac arrest within 1 hour.

122. The type of AED that provides complete operation by pushing a single "on" button is a:
    A. manual defibrillator.
    B. semimanual defibrillator.
    C. fully automated defibrillator.
    D. semi-automatic defibrillator.

123. The application of a shock to a patient **not** in cardiac arrest:
    A. will cause a dangerous disruption of the heart's conduction system.
    B. is not harmful to the patient because the energy used is minimal.
    C. will cause a dangerous increase in the patient's blood pressure.
    D. is not harmful to the patient because the heart is already damaged.

124. The AED is preferred over the use of a manual defibrillator for all of the following reasons **except:**
    A. a shock can be delivered within 1 minute of the AED attachment.
    B. a shock can be delivered quicker than a manual defibrillator.
    C. the AED delivers a less effective shock than the manual defibrillator.
    D. the AED is safer to use than a manual defibrillator.

125. The AED is indicated for which "pulseless" cardiac rhythm?
    A. asystole
    B. ventricular tachycardia

126. You are on-scene treating a cardiac arrest patient with the AED. Dispatch advises that ALS backup is not available. You should transport the patient when:
    A. a total of four shocks have been delivered.
    B. the AED has given one "No Shock" message.
    C. the AED has given three "No Shock" messages.
    D. a total of three shocks have been delivered.

127. Which of the following is **not** one of the four items associated with the American Heart Association's chain of survival?
    A. early access
    B. early medical control
    C. early defibrillation
    D. early CPR

128. Frequent practice with the AED is required to:
    A. meet local rules and operating regulations.
    B. meet federal training and recertification requirements.
    C. ensure the EMT-B can properly use the device.
    D. meet state training and recertification requirements.

129. Medical direction's involvement in an AED program may include all of the following **except:**
    A. ensuring the EMS system has all necessary AHA chain of survival links.
    B. engaging in an audit/quality improvement program.
    C. recommending alternative drug therapy in place of defibrillation.
    D. reviewing programs to ensure skill competency.

130. The EMS system's medical director should:

    A. review all incidents of AED use.

    B. not be involved in the operation of an AED program.

    C. be available by radio at all times for consultation.

    D. respond to the scene of all incidents when the AED is used.

131. Defibrillation is most successful for patients in cardiac arrest resulting from:

    A. stroke.

    B. hypoglycemia.

    C. a dysrhythmia associated with coronary artery disease.

    D. an auto accident involving head trauma and hypoventilation for the patient.

132. A 3-year-old child in cardiac arrest:

    A. requires immediate AED application.

    B. requires AED use only if in ventricular tachycardia.

    C. requires aggressive airway and ventilatory management.

    D. requires AED use if the cardiac arrest is due to trauma.

133. Nitroglycerin is contraindicated if the patient's blood pressure is less than:

    A. 80 mmHg diastolic.

    B. 90 mmHg systolic.

    C. 100 mmHg systolic.

    D. 100 mmHg diastolic.

134. Nitroglycerin could typically be repeated when the patient has taken:

    A. 2 doses without pain relief.

    B. 3 doses without pain relief.

    C. 4 doses without pain relief.

    D. 5 doses without pain relief.

135. A common side effect associated with nitroglycerin is:

    A. nausea.

    B. dyspnea.

    C. blurred vision.

    D. headache.

136. Select the statement that is true of the AED.

    A. It is easier to learn CPR than it is to learn how to operate an AED.

    B. AEDs are unable to detect loose leads and false or misleading rhythm readings.

    C. The semi-automatic AED requires no involvement by the operator.

    D. The American Heart Association has stated that both types of AEDs are equally effective.

137. Which of the following sign(s) of cardiac arrest must be present in order to attach the AED to the patient?

    A. no pulse and dilated pupils

    B. no respirations and no spontaneous movement

    C. unresponsive only

    D. no pulse, unresponsive, and no respirations

138. If after AED application and defibrillation the patient regains a pulse, and ALS backup is delayed you should:

    A. remain on-scene and await ALS.

    B. delay transport until the ALS is on the scene.

    C. delay transport until medical control advises otherwise.

    D. transport without delay.

139. You have responded to a call for a patient complaining of chest pain. You arrive on-scene and are evaluating a 65-year-old male patient who has complained of substernal chest pain for the last 10 minutes. The patient has a history of cardiac problems and is prescribed nitroglycerin. The patient is alert and oriented and states that he took 3 nitroglycerin tablets with no relief. The patient's blood

pressure is 124/90, the pulse is 90, and his skin is cool and clammy. The most appropriate treatment for this patient is to:

A. recheck the blood pressure and then administer up to 2 additional doses of nitroglycerin.

B. administer oxygen by non-rebreather and complete the initial assessment.

C. complete a detailed history and detailed physical exam.

D. administer 1 additional dose of nitro-glycerin.

140. The patient suddenly grabs his chest and closes his eyes. He is unresponsive to pain and verbal stimuli and is pulseless and breathless. You place the patient on the AED and analyze the rhythm. The AED advises "No Shock." You should next:

A. check the breathing.

B. resume CPR.

C. check the patient's pulse.

D. reanalyze the rhythm.

141. After your analysis of the rhythm the AED advises "Deliver Shock." It is important to:

A. check the patient's pulse before delivering the shock.

B. check with medical control before delivering the shock.

C. ensure that all personnel are clear of the patient.

D. ventilate twice before delivering the shock.

DIABETES/AMS 4.4

142. You arrive on-scene to find the apartment manager urging you to come inside. You survey the scene and find no immediate dangers so you proceed in. The manager tells you that he brought the patient his evening meal and found him on the floor unresponsive. You assess the patient, and your partner begins to

look around the apartment for any further clues. Your assessment reveals a male patient unresponsive to verbal stimuli, blood pressure 120/67, pulse rate 122, respiratory rate 18, and cool moist skin. Your partner comes back with a pill bottle of Micronase he found on the counter. From your assessment findings and the patient's medication, you suspect he is most likely suffering from:

A. a myocardial infarction.

B. a CVA.

C. hypoglycemia.

D. hyperglycemia.

143. Signs and symptoms of a patient with an altered mental status and a history of diabetes include:

A. rapid onset of an altered mental status.

B. tachycardia.

C. cool, moist skin.

D. all of the above.

144. In order to administer instant glucose, a patient must have:

A. an intact gag reflex and an ability to swallow.

B. a history of diabetic seizures.

C. a history of epilepsy controlled by medications.

D. an altered mental status with only a response to painful stimuli.

145. The proper administration of instant glucose includes:

A. allowing the patient to suck on the tube until the symptoms appear to resolve.

B. placing a pinch between the patient's cheek and gum every 3 to 5 minutes until the symptoms resolve.

C. placing the glucose on a tongue depressor, placing the depressor between the cheek and gum, and rubbing the area.

D. squirting approximately half the tube into the patient's mouth and allowing it to dissolve.

146. Your patient is suffering from an altered mental status. The patient has a history of diabetes that is controlled with medication. The patient, however, has snoring respirations and is responsive only to painful stimuli. You should:

    A. open the airway, place the patient on high-flow oxygen, and place a pinch of glucose between his cheek and gum.

    B. open the airway, place the patient on high-flow oxygen, place a small amount of glucose on a tongue depressor, and place it between the gum and cheek.

    C. open the patient's airway and transport rapidly.

    D. open the patient's airway, insert an airway adjunct, place the patient on high-flow oxygen, and continue your assessment.

147. A contraindication to the administration of oral glucose is:

    A. inability to swallow or unconsciousness.

    B. decreased level of consciousness.

    C. systolic BP less than 100 mmHg.

    D. headache and diaphoresis.

148. You are treating a patient who has an altered mental status, with a history of diabetes controlled by medication. Your priority in emergency medical care should be:

    A. provide positive pressure ventilation.

    B. administer oxygen by nasal cannula.

    C. establish and maintain an open airway.

    D. determine if the patient can swallow.

149. You are called to the scene for an altered mental status patient with a history of diabetes controlled by medication. When assessing the airway, you must also:

    A. perform a finger sweep of the mouth.

    B. place the patient in a Fowler position.

    C. determine if the patient can swallow.

    D. administer glucose per your protocol.

150. Your patient has a history of diabetes that is controlled by medication. The patient is unresponsive to verbal stimuli but responds to pain. Which of the following emergency care is most appropriate?

    A. initiate oxygen therapy, Trendelenburg position, administer oral glucose

    B. initiate oxygen therapy, administer oral glucose, position on his side

    C. maintain an open airway, administer oxygen by nasal cannula, Fowler position

    D. maintain open airway, administer high-flow oxygen, position on his side

151. Which of the following is the correct method to administer oral glucose to a patient with a history of diabetes controlled by medication?

    A. lift the tongue; squeeze a small amount under the tongue (sublingually)

    B. hold back the cheek; squeeze the oral glucose between the cheek and gum

    C. tip the patient's head backwards; squeeze a small amount into the mouth and ask the patient to swallow it

    D. place a small amount onto the tongue; ask the patient to swallow it at once

152. While you are administering oral glucose to an insulin dependent diabetic patient, the patient becomes unresponsive. You should immediately:

    A. reassess the patient's airway, breathing, and circulation status.

    B. place the patient in a semisitting position.

    C. try to remove the drug by gently scraping the cheek.

    D. administer an additional dose to quickly raise the blood glucose level.

153. A priority in managing the patient with an altered mental status is:

    A. the administration of oral glucose.

    B. maintenance of a patent airway.

C. obtaining an accurate and complete history.

D. completion of an early detailed physical exam.

154. Place the following treatment steps of the patient with an altered mental status in the most appropriate order.

   1. Administer oxygen
   2. Suction secretions
   3. Transport
   4. Position the patient
   A. 1,2,4,3
   B. 4,2,1,3
   C. 2,4,1,3
   D. 2,1,4,3

155. A patient who has an altered mental status still requires:

   A. a supine position with the feet elevated.
   B. hypoventilation at a rate of 8–12 per minute.
   C. an explanation of procedures performed.
   D. a lateral recumbent position with feet elevated.

156. When administering oral glucose, the EMT-B should:

   A. place ⅓ of the tube onto a tongue depressor and place between the cheek and gum.
   B. place ½ of the tube onto a tongue depressor and place between the cheek and gum.
   C. place ¾ of the tube onto a tongue depressor and place between the cheek and gum.
   D. place 1 full tube onto a tongue depressor and place between the cheek and gum.

STROKE

157. Signs of a stroke include:
   A. aphasia.

B. hemiplegia.

C. hemiparesis.

D. all of the above.

158. The difference between a stroke and a TIA (transient ischemic attack) is:

   A. a TIA usually only involves one side of the body while a CVA affects both sides.
   B. a stroke usually causes a TIA.
   C. the signs and symptoms of a TIA disappear within 24 hours and usually results in no permanent neurologic dysfunction.
   D. only patients suffering a stroke require transport and treatment.

159. You arrive on-scene and find your patient sitting on the porch. Upon assessment, you find the patient is unable to move his right arm and has decreased sensation in his right leg. The patient's vital signs are blood pressure 193/110, pulse 112, and respiration 22. Your treatment should include all of the following **except:**

   A. providing oxygen at 15 lpm.
   B. protecting the afflicted extremities from any injury.
   C. having the patient ambulate to regain sensation in his leg.
   D. rapidly transporting the patient to the nearest appropriate facility.

160. You arrive on-scene and find your patient supine on the floor. The patient's wife tells you that he just got back from running and complained of "the worst headache of my life" and then fell to the ground. You suspect what type of injury?

   A. myocardial infarction
   B. hemorrhagic stroke
   C. occlusive stroke
   D. TIA

161. A cerebral embolism could originate from:
    A. clotted blood from the inferior vena cava.
    B. fat particles from the left side of the heart.
    C. tumor fragments from the right ventricle.
    D. thrombophlebitis from deep vein thrombosis.

162. Which of the following may be a late sign or symptom of a stroke?
    A. unequal pupils
    B. headache
    C. seizures
    D. stiff neck

163. All of the following are signs or symptoms of neurologic deficit resulting from a stroke **except:**
    A. loss of bowel and bladder control.
    B. hemiplegia.
    C. severe intermittent abdominal pain.
    D. unequal pupils with loss of vision in one eye.

164. Your patient awoke this morning and felt dizzy. The patient also experienced nausea with vomiting. You note incomprehensible speech and unequal pupils. You suspect:
    A. myocardial infarction.
    B. stroke.
    C. hypoglycemia.
    D. traumatic brain injury.

ALLERGIES 4.5

165. All the following are signs and symptoms of an allergic reaction **except:**
    A. warm, tingling feeling in the face, mouth, feet, and tongue.
    B. decreased heart rate.
    C. tightness in the throat and/or the chest.
    D. urticaria and pruritis.

166. During an allergic reaction, which of the following is (are) effects on the respiratory system?
    A. swelling at the level of the larynx, causing airway compromise
    B. spasms of the bronchi, causing wheezing
    C. significant swelling of the tongue, causing airway compromise
    D. all of the above

167. Your patient was stung by a yellow jacket and now is complaining of difficulty swallowing, shortness of breath, and tightness in the chest. Your primary concern in this patient is to:
    A. provide aggressive airway management with positive ventilation if necessary.
    B. place him or her in a left lateral recumbent position.
    C. activate ALS due to rapid respiratory deterioration.
    D. apply the AED for impending cardiac arrest.

168. Your patient states she is "deathly" allergic to peanuts and she just ate a pie cooked with peanut oil. She appears to be itching all over and has watery eyes and hives on her arms. The patient has no other complaints. You would classify this as a _____ and treat it by _____.
    A. severe reaction, immediately administering epinephrine
    B. mild reaction, positive pressure ventilation and endotracheal intubation
    C. mild reaction, providing reassurance and supplemental oxygen
    D. severe reaction, providing reassurance and supplemental oxygen

169. It is important to treat all possible cases of allergic reactions as serious because:
    A. a mild reaction can rapidly progress to severe anaphylaxis.

B. infection from the stinger can cause loss of an extremity.

C. allergic reactions can mimic other more serious medical emergencies.

D. the patient may develop urticaria and pruritis.

170. A sign of anaphylactic shock that would require epinephrine administration is:

A. hypotension.

B. tachycardia.

C. hives.

D. flushed skin.

171. A sign of anaphylaxis is:

A. increased systolic blood pressure.

B. nasal flaring and tachypnea.

C. weakness to one side of the body.

D. all of the above.

172. Your patient took a new medication today and began experiencing difficulty breathing. When you arrive on-scene you hear a high-pitched sound as she breathes. This sound is indicative of:

A. lower bronchial obstruction.

B. main stem bronchi obstruction.

C. laryngeal swelling.

D. fluid in the alveoli.

173. When managing the patient with an allergic reaction, it is important to constantly reassess:

A. inspiratory rales.

B. hives.

C. itching.

D. stridorous respirations.

174. Epinephrine by auto-injector:

A. is carried on all EMS units.

B. is a sublingual injection.

C. does not require an order to administer it.

D. is prescribed to the patient.

175. You arrive on the scene and find a patient who states he is allergic to shellfish. He has hives, itching, and slightly flushed skin. His BP is 128/78, HR is 102, and RR is 18. Which of the following treatments would be inappropriate?

A. epinephrine administration by auto-injector into the thigh

B. high-flow oxygen by non-rebreather mask set at 15 lpm

C. positioning the patient in the position most comfortable for him or her

D. transporting early and providing treatment while en route to the hospital

176. You suspect your patient is suffering from an anaphylactic reaction and the airway is compromised by a swollen larynx. The most effective method of managing this obstruction is:

A. providing positive pressure ventilation.

B. positioning the patient's head.

C. inserting an oropharyngeal airway.

D. suctioning the upper airway often.

177. Which of the following is the correct administration procedure for a prescribed epinephrine auto-injector?

A. Push the auto-injector firmly against the patient's upper hip between the thigh and the lower back; hold in place for one second.

B. Push the auto-injector firmly against the patient's upper arm between the elbow and the shoulder; hold in place until half the vial is delivered.

C. Push the auto-injector firmly against the patient's thigh midway between the waist and the knee; hold in place until all the medication is delivered.

D. Push the auto-injector firmly against the patient's lower leg midway between the knee and the ankle; hold in place until all the medication is delivered.

178. You have administered epinephrine to an anaphylactic patient. She complains of a headache, dizziness, chest pain, and increased heart rate. These signs are indicative of:
    A. incorrect administration.
    B. overdose of epinephrine.
    C. side effects of epinephrine.
    D. allergic reaction to the drug.

179. Which of the following is a contraindication of epinephrine administration in anaphylaxis?
    A. there are no contraindications in anaphylaxis
    B. elderly patient
    C. infants and children
    D. stridorous respiration

POISONING/OVERDOSE 4.6

180. All of the following may be signs and symptoms of a poisoning **except:**
    A. severe headache.
    B. unequal pupils.
    C. slow heart rate.
    D. abdominal pain.

181. Your first priority in providing emergency medical care to a patient who has overdosed on an unknown medication is:
    A. administering activated charcoal.
    B. identifying the medication taken.
    C. administering high-flow oxygen.
    D. maintaining a patent airway.

182. While you are transporting a patient who has overdosed on sleeping pills, the respiratory rate decreases from 20 to 8 times a minute. Your immediate action should be to:
    A. administer activated charcoal.
    B. provide positive pressure ventilation.
    C. administer oxygen by non-rebreather mask.
    D. position the patient in the Trendelenburg position.

183. In which of the following poisoned patients is activated charcoal indicated?
    A. 8-year-old who mistakenly drank liquid bleach less than 1 hour ago
    B. 38-year-old who has inhaled carbon monoxide 3 hours ago
    C. 60-year-old who has overdosed on blood pressure pills 2 hours ago
    D. 3-year-old who has ingested liquid ammonia less than 10 minutes ago

184. Activated charcoal:
    A. increases urinary output, which forcefully eliminates the poison.
    B. speeds absorption into the body where it is eliminated quickly.
    C. adsorbs the contaminant, inhibiting absorption into the body.
    D. actively neutralizes most poisons, rendering them harmless.

185. Poisons may enter the body by:
    A. ingestion.
    B. inhalation.
    C. injection.
    D. all of the above.

186. You are assisting a patient who is having chest pain with sublingual administration of nitroglycerin. What route does the medication enter the body?
    A. inhalation
    B. ingestion
    C. absorption
    D. injection

187. A patient is suffering an anaphylactic reaction from a yellow jacket bite. What route did the venom enter the patient's body?
    A. absorption
    B. injection
    C. inhalation
    D. ingestion

188. Emergency care for a dry powder absorption poison would include:
   A. covering the patient's arm with a burn sheet to preserve the powder for the emergency room.
   B. immediately washing the powder off to prevent further exposure.
   C. brushing the powder off before irrigating the contaminated area.
   D. flushing the area with water and then brushing the area dry.

189. You are called to the scene for a possible chlorine leak. As you pull up to the scene you see two victims lying on the ground by a tool shed. Your immediate action(s) include:
   A. removing the victims from the scene to prevent further injury.
   B. immediately providing positive pressure ventilation to the victims to prevent further hypoxia.
   C. rapidly extricating the patients from the chlorine gas.
   D. moving to a safe environment uphill and upwind and contacting the fire department.

190. What position should you place the medical patient in to prevent aspiration?
   A. prone
   B. lateral recumbent
   C. Fowler's
   D. supine

191. In cases of poisoning, your best resource for information regarding treatment of the patient is:
   A. the patient's family physician.
   B. drug/chemical information booklet.
   C. local poison control center.
   D. handheld drug reference.

192. Any patient with a poisoning/overdose should be transported to be seen by a physician because:

   A. the effects of the poison may take minutes to hours to days to become evident.
   B. poisons can aggravate underlying medical conditions.
   C. usually the exact poison, amount, time frame taken over, and effect cannot be determined.
   D. all of the above.

193. Your patient has swallowed industrial drain cleaner in a possible suicide attempt. She responds only to deep painful stimuli. Your treatment for this patient would include all of the following **except:**
   A. maintaining a patent airway.
   B. flushing the mouth to remove any cleaner to prevent further contamination.
   C. providing supplemental oxygen and possibly positive pressure ventilation.
   D. inserting a nasal pharyngeal airway.

194. Which of the following is not always part of the treatment of an overdose patient?
   A. airway control management
   B. administration of activated charcoal
   C. reassessment of the airway and ventilation
   D. administration of oxygen

195. All of the following are trade names for activated charcoal **except:**
   A. CharMed.
   B. InstaChar.
   C. Actidose.
   D. Liqui-Char.

196. Activated charcoal is only indicated for poisoning that occurs by:
   A. ingestion.
   B. injection.
   C. absorption.
   D. inhalation.

197. Which is **not** a contraindication for the use of activated charcoal?
    A. The patient is unable to swallow.
    B. The patient has ingested ammonia.
    C. The patient is fully alert.
    D. The patient has ingested bleach.

198. Activated charcoal's medication form is:
    A. a fine powder for inhalation.
    B. a powder pre-mixed in water.
    C. a solid that is ingested.
    D. a liquid for injection.

199. The dose for activated charcoal is usually:
    A. 1 gram per kilogram of body weight.
    B. 5 milligrams per kilogram of body weight.
    C. 1 milligram per kilogram of body weight.
    D. 5 grams per kilogram of body weight.

200. When administering activated charcoal, the EMT-B should:
    A. avoid shaking the contents.
    B. notify medical control if the patient vomits.
    C. administer it prior to receiving an on- or off-line medical control.
    D. have the patient drink it from the bottle.

201. Activated charcoal acts by:
    A. binding to poisons while in the stomach.
    B. flushing the poison from the circulatory system.
    C. moving the substance quickly through the intestines.
    D. increasing the absorption in the small intestine.

202. The most common side effect of activated charcoal is:
    A. an increase in the blood pressure.
    B. a decrease in the blood pressure.
    C. blackened stool.
    D. rectal bleeding.

203. Why is it necessary to contact medical control early in the management of the overdosed or poisoned patient?
    A. It is necessary to provide quality assurance information.
    B. It is necessary to control medical liability costs.
    C. It is required by most state laws.
    D. It is necessary in order to obtain the most current treatment orders.

204. Which of the following does not indicate an emergency that is due to drug or alcohol?
    A. empty liquor bottles
    B. hospital discharge orders
    C. digital clubbing
    D. prescription bottles

205. The "Talk-Down Technique" for managing a violent drug or alcohol patient is not useful for patients who have taken:
    A. phencyclidine.
    B. cocaine.
    C. crack.
    D. marijuana.

ENVIRONMENTAL 4.7

206. What is the most significant mechanism of heat loss (approximately 60%) that involves the transfer of heat from the surface of one object to another without physical contact?
    A. convection
    B. conduction
    C. evaporation
    D. radiation

207. Taking into consideration the process of conduction and water chill, how much faster than any other mechanism will wet clothing conduct heat away from the body?
    A. 100 times faster
    B. 200 times faster
    C. 240 times faster
    D. 275 times faster

208. All of the following are early signs of hypothermia **except:**
    A. muscle stiffness.
    B. slow heart rate.
    C. uncoordination.
    D. rapid heart rate.

209. When a patient is surrounded by water that has the same temperature as that of the ambient air:
    A. the core temperature will drop 25 to 30 times faster in the water than in the ambient air.
    B. the core temperature will stay the same as the temperature of the ambient air regardless of the temperature of the water.
    C. the core temperature will drop 100 times faster in the water than in the ambient air.
    D. the core temperature will not drop as fast because the water will act as an insulator of body heat.

210. Characteristics that predispose the elderly to heat emergencies include:
    A. poor thermoregulation.
    B. the tendency for the elderly to retire to communities in hotter climates.
    C. poor fluid intake and hydration status.
    D. all of the above.

211. Treatment for a patient suffering from a heat emergency with hot dry skin includes all of the following **except:**
    A. removing the patient from the hot environment.
    B. cooling the patient with cool water, ice packs, and fans.
    C. administration of high-flow oxygen.
    D. covering the patient with blankets to prevent too rapid of cooling.

212. It is late September and you are called to the scene of a popular teenage beach. Your 16-year-old patient had attempted to swim out to the deep water buoy in rough tides. The lifeguards rescued the boy after he had been "under" for approximately 10 minutes. The patient only responds to deep painful stimuli. All of the following would be likely causes of the patient's condition **except:**
    A. myocardial infarction from exertion.
    B. possible hypothermia from cold water temperatures.
    C. decreased level of consciousness from anoxia.
    D. pulmonary edema and pneumonia resulting from possible salt water aspiration.

213. The call comes in as a drowning at the local beach. Bystanders pulled a young man from the water who is now sitting on the beach coughing up small amounts of water. He states that he does not believe he needs to go to the hospital because he only swallowed a small amount of water. What should you do?
    A. Agree with the patient because a small amount of water is not harmful.
    B. Explain to the patient that if he wants to he can go to the hospital in his friend's car.
    C. Explain to the patient the implications involved with a near drowning and attempt to convince the patient to allow you to transport him to be evaluated in the emergency department.
    D. Have him make an appointment to see his family physician the next day after the incident.

214. Infants and young children lose heat quicker than adults because:
    A. they are smaller in size with a larger surface area.
    B. they can not protect themselves from temperature changes by putting on or taking off their clothes.
    C. they usually have less body fat proportionately than adults.
    D. all of the above.

215. Which of the following is an appropriate treatment for the patient with generalized hypothermia?
    A. Transfer, move, or handle the patient as you would any other patient.
    B. Provide only one set of three defibrillations if the patient is in cardiac arrest.
    C. Rub or massage the patient's arms or legs.
    D. Hyperventilate the patient at a rate of 24 per minute.

216. When managing a hypothermic patient, you can not detect a pulse or respiration, but the patient moves; you should:
    A. start CPR immediately.
    B. start CPR and apply the AED immediately.
    C. begin positive pressure ventilation.
    D. apply the AED to determine the patient's rhythm.

217. When actively rewarming the hypothermic patient, the patient's temperature should not be increased by more than _____ degree(s) F per hour.
    A. $\frac{1}{2}$
    B. 1
    C. 2
    D. 3

218. Which of the following is appropriate management for a patient with immersion hypothermia?
    A. Instruct the patient to swim and tread water as vigorously as possible.
    B. Lift the patient from the water in a horizontal position.
    C. Lift the patient from the water in a vertical position.
    D. Leave the wet clothing on the patient to insulate him or her from heat loss upon removal from the water.

219. Appropriate emergency management of a localized cold injury includes:
    A. massaging the affected skin.
    B. removing jewelry.
    C. applying of a salve or ointment to open wounds.
    D. breaking blisters that are present on the surface of the skin.

220. Rewarming of localized frozen tissue:
    A. is safe to perform on all patients.
    B. can be safely performed by using dry heat.
    C. requires water of 120 to 130 degrees F.
    D. is extremely painful for the patient.

221. Which of the following treatments for bites and stings is appropriate?
    A. Remove the stinger using tweezers or your fingers.
    B. Elevate the injection site above the level of the heart.
    C. Wash the area around the bite or sting site with soap.
    D. Apply a hot pack to the injection site to relieve swelling.

222. It is mid-summer and you have been dispatched to a local park for a man down. You arrive and observe a workman who appears to be in his 40s lying supine. He is in the full sun and is next to a ditch. A co-worker informs you that the patient was digging the ditch and just passed out. The patient's eyes are closed and he does not respond to your voice or painful stimuli. His respirations are deep and rapid. His pulse is 110 per minute, regular, and strong. His skin is hot and slightly moist. The co-worker further informs you that the patient had complained of a headache and nausea for at least 30 minutes prior to passing out. Which action should be taken first?
    A. Administer oxygen at 15 lpm.
    B. Apply cold packs to the patient's body.

C. Remove the patient's clothing.

D. Move the patient to a cooler environment.

223. The patient in #222 would be considered:

A. a high priority transport.

B. a medium priority transport.

C. a low priority transport.

D. a patient not requiring transport.

224. The patient in #222 is most likely suffering from a _____. This is common on days in which the temperature is greater than _____ degrees F with a relative humidity greater than _____ %.

A. vascular accident, 80, 90

B. heat seizure, 80, 65

C. heat emergency, 80, 65

D. heat emergency, 90, 75

225. Which of the following is **not** a predisposing factor that increases the risk of hypothermia?

A. alcohol use

B. family history

C. medical conditions

D. patient's age

226. The first compensatory mechanism the body uses to try to maintain body temperature is:

A. increased heart rate.

B. increased respirations.

C. shivering and goose bumps.

D. increased fine motor function.

227. You are treating a responsive patient who is experiencing a heat emergency. The patient's skin is moist, pale and cool. Which treatment is **incorrect** for this patient?

A. Have the patient drink cool water if not nauseated.

B. Place the patient in a Fowler's position.

C. Cool the patient with wet compresses.

D. Administer oxygen by non-rebreather mask at 15 lpm.

228. You are assessing a responsive patient who has been bitten by a rattlesnake. Which treatment would be **inappropriate?**

A. Apply cold packs to the injection site.

B. Lower the injection site below the level of the heart.

C. Wash the area around the injection site.

D. Apply a constricting band above the injection site.

229. How should a stinger be removed?

A. Remove the stinger by squeezing it with a pair of tweezers.

B. Remove the stinger by scraping an edge of a knife against it.

C. Remove the stinger by compressing it between your fingers.

D. Do not remove the stinger because increased tissue damage may result.

SCENARIO

Questions 230–232 refer to the following scenario:

You and your partner Ashley are restocking the ambulance after a serious automobile accident on I 95. The station alerting system sounds, "Medic one respond to an allergic reaction at 1729 17th Avenue. Time out 13:52." As you approach the scene you are met at the street by a frantic husband who states, "It's my wife; she was stung by a bee and now she can't breathe." You and Ashley enter the house and find a 36-year-old female sitting on a kitchen chair. She is in a tripod position and looks at you and Ashley with fright-filled eyes. She is breathing approximately 40 times a minute. Ashley states she can hear audible wheezes; the skin is flushed and dry with urticaria (hives) covering the chest and back. The patient begins to slump over the chair. Her pulse rate is 134 beats per minute.

230. From the information provided, select the most appropriate immediate treatment for this patient:
    A. Place a constricting band above injection site.
    B. Immediately wash the injection site.
    C. Provide positive pressure ventilation.
    D. Administer oxygen by non-rebreather mask.

231. The patient's husband locates and gives you the patient's epinephrine auto-injector. You should do which of the following next?
    A. Obtain an order from medical direction to administer the patient's prescribed epinephrine by auto-injector.
    B. In this situation, there is no need to administer the epinephrine auto-injector.
    C. This patient is not having an anaphylactic reaction and should not receive epinephrine by auto-injector.
    D. Administer epinephrine by auto-injector after you have applied constricting bands below the injection site.

232. After you have administered epinephrine by auto-injector, the patient becomes very pale and the heart rate increases to 150 per minute. The patient becomes very anxious and states she feels as if she is going to vomit. The signs and symptoms indicate:
    A. an epinephrine overdose.
    B. a common side effect of epinephrine.
    C. the patient's condition is worsening.
    D. incorrect administration of epinephrine.

BEHAVIORAL 4.8

233. The manner in which a person acts including any and all physical and mental activity is a definition of:
    A. anxiety.
    B. behavior.
    C. depression.
    D. morals and ethics.

234. A behavioral emergency is best defined as:
    A. behavior that is unethical.
    B. behavior that does not represent what the prudent person would do in certain situations.
    C. behavior that is "abnormal" in the given situation and intolerable to the patient, community, or family.
    D. any situation that requires a psychiatrist consultation.

235. A patient thought to be suffering from a behavioral emergency might be actually suffering from:
    A. hypoglycemia.
    B. hypoxia.
    C. head injury.
    D. all of the above.

236. You are called to the scene for a patient who was struck by an automobile. There are no witnesses and the driver states that the patient came out of nowhere. En route to the hospital the patient states that all he wanted to do was to die. Your reaction to this comment should be to:
    A. assume the patient has suffered severe head trauma and is incoherent.
    B. assume the patient is intoxicated and doesn't know what he is saying.
    C. pay no attention to the remark because the patient may be delirious from the accident or suffering a head injury.
    D. report the statement to the nurse and physician as the accident may have been a suicide attempt.

237. Risk factors that are suggestive of suicidal tendencies include:
    A. recent marriage.
    B. ages of 17 through 30.
    C. loss of a significant loved one.
    D. recent promotion with additional stress.

238. What percentage of patients that have succeeded in committing suicide have made previous attempts?
   A. approximately 90%
   B. approximately 80%
   C. approximately 50%
   D. approximately 40%

239. During the assessment of a despondent patient, you notice multiple cuts on the victim's wrists and arms. You should be concerned that the patient:
   A. may have been involved in a fight.
   B. may have been tied up for a period of time.
   C. may have attempted suicide.
   D. is an IV drug user and possibly HIV positive.

240. When you are determining suicidal tendencies, the patient with a realistic and concrete plan is (as) _____ determined to commit suicide than (as) the person who has no plan or one that is vague.
   A. less
   B. more
   C. equally
   D. Neither is determined to commit suicide.

241. When a patient tells you that he or she has thought of harming himself or herself with a gun you should:
   A. do nothing because this is just a way to gain attention.
   B. make sure that the patient is not armed and is of no danger to you.
   C. ask the patient to show you the gun as this will prove his or her intentions.
   D. attempt to console the patient and find out why the patient wants to hurt himself or herself.

242. You are called to a private residence for an unknown emergency. You walk into the residence and find an elderly man sitting among bottles of whiskey, crying over a picture. You observe a pistol in the patient's waistband. Your first action should be to:
   A. ask the patient why he is so sad.
   B. determine if the patient wants to kill himself.
   C. slowly and calmly back out of the room.
   D. charge the patient and pin him down.

243. In #242 all of the following are risk factors of suicide **except:**
   A. the patient sitting amongst whiskey bottles, possibly indicating a substance abuse problem.
   B. the patient's age. Older individuals usually are more mature and less likely to commit suicide.
   C. the patient's sex. Males are more likely to commit suicide than are females.
   D. the patient's firearm.

244. When assessing a patient who you believe is a risk for violence, you should:
   A. assess the patient with adequate help to restrain the patient if he or she becomes violent.
   B. make sure that all potential weapons or unsafe objects are outside of his or her reach.
   C. ask the patient if he or she wants to kill himself or herself.
   D. all of the above.

245. If you suspect that your patient is a suicide risk and does not want to go to the hospital, the EMT-B should do all the following **except:**
   A. call medical control and ask for permission to restrain the patient.
   B. have the patient wait alone in the bedroom while you call the patient's doctor.
   C. contact dispatch for additional helpers for the situation if restraint is necessary.
   D. request the police department if medical control orders you to transport.

246. Which of the following factors show a strong correlation with attempted suicide?
    A. male patient in his mid 20s
    B. arrest or imprisonment even for minor offenses
    C. recent marriage
    D. promotion in current job

247. Which of the following can cause a patient to exhibit signs of aggression?
    A. fear
    B. anxiety
    C. hypoglycemia
    D. all of the above

248. When asking a patient about suicidal intentions, you should do all of the following **except:**
    A. remain nonjudgmental.
    B. explain to the patient that his or her thoughts are irrational.
    C. ask the patient if he or she wants to kill himself or herself.
    D. be honest at all times.

249. You have restrained a patient who was exhibiting violent behavior toward his family. While en route to the hospital, the patient calms down and wants the restraints removed. The EMT-B should:
    A. remove the restraints if the patient states he is no longer violent.
    B. not remove the restraints for the EMT-B's safety.
    C. remove the leg restraints only and see how the patient responds.
    D. remove the wrist restraints only for a short time and monitor the patient's behavior.

ABDOMINAL PAIN

250. Which of the following patients complaining of abdominal pain would concern you the most? The one who:

    A. walks out to the ambulance informing you he has the worst "belly ache."
    B. is sitting upright in a chair, moaning in pain, and drinking antacid.
    C. is rolling about on the floor complaining of pain.
    D. is lying on the floor very still and quiet with his or her knees drawn up to his or her chest.

251. Organs of the right upper quadrant include:
    A. pancreas, spleen, and part of the liver.
    B. most of the liver, gallbladder, and part of the large intestine.
    C. small intestine, stomach, and spleen.
    D. most of the liver, spleen, and gallbladder.

252. Your patient was diagnosed with cholecystitis (gallbladder attack) 3 days ago. The patient now presents with nausea and vomiting and pain in the right shoulder. The pain in the shoulder can be classified as:
    A. referred pain.
    B. visceral pain.
    C. pancreatic pain.
    D. somatic pain.

253. You arrive on-scene to find an approximately 60-year-old male patient writhing on the floor. The patient is complaining of a tearing pain radiating to his lower back; the patient has absent femoral pulses and has a pulsatile mass just superior to his umbilicus. You suspect which of the following?
    A. myocardial infarction
    B. abdominal aortic aneurysm
    C. acute pancreatitis
    D. ruptured appendix

254. You are called to a residential neighborhood at 12:30 A.M. Your patient has just finished eating a super sized meal of deep fried fish. The patient now is complaining of a "crampy" pain in the RUQ and has had two episodes of nausea and vomiting with a

green emesis. You suspect that your patient is suffering from:

A. a peptic ulcer.

B. an intestinal obstruction.

C. cholecystitis.

D. appendicitis.

255. Pain that is felt in a body part removed from its point of origin is called:

A. epigastric pain.

B. abdominal pain.

C. retroperitenal pain.

D. referred pain.

256. Which of the following is **not** a probable cause of abdominal pain?

A. esophageal varices

B. intestinal obstruction

C. enccphalitis

D. appendicitis

257. You are treating a patient for severe acute abdominal pain. The patient presents with signs of hypoperfusion. In which position should you place this patient?

A. left lateral (recovery)

B. sitting with feet extended

C. supine with feet elevated

D. position of most comfort

258. You are treating a patient with an acute abdomen without signs of shock. The patient should be placed in which position?

A. supine with feet elevated

B. position of most comfort

C. left lateral recumbent

D. semi-Fowler with knees bent

259. Which of the following is **inappropriate** for the patient being treated for an acute abdomen?

A. performing an ongoing assessment every 5 minutes for unstable patients

B. administering sips of water to the thirsty patient

C. administering high-flow oxygen at 15 lpm via a non-rebreather mask

D. positioning the hypoperfusion patient in a supine position with feet elevated

OB-GYN 4.9

260. In a normal pregnancy which female reproductive organ houses the developing fetus until the child is born?

A. cervix

B. placenta

C. uterus

D. fallopian tubes

261. This is the sole organ through which the fetus receives oxygen and nourishmcnt, and discharges carbon dioxide and other waste products.

A. amniotic sac

B. placenta

C. cervix

D. fallopian tubes

262. You arrive at the local doctor's office and find your patient lying on the bed, moaning in pain. The nurse tells you that the patient is 9 months pregnant and that she is having contractions 2 minutes apart and lasting 45 seconds. The nurse adds that the patient has the need to move her bowels. As your partner prepares the OB kit, your next immediate action should be to:

A. prepare to transport because her labor may last for hours.

B. examine her vaginal area for crowning.

C. place the patient on the cot and transport rapidly.

D. place the patient's legs together to delay the delivery.

263. Approximately how far from the infant's abdomen should the first clamp be placed on the umbilical cord?
    A. 12 inches
    B. 10 inches
    C. 6 inches
    D. 2 inches

264. What are the minimum requirements for body substance isolation when you are preparing to perform a delivery?
    A. gloves, eye protection, and head nets
    B. mask, gloves, and foot protectors
    C. gown, gloves, and mask
    D. mask, gown, gloves, and eye protection

265. Approximately how far from the first cord clamp should the second cord clamp be placed on the umbilical cord?
    A. 1 inch
    B. 3 inches
    C. 6 inches
    D. 10 inches

266. The treatment sequence for neonatal resuscitation is:
    A. position, warm, dry, suction, tactile stimuli, oxygen, BVM, chest compressions.
    B. dry, warm, position, stimulate, suction, oxygen, BVM, chest compressions.
    C. dry, warm, position, suction, stimulate, oxygen, chest compressions, BVM.
    D. dry, warm, position, suction, stimulate, oxygen, BVM, chest compressions.

267. What are the indications for chest compressions in the neonate?
    A. when the blood pressure drops below 90 mmHg
    B. when the patient's pulse drops below 130 bpm for over 1 minute
    C. when the heart rate despite ventilation is below 60 bpm
    D. when the heart rate falls below 100 bpm

268. A foul smelling, greenish brown thick viscous fluid that may be present in the amniotic fluid is:
    A. afterbirth.
    B. meconium.
    C. dried blood.
    D. the bloody show.

269. Meconium is an indication of:
    A. precipitative delivery.
    B. poor prenatal care.
    C. fetal distress.
    D. congenital deformities.

270. When you suspect meconium in the amniotic sac or in the infant's airway, you should:
    A. stimulate the infant immediately to allow full expansion of the infant's lungs to prevent fetal hypoxia.
    B. immediately warm and stimulate the patient because the meconium can depress the infant's ability to warm itself.
    C. help stimulate the baby's cough reflex to allow removal of the meconium from the lungs.
    D. immediately suction the airway first before any other treatment including stimulation.

271. When the head of the newborn is delivered, the EMT-B should gently place a gloved hand over the head to prevent an explosive delivery during a forceful contraction and tearing the perineum. The perineum is the:
    A. area between the vagina and the anus.
    B. organ that the umbilical cord is attached to.
    C. opening of the uterus.
    D. lateral aspects of the vagina.

272. You are delivering a baby and notice a thick viscous fluid all over the baby and a foul

smell. Your immediate reaction and treatment should be to:

A. finish the delivery and activate ALS immediately.

B. begin to suction the baby's mouth and nose immediately.

C. wait for the placenta to deliver before you begin cleaning the baby off.

D. do nothing as this is a normal event.

273. You just delivered a baby who required positive pressure ventilation. You assess the baby and determine that the infant's heart rate is 138/minute, respirations are 38/minute and full volume, and the skin is pink. You should:

A. stop PPV immediately so the infant does not become dependent on your assistance.

B. gradually decrease rate and volume of each ventilation until the infant takes over.

C. hyperventilate the patient for 1 full minute before ceasing ventilations.

D. stop ventilating, and reassess the ventilation status and heart rate in 1 minute.

274. What is the compression to ventilation ratio for infant CPR?

A. 120 compressions to 30 ventilations per minute

B. 30 compressions to 90 ventilations per minute

C. 100 compressions to 30 ventilations per minute

D. 90 compressions to 30 ventilations per minute

275. The correct depth for chest compressions in a newborn is:

A. ½ the depth of the chest.

B. ¼ to ¾ inches in depth.

C. ¼ to ½ inches in depth.

D. ⅓ the depth of the chest.

276. You begin to assist ventilations in a newborn. How often should you reassess your treatment and the patient's response?

A. every 30 seconds

B. every minute

C. every 2 minutes

D. every 3–5 minutes

277. The condition that may result when the combined weight of the enlarged uterus and fetus reduces the blood return to the heart while the patient is lying on her back is called:

A. gravid uterus syndrome.

B. hypertensive uterine syndrome.

C. fatal hypoperfusion syndrome.

D. supine hypotensive syndrome.

278. Vaginal bleeding should be managed by:

A. placing the patient in a Fowler's position.

B. placing a pad over the vaginal opening.

C. packing pads into the vagina to control excessive blood loss.

D. placing additional pads on top of blood soaked pads.

279. Delivery of the fetus before it is viable is termed:

A. placenta previa.

B. abruptio placenta.

C. breech presentation.

D. spontaneous abortion.

280. When managing a normal delivery:

A. put on eye protection only when preparing to deliver.

B. hold the mother's legs together to prevent an explosive delivery.

C. always take the maximum BSI precautions.

D. it is acceptable to allow the mother to use the bathroom when she has the urge to defecate.

281. Recommended equipment for a sterile obstetric kit includes all of the following **except:**
    A. bulb syringe.
    B. sanitary napkins.
    C. bag-valve-mask.
    D. cord clamps.

282. As soon as the head is delivered:
    A. quickly provide aggressive uterine massage.
    B. suction the mouth first and then the nose.
    C. begin bag-valve-mask ventilation.
    D. suction the nose first and then the mouth.

283. During delivery of the infant's head, excessive pressure should be:
    A. utilized to remove the cord from around the infant's neck.
    B. used to puncture the amniotic sack.
    C. used over the perineum to reduce the risk of tears.
    D. avoided over the fontanel area of the head.

284. Following delivery of the infant's head, the EMT-B should immediately:
    A. create a sterile field around the vaginal opening.
    B. determine if the umbilical cord is around the neck of the baby.
    C. record the time of delivery on the medical report.
    D. deeply suction the back of the infant's mouth.

285. Up to _____ cc's of blood loss is normal during childbirth and typically well tolerated by the mother.
    A. 100
    B. 300
    C. 500
    D. 700

286. Uterine massage is performed to:
    A. increase the uterus size by smooth muscle relaxation.
    B. stimulate milk production.
    C. reduce uterine contractions.
    D. contract the uterine smooth muscle.

287. In a multiple birth (twins, triplets):
    A. each infant always has its own placenta.
    B. each infant always shares a placenta.
    C. infants may have their own placenta or share one.
    D. the placenta is abnormally large.

288. In multiple births about _____ of the deliveries of the second infant will be breech.
    A. ½
    B. ⅕
    C. ¾
    D. ⅓

289. Place in the correct sequence the following steps for treatment of the patient with an injury to the external female genitalia.
    1. ensure airway, breathing, and circulation
    2. provide transportation
    3. care for bleeding from the vagina
    4. administer oxygen

    A. 1, 3, 4, 2
    B. 3, 1, 4, 2
    C. 1, 4, 3, 2
    D. 4, 1, 3, 2

290. You have responded to a vehicle accident. Upon arrival you observe a pregnant patient who is the unrestrained driver of the vehicle. She was involved in a low speed accident in a parking lot at the grocery store. She tells you that she struck the back end of a car while traveling about 15 miles per hour. She is about a week from her due date. The patient refuses transport. When assessing her for evidence of bleeding from trauma, you should:
    A. expect the blood pressure to fall quickly.

B. not bother checking peripheral perfusion.

C. realize that signs of shock may be subtle and the patient can deteriorate quickly.

D. rely on the blood pressure as the best evidence of blood loss.

291. The patient in #290 begins complaining of lower abdominal pain. Which of the following questions would be **least** important when obtaining a history of the present illness from this patient?

A. How intense is the pain?

B. What is the quality of the pain?

C. Is the pain constant?

D. Do you take any over-the-counter medications?

292. The third trimester pregnant patient complains of intermittent abdominal pain that occurs about every 2 minutes and that last for about a minute. The patient's abdomen is very rigid on palpation. The patient tells you that she needs to use the bathroom. The EMT-B should:

A. allow the patient to use the bathroom.

B. rapidly transport; early signs of shock are present.

C. evaluate the patient for signs of crowning.

D. perform a rapid episiotomy.

293. Your initial suctioning of a newborn's mouth and nose with a bulb syringe should be performed:

A. immediately following the cutting of the umbilical cord.

B. as soon as the entire delivery of the infant is completed.

C. as soon as the head is delivered.

D. directly after the torso is delivered.

294. When initially removing fluids from a newborn's airway during the birth process, you should:

A. place the bulb syringe into position and then compress the bulb.

B. suction the mouth first and then suction the nose.

C. advance the tip of the bulb syringe until it touches the back of the pharynx.

D. stimulate the newborn prior to removing fluid with the bulb syringe.

295. You are treating a nontrauma pregnant patient who is close to full term. To prevent hypotensive syndrome during transport, you should:

A. place the patient on her back with knees bent.

B. manually displace the uterus to the right.

C. place the patient in a supine position.

D. place the patient in a supine position with her right hip elevated.

296. You are treating a patient who is 8 months pregnant. The patient is suffering from a generalized seizure. Your immediate treatment should be to:

A. transport the patient immediately using lights and siren.

B. administer high-flow oxygen by non-rebreather mask.

C. position this postictal patient lying on her left side.

D. suction any blood or secretions from the patient's mouth.

297. Which emergency medical treatment is **inappropriate** when assisting the delivery of a newborn?

A. Tear the amniotic sac with your fingers if it has not ruptured during crowning.

B. If bleeding appears heavy after delivery, massage the mother's abdomen.

C. Place the first umbilical clamp approximately 6 inches from the infant.

D. Apply pressure to the fontanel to prevent an explosive delivery.

298. Which statement is **correct** regarding the delivery of the placenta?
    A. When the placenta appears in the vaginal opening, grasp it and guide it from the vagina.
    B. Pull the placenta and all attached membranes from the vagina.
    C. Remain on scene until the placenta and attached membranes are delivered.
    D. Place the placenta and membranes into a biohazard bag and dispose properly.

299. In which emergency setting is it permissible to insert your gloved hand into the pregnant patient's vagina?
    A. a prolapsed cord
    B. abruptio placenta
    C. arm or leg presentation
    D. multiple births

300. Your pregnant patient is in active labor and you encounter a limb presentation where the fetus's arm is protruding from the vagina. You should:
    A. place the mother in a head-down supine position with her pelvis elevated.
    B. gently pull the limb until the fetus is in the proper position for delivery.
    C. place your gloved hand into the vagina and maneuver the fetus into position.
    D. push the limb back into the vagina while pushing on the mother's abdomen.

301. Which of the following indicates that an infant is premature?
    A. The infant has coarse hair.
    B. There are many creases across the sole of the foot.
    C. There is no cartilage in the infant's outer ear.
    D. The infant weighs 6½ pounds at birth.

302. You are caring for a newborn who was born during the 36th week of pregnancy. Which of the following emergency treatments is a priority for this patient?
    A. Provide high-flow oxygen by nonrebreather mask.
    B. Place the infant in warmed blankets.
    C. Suction secretions with a tonsil tip catheter.
    D. Cover the infant except for the head.

SCENARIO

Questions 303–305 refer to the following scenario:

You and your partner Jim are refueling your vehicle when dispatch alerts you of a woman in active labor. You quickly secure the fuel pump and respond to the emergency. Upon arrival at the scene, you find a 23-year-old female lying supine on her bed. The amniotic sac has ruptured and she feels as if she must push. Jim quickly inspects the vagina for crowning and finds the pulsating umbilical cord protruding.

303. In which position should you and Jim place this patient?
    A. prone with chest elevated with pillows
    B. supine with the hips elevated with pillows
    C. semisitting with knees bent slightly
    D. lying flat on right side with knees bent

304. While rapidly transporting this patient to the hospital, you notice the baby's head appears to be pushing against the pulsating umbilical cord. You should immediately:
    A. place a gloved hand into the vagina and gently push the head back and away from the cord.
    B. with your gloved hand, gently pull the cord away from the baby's head.
    C. with your gloved hand, gently push the pulsating cord back into the vagina.
    D. place a gloved hand into the vagina and push the vaginal wall away from the cord.

305. After applying pressure against the fetal head, you observe that the mother is breath-

ing 42 times a minute with shallow breathing. You should immediately:

A. provide oxygen by nasal cannula at 6 lpm.

B. provide oxygen by non-rebreather mask at 15 lpm.

C. open the airway and begin positive pressure ventilation.

D. place the patient supine and elevate her right hip.

SEIZURE

306. A sudden and temporary alteration in behavior caused by the massive electrical discharge from a neuron or group of neurons in the brain is a:

A. stroke.

B. seizure.

C. TIA.

D. cerebral hemorrhage.

307. The pattern or sequence of events for a generalized tonic-clonic seizure include:

A. seizure, aura, postictal state.

B. aura, clonic phase, tonic phase, postictal state.

C. aura, tonic phase, myotonic phase, postictal state.

D. aura, tonic phase, clonic phase, postictal state.

308. Which of the following are possible causes of seizures?

A. infection

B. high fever

C. hypoxia

D. all of the above

309. Treatment for a patient who is actively seizing includes:

A. protecting and positioning the patient, maintaining an airway, administering oral glucose, suctioning the airway, and applying supplemental oxygen.

B. protecting and positioning the patient, prying the mouth open to insert an oral airway, suctioning the airway, applying supplemental oxygen, and rapid transport.

C. protecting and positioning the patient, maintaining an airway, suctioning the airway, assisting ventilations if necessary, applying supplemental oxygen, and transporting.

D. protecting and positioning the patient, maintaining an airway, suctioning the airway, assisting ventilations if needed, applying supplemental oxygen, waiting for the patient to regain consciousness to sign a refusal form.

310. A patient having seizures lasting more than 5 minutes in length or seizures that occur without a period of consciousness between is considered to be suffering from:

A. a grand mal seizure.

B. tonic-clonic seizures.

C. status epilepticus.

D. a prolonged hysterical seizure.

311. The tonic phase of a seizure is identified by:

A. loss of consciousness.

B. rigid muscles.

C. jerky muscle movement.

D. all of the above.

312. The tonic-clonic phase of a seizure results in all of the following **except:**

A. muscle spasms that alternate with a period of relaxation.

B. loss of bowel and bladder control.

C. prolonged period of jerky movement.

D. breathing that may be shallow or absent.

313. The preferred airway adjunct for an actively seizing patient with clenched teeth is the:
    A. nasopharyngeal airway.
    B. oropharyngeal airway.
    C. endotracheal tube.
    D. combitube.

314. Common patient medications used for the treatment of epilepsy include:
    A. valproic acid.
    B. phenytoin.
    C. phenobarbital.
    D. all of the above.

315. A patient who suffers two or more consecutive seizures without a period of consciousness between them or a seizure that lasts longer than 5 minutes has a condition referred to as:
    A. continual epilepsy.
    B. continual seizure.
    C. status epilepticus.
    D. status seizure.

316. Which of the following statements is true regarding syncope?
    A. The episode usually occurs when the patient is supine.
    B. The patient does not remember feeling faint or lightheaded.
    C. The patient becomes responsive immediately after being positioned supine.
    D. The patient remembers an abnormal sound, odor, or visual disturbance.

317. The patient with a history of epilepsy suddenly states she is experiencing a metallic taste in her mouth. She says it is an aura. She will next likely suffer:
    A. a postictal state.
    B. a petit mal seizure.
    C. a generalized tonic-clonic seizure.
    D. a focal motor seizure.

318. The convulsion phase that presents with typical violent and jerky seizure activity is known as the _____ phase.
    A. hypertonic
    B. tonic-clonic
    C. tonic
    D. postictal

319. Which stage of a seizure is known as the recovery phase during which the patient's mental status progressively improves over time?
    A. postictal phase
    B. tonic phase
    C. clonic phase
    D. aura phase

320. A syncopal episode usually begins while the patient is in which position?
    A. lying
    B. kneeling
    C. standing
    D. sitting

321. You are treating a patient who has experienced a syncopal episode. You should place this patient in which position?
    A. sitting with head between the knees
    B. supine with the legs elevated
    C. prone with the head elevated
    D. Fowler with the feet elevated

322. A bystander states your patient was standing when he became dizzy and then unresponsive. After the patient was assisted to the floor he immediately became responsive again. The skin is pale and moist. You suspect:
    A. a generalized seizure.
    B. a syncopal episode.
    C. a heart attack.
    D. hypoglycemia.

323. A patient that is postictal following a tonic-clonic seizure is displaying obvious right-sided weakness upon assessment. There is no obvious trauma to the patient. The family states that is a normal seizure for the patient. You should suspect which of the following?

A. A stroke occurred during the seizure.

B. A heart attack caused the seizure.

C. The patient struck his or her head during the seizure.

D. The weakness is a normal response after the seizure.

324. A febrile seizure would be considered serious if it lasted greater than:

A. 3 minutes.

B. 5 minutes.

C. 10 minutes.

D. 15 minutes.

325. A patient with a history of epilepsy complains of a sharp pain in his abdomen prior to suffering a tonic-clonic seizure. The abdominal pain would best be described as:

A. abdominal bleeding that caused the seizure.

B. an aura that indicated the seizure was imminent.

C. a postictal symptom associated with the seizure.

D. a result of the medication to control the seizure.

GENERAL PHARMACOLOGY 4.1

1.

B. Activated charcoal, oral glucose, and oxygen are medications that should be carried on all EMT-B units. An epinephrine auto-injector is not typically carried on the ambulance, but is carried by the patient. The EMT-B is allowed to assist with the administration of the epinephrine auto-injector. (4-1.1) (EC 332-333 PEC 285)

2.

D. The EMT-B can assist with the administration of epinephrine for anaphylaxis, a MDI for respiratory emergencies, and nitroglycerin for cardiac emergencies, if the prescription is for the patient, there are no contraindications, and medical control authorizes the procedure. (4-1.3) (EC 333-335 PEC 285)

3.

A. The EMT-B is not allowed to help assist in the administration of Decadron for respiratory emergencies. The EMT-B can help assist with the other medications. (4-1.3) (EC 333-335 PEC 285)

4.

B. Actidose and SuperChar are trade names for activated charcoal. Activated charcoal is used to bind with certain poisons in the stomach to limit the amount of poison being absorbed by the gastrointestinal tract. (4-1.2) (EC 332-333 PEC 285)

5.

C. The generic name for Alupent is metaproterenol. Albuterol is the generic name for Proventil and isoetharine is the trade name for Bronkosol. (4-1.2) (EC 332-333 PEC 285)

6.

D. Salmeterol xinafoate is the generic name for Serevent, a common respiratory medication that the EMT-B can assist with the administration of. (4-1.4) (EC 333-335 PEC 285)

7.

C. When the treatment involves medication administration, any time that you have a question, medical control should be contacted for clarification and further orders. (4-1.4) (EC 333-335 PEC 285)

8.

D. All are true. The generic name is a shortened name assigned to the drug before it is officially listed. The generic name will be listed in the U.S. Pharmacopoeia. It also is commonly similar to the chemical name. (4-1.4) (EC 333-335 PEC 285)

9.

A. The only approved medication is LiquiChar. The trade name for activated charcoal. The other three are medications that the EMT-B can assist the patient with administration of, but are not to be carried as standard medications on the ambulance in most systems. (4-1.1) (EC 332-333 PEC 285)

10.

D. The EMT-B may assist the patient with administration of metered-dose inhalers such as albuterol, metaproterenol and isoetharine. Epinephrine by auto-injector may be administered; however, the patient must have a prescription for the medication. Inderal is not to be administered by the EMT-B. (4-1.1) (EC 332-333 PEC 285)

11.

C. After assisting with the administration of any medication, it is important to recheck the patient for improvement or deterioration. This is achieved by conducting an ongoing assessment. Report any changes to medical control and document these changes in the PCR. (4-1.3) (EC 333-335 PEC 285)

12.

B. The oral route is by mouth. The drug is swallowed and absorbed from the stomach or intestinal tract. Nitroglycerin is administered sublingually by either spray or tablet. (4-1.5) (EC 336 PEC 287-288)

RESPIRATORY 4.2

13.

C. The respiratory system includes the larynx, the trachea, and the lungs. The esophagus is part of the gastrointestinal system. (4-2.1) (EC 344-345 PEC 295-296)

14.

D. Functions of the nose include warming, filtering, and humidifying inspired air. (4-2.1) (EC 344-345 PEC 295-296)

15.

B. The epiglottis is a flap of cartilage that acts like a valve directing air into the trachea and food into the esophagus. (4-2.1) (EC 344-345 PEC 295-296)

16.

C. The major muscle of respiration is the diaphragm. It accounts for 60% of the respiratory effort. (4-2.1) (EC 344-345 PEC 295-296)

17.

A. A sympathetic response to hypoxia is an increase in the heart rate. (4-2.1) (EC 344-345 PEC 295-296)

18.

D. Cyanosis caused by inadequate oxygen to peripheral circulation, tachypnea as an initial sympathetic response, and bradycardia, a late sign of severe hypoxia are all signs of inadequate oxygenation. (4-2.2) (EC 345-346, 347, 349-350 PEC 297-302)

19.

C. To determine the tidal volume, the EMT-B must assess the chest rise and fall, auscultate breath sounds for air movement, and determine the respiratory rate. By determining the tidal volume, the EMT-B can determine if the patient is breathing adequately. (4-2.2) (EC 345-346, 347, 349-350 PEC 297-302)

20.

C. Cyanosis to the oral mucosa indicates inadequate oxygenation. A respiratory rate between 12 and 20 breaths per minute, breath sounds that are equal and clear bilaterally, and equal rise and fall of the chest are all parameters of normal respirations. (4-2.2) (EC 345-346, 347, 349-350)

21.

B. The size of the tongue in an infant proportionately is considerably larger than that of an adult. (4-2.9) (EC 346, 348 PEC 307-310)

22.

D. The narrowest portion of the upper airway in a patient under 10 years of age is at the cricoid ring, which is below the vocal cords. The narrowest portion of an adult's airway is at the level of the vocal cords. (4-2.9) (EC 346, 348 PEC 307-310)

23.

B. The infant is exhibiting signs of a partial airway obstruction. The stridorous respirations and the infant's color indicate oxygenation/ventilation is still occurring. (4-2.9) (EC 346, 348 PEC 307-310)

24.

C. If you suspect a partial airway obstruction, it is most important to keep your patient calm, instruct him or her to cough, and provide high-flow oxygen via a nonrebreather mask. (4-2.10) (EC 348 PEC 309-310)

25.

C. In a complete airway obstruction the patient will not be able to cough, whereas in the partial airway obstruction the patient will cough forcefully in an attempt to remove the object. (4-2.10) (EC 348 PEC 309-310)

26.

A. Inspiration occurs due to the contraction of the diaphragm, causing it to move downward, and the contraction of the intercostal muscles, pulling the ribs outward and resulting in an increased thoracic cavity size, which allows air to rush in. (4-2.1) (EC 344-345 PEC 295-296)

27.

D. Respiration is the molecular process of exchange of oxygen and carbon dioxide. Ventilation is the mechanical process of moving oxygen into the lungs and carbon dioxide out of the lungs. Oxygenation is the process of supplementing the oxygen content or providing oxygen therapy. (4-2.1) (EC 344-345 PEC 295-296)

28.

D. The pharynx is a common passage way for food, water, and air. (4-2.1) (EC 344-345 PEC 295-296)

29.

D. The occiput (back of the head) in the young child is disproportionately larger when compared with the child's body. The large occiput causes the flexion and leads to airway obstruction. To alleviate this problem in young children and infants, pad under the shoulders to bring the thorax up to the level of the head. (4-2.1) (EC 344-345 PEC 295-296)

30.

D. The parietal pleura is in contact with the thoracic cavity, while the visceral pleura covers the lungs itself. The visceral pericardium covers the heart. The peritonium is a lining in the abdominal cavity. (4-2.1) (EC 344-345 PEC 295-296)

31.

D. In order for the EMT-B to assist in the administration of a medication, he or she must have protocol or online medical direction authorizing the action. Also, the medication must be prescribed to the patient. (4-2.5) (EC 346-348, 350-351 PEC 302-307)

32.

D. The pharynx is divided into two major subdivisions, the oroparhynx and the nasopharynx. The larynx and the trachea are separate parts of the upper airway. (4-2.1) (EC 344-345 PEC 295-296)

33.

C. The larynx is a cartilaginous structure responsible for phonation. The larynx is commonly referred to as the voice box. (4-2.1) (EC 344-345 PEC 295-296)

34.

C. The EMT-B can only help administer the medication if it is prescribed for that patient. In this situation explain your protocol to the family physician and defer further questioning to the medical director or on-line medical control. (4-2.5) (EC 346-348, 350-351 PEC 302-307)

35.

D. Before helping with medication administration, the EMT-B must perform a thorough assessment and life-saving measures. (4-2.5) (EC 346-348, 350-351 PEC 302-307)

36.

B. An indication of severe respiratory failure is a silent chest. The diminished breath sounds and decreased wheezes are caused by increasing bronchoconstriction and a severely decreased tidal volume. (4-2.7) (EC 346 PEC 298)

37.

B. When the EMT-B is performing positive pressure ventilation, the patient should have equal chest rise and fall, clear breath sounds bilaterally, and an improving mental status. A sign of hypoxia is an elevated heart rate or one

that remains elevated. (4-2.3) (EC 341-348, 350-351 PEC 302-307)

38.

C. Stridor is caused by a 75% blockage of the upper airway. Wheezing is caused by lower airway bronchial constriction. Rales are due to fluid filled or collapsed terminal airways and alveoli. (4-2.3) (EC 341-348, 350-351 PEC 302-307)

39.

B. Asthma is an example of a lower airway disease. Epiglottitis is a bacterial infection causing inflammation of the upper airway at the level of the epiglottis and subglottic area. (4-2.10) (EC 348 PEC 309-310)

40.

A. Patients that present in a tripod position are usually in severe respiratory distress. The tripod position is when patients sit upright and lean forward, supporting themselves with their arms, with elbows locked between their dangling legs. Occasionally you may find a severe respiratory distress patient lying supine or in a reclining position; these patients may be too exhausted to support themselves. (4-2.2) (EC 345-346, 347, 349-350 PEC 297-302)

41.

D. Apnea is the term used to describe the patient in respiratory arrest. Dyspnea is the term used to describe the patient who is having difficulty breathing. Bradypnea is the term used to describe the patient breathing at a rate that is less than the normal. Tachypnea describes the patient breathing faster than the normal respiratory rate. (4-2.2) (EC 345-346, 347, 349-350 PEC 297-302)

42.

B. The patient with cyanosis—a bluish-gray skin color on the neck or chest, an ominous sign of respiratory distress—requires immediate emergency intervention. The patient that can speak full sentences is most likely not in severe respiratory distress. The patient that can only speak one or two words in between breaths is in severe respiratory distress. Normal respiratory rates for children are 15 to 30 times each minute. It is normal for infants to use their abdominal muscles when breathing. (4-2.7) (EC 346 PEC 298)

43.

D. Stridor is a high-pitched inspiratory sound that is caused by a narrowing of the upper airway. Stridor indicates that the airway is partially obstructed. Obstruction can be caused by a foreign body or swelling of the larynx. (4-2.10) (EC 348 PEC 309-310)

44.

C. Hypotension, low blood pressure, is a late sign of respiratory distress in infants and children. When you encounter these late signs in the infant or child, you must immediately provide positive pressure ventilation. (4-2.2) (EC 346-346, 347, 349-350 PEC 297-302)

45.

B. If you are unsure if the patient's condition warrants positive pressure ventilation, it is better to provide the ventilation than to delay the treatment. Delaying the treatment may worsen the respiratory condition and may lead to respiratory arrest and even death. Administering high-flow oxygen will not provide an adequate tidal volume. A nasopharyngeal airway alone will not help the patient with breathing difficulty. Placing the patient in the Trendelenburg (shock) position may worsen the patient's condition. (4-2.6) (EC 346, 348, 350 PEC 296, 298, 302, 309)

46.

B. You should provide oxygen by non-rebreather mask at 15 lpm. The patient is talking, which indicates an adequate tidal volume. His respiratory rate is adequate. The nasal cannula only delivers 44% oxygen at 6 lpm and should be used only if the patient will not tolerate the non-rebreather mask. Never withhold oxygen for the patient complaining of shortness of breath. (4-2.6) (EC 346, 348, 350 PEC 296, 298, 302, 309)

47.

A. Loss of muscle tone is a late sign of respiratory failure in an infant and must be managed immediately with positive pressure ventilation. Cyanosis of the extremities is an early sign of breathing difficulty in the infant. Tachycardia is an early sign, whereas bradycardia (slow heart rate) is a late sign of respiratory failure in the infant. Prolonged exhalation and nasal flaring are early signs of breathing difficulty. (4-2.2) (EC 345-346, 347, 349-350 PEC 297-302)

48.

B. If the child will not tolerate a non-rebreather mask, you should have the parent hold the child and administer oxygen by holding the mask near but not on his face. Never withhold oxygen from any patient complaining of difficulty breathing. You should always speak to children softly; however, holding the mask on their face will

only add to their stress. Always reassure your patient. Administering oxygen by nasal cannula is not appropriate in this situation. In addition, the liter flow is too high. (4-2.9) (EC 346, 348 PEC 307-310)

49.

C. Suspect the child has epiglottitis if he has a fever, sore throat, is sitting upright with his neck jutted out, and drooling. Epiglottitis is a true emergency and should be treated with high-flow oxygen and immediate transport to the hospital. You should consider advanced life support backup. Epiglottitis is a condition that causes the epiglottis to swell and the larynx to spasm, blocking the opening into the trachea. (4-2.9) (EC 346, 348 PEC 307-310)

50.

A. The action of the aerosolized medication in a metered-dose inhaler (MDI) is a beta agonist, which relaxes the smooth muscle that lines the bronchioles. This drug, when administered, is inhaled and must travel deep into the lower airway where it is deposited on receptor sites on the bronchioles. The beta agonist relaxes the smooth muscle and dilates the airway, relieving the bronchoconstriction. (4-2.8) (EC 354 PEC 304-305)

51.

B. Do not administer a metered-dose inhaler (MDI) if the patient is not responsive enough to use the device. The MDI will only be effective if the patient is able to take a deep breath. (4-2.8) (EC 354 PEC 304-305)

52.

C. You should instruct the patient to inhale slowly and deeply over about 5 seconds as you or the patient depresses the canister. Depressing the canister and then taking a rapid, deep breath will cause the majority of the medication to be deposited in the mouth and upper airway and not on the receptor sites deep in the lower airway. Prior to administering the MDI you must have either on-line or off-line direction from medical control. After the drug is administered, you should coach the patient to hold his or her breath for 10 seconds. After holding his or her breath, the patient should be instructed to exhale slowly through pursed lips. (4-2.5) (EC 346-348, 350-351 PEC 302-307)

53.

D. Ipratropium bromide (Atrovent®) is not a beta agonist and does not provide immediate action when inhaled. This drug should not be administered by the EMT-B. The other drugs are common beta agonists that are supplied in the MDI and can be given by the EMT-B after obtaining orders from medical direction. (4-2.8) (EC 354 PEC 304-305)

54.

A. These are common side effects of the drug. Tachycardia, tremors, shakiness, nervousness, dry mouth, nausea, and vomiting are all common side effects of the drug. Continue to reassess the patient looking for signs of improvement or deterioration. (4-2.8) (EC 354 PEC 304-305)

55.

A. The barking seal sound when the patient coughs is the hallmark sign of croup. Croup results in the swelling of the larynx, trachea, and bronchi. It is common for the condition to worsen at night. Apply oxygen, humidified if possible. (4-2.10) (EC 348 PEC 309-310)

56.

A. Audible wheezes with diminished breath sounds are signs and symptoms of lower airway disease, such as asthma. A cough that produces a sound like a barking seal is indicative of croup, which is an upper airway problem. Fever with stridorous airway sounds and drooling are signs of epiglottitis, which occurs in the upper airway. Stridorous airway sounds that come on suddenly without other signs of sickness are likely from a partially blocked airway from a foreign body. (4-2.10) (EC 348 PEC 309-310)

57.

C. The wheezing breath sounds should lead you to suspect lower airway disease. This patient has been prescribed medication, which is delivered through a metered-dose inhaler. Knowing that Proventil® is a beta agonist that relaxes the bronchiole smooth muscle, you highly suspect that the child has a lower airway disease. Epiglottitis and croup are both upper airway conditions. (4-2.10) (EC 348 PEC 309-310)

CARDIOVASCULAR

58.

C. Blood is pumped from the right atrium to the right ventricle to the lungs back to the left atrium to the left ventricle and through the aorta and finally to the body. (4-3.1) (EC 367 PEC 324-327)

59.

B. Oxygen, carbon dioxide, and other nutrients are exchanged in the capillaries. (4-3.1) (EC 367 PEC 324-327)

60.

C. The right side of the heart is a low pressure pump that pumps the blood to the lungs and then to the high pressure left side that pumps the blood to the body. (4-3.1) (EC 367 PEC 324-327)

61.

D. The AED should only be applied to patients older than 8 years of age and > 25 kg (55 lbs.) who are unresponsive, pulseless, and apneic and not victims of a traumatic incident. (4-3.3) (EC 380-381, 384-385, 388, 390 PEC 355)

62.

C. A patient who is having difficulty breathing or who is suffering from CHF should be placed with the head of the cot in an upright and elevated position. (4-3.7) (EC 369 PEC 334)

63.

C. Ventricular fibrillation is the most common presenting rhythm in the first eight minutes of cardia arrest. (4-3.11) (EC 378, 380 PEC 351)

64.

C. Defibrillation is the most effective treatment of ventricular fibrillation. Defibrillation should not be delayed to perform CPR, hyperventilate, or transport the patient. (4-3.10) (EC 380 PEC 351)

65.

B. Prehospital ALS is an important link in the chain of survival. Patients need to receive definitive care that can be provided by ALS units in the field. (4-3.13) (EC 380-381, 392 PEC 351-352, 361)

66.

D. The semi-automatic defibrillator requires the operator to turn the unit on and push a button to shock the patient. The automatic defibrillator only requires the EMT-B to push the "on" button. (4-3.16) (EC 383-394, 396 PEC 352-353)

67.

D. When the EMT is by himself, he should deliver up to three shocks and then leave to activate the EMS system. This allows for early defibrillation and early access to ALS care. (4-3.26) (EC 383, 385-394 PEC 361)

68.

D. If your patient regains a pulse, a total of six shocks have been given, or the AED has given three "No Shock" messages, you should begin transport. (4-3.27) (EC 393 PEC 361)

69.

C. Defibrillation has already been proven to be the most effective treatment for ventricular fibrillation. Reducing the time to defibrillation, working with ALS units more effectively, and determining if further training is needed are aspects that can be reviewed. (4-3.22) (EC 397-399 PEC 352)

70.

B. If the EMT-B is trained and proficient in the use of the AED, the first defibrillation can be administered within 1 minute of the arrival of the AED at the patient's side. (4-3.21) (EC 397 PEC 352)

71.

D. Nothing should take precedence over applying and activating the AED, except scene safety issues. Proper training and application of the AED can decrease the time to defibrillation. (4-3.17) (EC 385-399 PEC 356-361)

72.

D. Weak or dead batteries are the most common cause of failure of the AED. Because of this it is imperative to check the batteries each and every shift. (4-3.34) (EC 399 PEC 364)

73.

C. The completion of the checklist assures the EMT-B that the machine is in working order. What it does not assure is that the operator is proficient in the use of the AED. (4-3.34) (EC 399 PEC 364)

74.

D. Studies have shown that to be most effective the defibrillation should occur within 4 minutes. (4-3.22) (EC 397-399 PEC 352)

75.

A. The studies have proven that if bystander CPR is started immediately defibrillation can be successful for up to 10 minutes after cardiac arrest. (4-3.30) (EC 392 PEC 351-352, 361, 364)

76.

D. CPR should only be performed after the first three shocks have been delivered and the pulse has been checked. CPR should not be performed in between shocks because it would delay the time to defibrillation. (4-3.20) (EC 384 PEC 357, 360)

77.

C. When using the semi-automatic defibrillator, the operator must stay clear of the patient so the machine will

reanalyze the rhythm and determine if another shock is necessary. (4-3.19) (EC 383 PEC 355)

78.

C. The AED should be placed only on an unresponsive, pulseless, apneic, patient. (4-3.18) 9EC 383 PEC 356)

79.

B. When two rescuers are present, one can prepare the AED and place it on the patient's chest while the other EMT performs CPR. (4-3.28) (EC 392 PEC 360)

80.

D. A single rescuer needs to protect himself with BSI, determine if the patient is unresponsive, apneic, and pulseless, apply the AED, and analyze the rhythm. (4-3.20) (EC 384 PEC 357, 360)

81.

D. If the patient becomes pulseless and apneic pull the ambulance off the road and turn the engine off. This prevents interference from the engine. Analyze the rhythm and deliver three stacked shocks if they are indicated. (4-3.27) (EC 393 PEC 361)

82.

C. If a patient regains a pulse and then loses it again, the EMT-B should proceed and begin the series all over again. (4-3.27) (EC 393 PEC 361)

83.

C. The post-resuscitation patient should be reassessed at least every 5 minutes or whenever the patient's condition changes. (4-3.32) (EC 392 PEC 359, 360, 361)

84.

B. The fully automatic defibrillator will deliver the shocks without the operator having to press a shock button. (4-3.21) (EC 397 PEC 352)

85.

D. All the information is important and should be included on the log. (4-3.38) (EC 399-400 PEC 364)

86.

C. Whenever you are ordered to perform a procedure outside your protocol, revert back to the standing orders and/or contact medical control for advice. (4-3.36) (EC 399 PEC 364)

87.

D. To reduce anxiety, which may help reduce the chest pain, the patient should be placed in the position that is most comfortable for him or her. (4-3.7) (EC 369 PEC 334)

88.

B. The batteries in an AED should be checked every day to prevent failure. (4-3.34) (EC 399 PEC 364)

89.

C. Whenever the AED advises "No Shock," the operator should perform CPR for 1 minute, reassess for a pulse and then reanalyze the rhythm. (4-3.25) (EC 388-391 PEC 356-361)

90.

D. The AED should only be used with an unresponsive, pulseless, apneic adult patient greater than 8 years of age. (4-3.4) (EC 393-394 PEC 355)

91.

C. The proper sequence of events when using an AED is to take BSI precautions; determine unresponsiveness, pulselessness, and apnea; have your partner initiate CPR while you prepare the AED; attach the AED and stop CPR; clear the patient and initiate the rhythm analysis; and deliver a defibrillation if indicated. (4-3.25) (EC 388-391 PEC 356-361)

92.

A. The EMT-B must reassess vital signs and determine if the nitroglycerin has had an effect by determining the severity of pain and if any relief has occurred. (4-3.42) (EC 373 PEC 338)

93.

D. The right side of the heart receives unoxygenated blood from the body and pumps it to the lungs and finally into the left side of the heart to be circulated throughout the body. (4-3.1) (EC 367 PEC 324-327)

94.

B. All patients that complain of chest pain or discomfort should receive oxygen at 15 lpm by non-rebreather mask. Chest pain or discomfort is commonly caused by the lack of oxygen to the cardiac tissue. When cardiac tissue becomes inadequately oxygenated, the area affected becomes hypoxic, causing pain. High-flow oxygen can help reduce damage to the tissue and significantly increase survival of the patient. (4-3.2) (EC 369, 372 PEC 333-337)

95.

D. You should first provide high-flow oxygen by non-rebreather mask. The high-flow oxygen will help to decrease tissue damage to the heart. High-flow oxygen should be administered early in your treatment. You should place the patient in the position in which he or she is comfortable. This will help reduce anxiety. You should assist the patient with his or her prescribed nitroglycerin only after a medical assessment is conducted and the necessary order from medical direction has been obtained. (4-3.2) (EC 369, 372 PEC 333-337)

96.

D. First perform a general impression and assess the mental status. You must then ensure an adequate airway. Next, assess the breathing for adequacy. Determine if the patient is breathing normally or with increased effort. Following the breathing assessment, check the pulse. Is circulation adequate? Finally, assess the skin. Is the patient pale, cyanotic, cool, clammy? This quick assessment will help you to rapidly determine the patient's condition. (4-3.8) (EC 372, 392 PEC 331)

97.

A. Approximately 20% of heart attacks are silent. There is no chest pain associated with the event. Silent heart attacks occur more frequently in the elderly because of diminished sensation of pain. Other assessment findings such as shortness of breath, nausea, vomiting, anxiety, abnormal blood pressure, abnormal pulse, dizziness, and feeling of impending doom should raise your suspicion of a silent heart attack. (4-3.2) (EC 369, 372 PEC 333-337)

98.

B. Nitroglycerin spray and tablets are administered sublingually. Sublingual pertains to spraying or placing a tablet under the tongue, which is then absorbed into the blood stream. Nitroglycerin paste is administered through the skin but is not considered appropriate for the EMT-B to administer. Nitroglycerin can also be administered by intravenous drip in the hospital and by paramedics. (4-3.41) (EC 372 PEC 338)

99.

A. This patient's blood pressure is 98/52 mmHg, which is too low to administer nitroglycerin. You should not administer nitroglycerin to patients with a systolic blood pressure less than 100 mmHg. Other contraindications include patients with a suspected head injury, infants and children, and a patient who has already taken greater than three doses. (4-3.41) (EC 372 PEC 338)

100.

B.Blurred vision is not a common side effect of nitroglycerin. Because nitroglycerin dilates blood vessels, the patient may experience a headache, drop in blood pressure, and a reflexive tachycardia. (4-3.42) (EC 373 PEC 338)

101.

C. Your first concern is to ensure the patient has an adequate airway. You should then assess the breathing and circulation. It is crucial to provide immediate oxygenation or positive pressure ventilation if the ventilation status is inadequate. Early recognition and treatment of the patient with cardiac compromise will help increase the patient's survival. (4-3.8) (EC 372, 392 PEC 331)

102.

C. Early diagnosis is not a part of the chain of survival. Early access is crucial. The sooner CPR is provided, the greater the chances of survival. Early defibrillation may restore a functional heart beat to the patient, thus providing better circulation of oxygen. Early advanced life support will provide medications and other techniques that increase the survival of the patient and reduce the chance of the patient refibrillating. (4-3.10) (EC 380 PEC 351)

103.

D. Ventricular fibrillation quickly degenerates into asystole (no electrical activity in the heart or "flat line"). The most effective defibrillation with successful conversion typically occurs within 4 minutes of the onset of cardiac arrest. As time elapses without defibrillation, the success rate falls significantly. (4-3.11) (EC 378, 380 PEC 351)

104.

C. Your goal as an EMT-B is to minimize the time from delivery of AED shocks to the arrival of advanced cardiac life support (ACLS). If a paramedic unit is not available to respond to the scene or meet with your unit while en route to the hospital, you must transport to the hospital. Do not delay ACLS. Remember early advanced life support is a link in the chain of survival. (4-3.13) (EC 380-381, 392 PEC 351-352, 361)

105.

D. The correct placement of the defibrillator pads is (−) placed on the right upper border of the sternum with the top of the (−) just below the clavicle. The (+) pad is placed over the left lower ribs at the anterior axillary line. An alternative placement is anterior and posterior. In A/P placement, the (−) is placed posterior near the center of the back, while the (+) is placed anterior over the apex of the heart. (4-3.23) (EC 397 PEC 352)

106.

A. When the AED delivers a shock and then gives a "No Shock massage" you must check for a pulse immediately. This message can indicate that the patient has regained a pulse or that the rhythm has changed to one where a shock is not necessary. If the patient has not regained a pulse, begin CPR immediately. (4-3.29) (EC 392 PEC 355, 357, 359)

107.

C. The semi-automated and fully automated AED are very similar; however, the fully automated AED will automatically deliver a shock if it senses that one is appropriate. The AED should not be used on children under the age of 8. Neither the fully automated or semi-automated AED can effectively analyze the rhythm during CPR. Both AEDs recognize systole and will not deliver a shock in this case. (4-3.16) (EC 383-394, 396 PEC 352-353)

108.

D. The AED can not effectively analyze the rhythm during CPR. The compression of the heart muscle produces electrical activity that produce artifact. The AED reads this rhythm and is unable to determine if a shock is needed. The semi-automated AED will only deliver a shock when the defibrillate button is pressed by the EMT-B. (4-3.20) (EC 384 PEC 357, 360)

109.

B.Manual defibrillators use paddles that must be held against the patient's chest. The AED uses external adhesive pads that attach to the patient and deliver a "hands-free" shock, which is considered safer for EMS personnel. AED produces the same amount of energy as the manual defibrillators. AEDs can shock the rescuers if someone is touching the patient when the shock is delivered. You should not use the device while you, the patient, or the device is wet. Dry the patient, device, and yourself after moving to a dry environment. (4-3.19) (EC 383 PEC 355)

110.

D. The AED is a sensitive device that can be influenced by outside interference. When the AED is performing an analysis of the patient between shocks, you should not touch the patient. Touching the patient may interfere with the analysis. (4-3.19) (EC 383 PEC 355)

111.

A. When the AED is to be used while transporting the cardiac arrest patient to the hospital, you must stop the ambulance and shut the motor off. The vibration from the motor can be picked up by the sensitive device and interfere with the analysis of the rhythm. (4-3.19) (EC 383 PEC 355)

112.

B. Interior lights of a vehicle are not likely to interfere with the AED's analysis of the rhythm. The AED is a sensitive instrument; therefore, movement of the patient may interfere with the analysis of the rhythm. Vehicle engine interference may increase the likelihood of a false interpretation of the patient's rhythm by the AED. (4-3.19) (EC 383 PEC 355)

113.

B. Your next action after checking the pulse following successful defibrillation is to assess the patient's breathing. If breathing is adequate, provide oxygen at 15 lpm via non-rebreather mask. If the breathing is inadequate, provide positive pressure ventilation with supplemental oxygen. (4-3.32) (EC 392 PEC 359, 360, 361)

114.

B. Most AED failures are a result of poor maintenance, especially poor battery maintenance. The AED and its batteries should be serviced on a regular schedule. The AED should be checked at the beginning of every shift. Always carry extra charged batteries. (4-3.34) (EC 399 PEC 364)

115.

B. All patients that complain of chest pain or have the symptoms of a silent heart attack should be treated with high-concentrations of oxygen, even if they deny any shortness of breath. Chest pain is caused by lack of oxygen reaching the cardiac tissue. High-concentration oxygen may decrease the size of the injury to the heart muscle, as well as decrease the chest pain. (4-3.2) (EC 369, 372 PEC 333-337)

116.

A. Placing the patient in a position of comfort will reduce anxiety and stress. Let the patient dictate the position that is most comfortable for him. (4-3.7) (EC 369 PEC 334)

117.

C. You should reassure Big Joe that these changes are common side effects of the drug. It is unlikely that this patient would be sensitive to this drug. Signs of anaphylaxis are itching, hives, redness, and increased difficulty breath-

ing. Do not administer another nitroglycerin tablet until you reassess the patient's vital signs. (4-3.41) (EC 372 PEC 338)

118.

C. The AED should only be used on patients over the age of 8 and/or weighing more than 25 kg. The patient must be breathless, pulseless, and unresponsive. It is not typically indicated for the patient in cardiac arrest resulting from trauma. (4-3.4) (EC 393-394 PEC 355)

119.

D. The AED should not be utilized on patients less than 8 and/or weighing less than 25 kg. (4-3.4) (EC 393-394 PEC 355)

120.

A. Patients suffering from cardiac emergencies fall into two general categories: the cardiac arrest patient and the responsive patient with signs and symptoms of a cardiac emergency. (4-3.5) (EC 369-372 PEC 333-334)

121.

C. All patients with chest pain or cardiac compromise will not go into cardiac arrest. Monitor the chest pain patient closely. If the patient becomes unresponsive, pulseless, and breathless application of the AED is indicated. (4-3.2) (EC 369, 372 PEC 333-337)

122.

C. The automatic defibrillator requires the operator to push a single button and the device does the rest. It analyzes the rhythm, determines if ventricular fibrillation (or pulseless ventricular tachycardia) is present, and then delivers shocks. The semi-automatic defibrillator requires the operator to turn the unit on, possibly push a button to analyze the rhythm, and then push a button to provide a shock. (4-3.17) (EC 385-399 PEC 356-361)

123.

A. Prevent the administration of an inappropriate defibrillation to a patient by ensuring that he or she is unresponsive, pulseless, and breathless before attaching the device. A patient's heart may be damaged by the inappropriate administration of a defibrillation. (4-3.18) (EC 383 PEC 356)

124.

C. The AED is preferred for use over the manual defibrillator for its speed of operation and safety features. The AED delivers a more effective shock than the paddles of a manual defibrillator. The adhesive pads of the AED provide a larger surface area upon which the shock is delivered. (4-3.16) (EC 383-394, 396 PEC 352-353)

125.

B. The AED is used to treat ventricular tachycardia without a pulse and ventricular fibrillation. (4-3.3) (EC 380-381, 384-385, 388, 390 PEC 355)

126.

C. If ALS backup is unavailable the patient should be transported when one of the following occurs: the patient's pulse returns; a total of six shocks have been delivered; or the AED has given three consecutive "No Shock" messages. (4-3.26) (EC 383, 385-394 PEC 361)

127.

B. The missing link in the AHA's chain of survival is early ACLS. Successfully resuscitating a cardiac arrest patient requires all four of the items in this chain. (4-3.35) (EC 378-381 PEC 350-352)

128.

C. Frequent practice ensures that the AED will be properly applied and operated. Practice also ensures that the EMT-B will properly utilize the device when needed. (4-3.33) (EC 383, 399 PEC 364)

129.

C. Medical direction is responsible for all aspects of AED services. EMTs utilize the AED under the medical director's control. Defibrillation is the most effective method to terminate v-fib. There is no alternative. The other items listed are all elements that should involve the medical director. (4-3.36) (EC 399 PEC 364)

130.

A. Medical direction for the AED program must be involved and available for advice. It would be appropriate if medical direction could respond to each AED incident but this is generally not practical. Medical direction or a designated representative should review all incidents of AED use. These reviews may identify potential areas requiring improvement. (4-3.36) (EC 399 PEC 364)

131.

C. Defibrillation or the use of the AED is most useful for patient's in cardiac arrest resulting from dysrhythmias associated with coronary artery disease. The other patients have etiologies of cardiac arrest that require alternative management. (4-3.3) (EC 380-381, 384-385, 388, 390 PEC 355)

132.

C. A 3-year-old child is not a candidate for AED. The most likely cause of arrest is a respiratory or airway compromise. The child requires aggressive airway and ventilatory management. (4-3.2) (EC 369-372 PEC 333-337)

133.

C. Nitroglycerin lowers a patient's blood pressure. For this reason nitroglycerin is contraindicated if the patient's systolic blood pressure is less than 100 mmHg. (4-3.42) (EC 373 PEC 338)

134.

A. Nitroglycerin should be administered to a total of 3 doses. Recheck the blood pressure after each dose to ensure that it remains at least 100 mmHg systolic. (4-3.41) (EC 372 PEC 338)

135.

D. Nitroglycerin dilates the coronary blood vessels. This increase in blood vessel size occurs in vessels in other parts of the body as well. This dilation causes an increase in blood volume in the cranium, causing a common complaint of headache. (4-3.41) (EC 372 PEC 338)

136.

D. It is easier to learn how to operate an AED than it is to learn CPR. AEDs are able to detect loose leads or false readings of the EKG. The AHA has endorsed the AED as being safe and effective. (4-3.11) (EC 378, 380 PEC 351)

137.

D. All three signs of cardiac arrest must be present to apply the AED: no respirations, no pulse, and the patient must not respond to verbal or pain stimuli (unresponsive). (4-3.12) (EC 367-372 PEC 348, 356)

138.

D. If ALS backup is delayed, the patient in most circumstances should be transported immediately after regaining a pulse. (4-3.27) (EC 393 PEC 361)

139.

B. The patient has reached the maximum of 3 total doses of nitroglycerin. Additional doses should only be administered after medical direction consultation. (4-3.40) (EC 370, 372 PEC 334, 335, 336)

140.

C. If the AED advises "No Shock," immediately check the pulse. If the pulse is present, check the respirations. If no pulse is present, continue CPR for 1 minute and then reanalyze the rhythm. (4-3.25) (EC 388-391 PEC 356-361)

141.

C. Before delivery of the shock, ensure that rescuers and bystanders are all clear of the patient and that no one is in contact with the patient. (4-3.25) (EC 388-391 PEC 356-361)

DIABETES/AMS

142.

C. Micronase is an oral hypoglycemia agent. This patient is exhibiting signs of hypoglycemia. (4-4.1) (EC 423, 428 PEC 373-380)

143.

D. A patient suffering from hypoglycemia will exhibit a rapid onset of signs and symptoms with an altered mental status due to the glucose deficiency; tachycardia; and pale, cool, clammy skin. (4-4.2) (EC 428 PEC 376, 378-380)

144.

A. A patient must have an intact gag reflex and the ability to swallow in order to receive instant oral glucose. (4-4.2) (EC 428 PEC 376, 378-380)

145.

C. The entire tube of glucose should be placed on a tongue depressor and placed between the gum and the cheek to dissolve in the patient's mouth. Rubbing the area may increase the absorption rate. (4-4.2) (EC 428 PEC 376, 378-380)

146.

D. Due to the decreased level of consciousness and snoring respirations, this patient should receive nothing by mouth. The treatment would be to open the airway, provide oxygen therapy, and continue the assessment. (4-4.3) (EC 423, 428, 430, 431, 436 PEC 371, 372, 378, 380, 387, 389, 391)

147.

A. The patient who is unable to protect his or her own airway should not receive oral glucose. (4-4.3) (EC 423, 428, 430, 431, 436, PEC 371, 372, 378, 380, 387, 389, 391)

148.

C. Your priority medical care is to establish and maintain an open airway. After you evaluate the patient's breathing you may need to administer positive pressure ventilation. Administer oxygen by non-rebreather mask at 15 lpm if the patient is breathing adequately. Determine if the patient is alert enough to swallow following airway assessment and management. (4-4.3) (EC 423, 428, 430, 431, 436, PEC 371, 372, 378, 380, 387, 389, 391)

149.

C. Immediately after management of the airway, including oxygen therapy, you should determine if the patient is alert enough to swallow. (4-4.3) (EC 423, 428, 430, 431, 436, PEC 371, 372, 378, 380, 387, 389, 391)

150.

D. The treatment for this patient is to maintain an open airway, administer high-flow oxygen, suction if necessary, assist ventilation if necessary, position the patient on his side, and transport. Do not administer the oral glucose. Three criteria must be met before administering oral glucose: (1) The patient must have an altered mental status; (2) The patient must have a history of diabetes controlled by medication; and (3) The patient must be alert enough to swallow. This patient only responded to tactile stimulation and would not be able to protect his own airway. (4-4.4) (EC 428 PEC 379)

151.

B. There are two acceptable ways to administer oral glucose. Hold back the cheek and squeeze a small amount between the cheek and gum. Place a small portion onto a tongue depressor; pull back the cheek, depositing the medication between the cheek and gum by sliding the depressor in place. (4-4.4) (EC 428 PEC 379)

152.

A. If the patient becomes unresponsive while you are administering oral glucose, remove the tongue depressor and reassess the airway, breathing, and circulation. Placing the unresponsive patient in a semisitting position may compromise the airway. Do not try to remove the glucose from the patient's cheek. This is a small amount and will not likely compromise the airway. Do not administer additional glucose to the unresponsive patient. (4-4.4) (EC 428 PEC 379)

153.

B. Airway maintenance is the priority of care in the patient suffering from an altered mental status.

(4-4.3) (EC 423, 428, 430, 431, 436 PEC 371, 372, 378, 380, 387, 389, 391)

154.

D. Airway management is the priority in patient care followed by positioning and transport. (4-4.3) (EC 423, 428, 430, 431, 436 PEC 371, 372, 378, 380, 387, 389, 391)

155.

C. This patient should be positioned in a left lateral recumbent position with the feet flat. Continually reassure and explain procedures to the patient, even though he or she is unresponsive. (4-4.3) (EC 423, 428, 430, 431, 436 PEC 371, 372, 378, 380, 387, 389, 391)

156.

D. The proper administration includes placing the full tube onto a tongue depressor and depositing it between the cheek and the gum. (4-4.5) (EC 428 PEC 375, 378, 379, 380, 382)

STROKE

157.

D. Aphasia is the inability to speak. Hemiplegia is paralysis to one side of the body. Hemiparesis is weakness to one side of the body. All are signs of a stroke. (EC 433-436 PEC 401-402)

158.

C. TIAs are often called "mini strokes" They differ in that the effects are only temporary. The signs and symptoms resolve within 24 hours and leave no permanent cognitive, temporary, or motor deficits. (EC 433-436 PEC 396)

159.

C. This patient is exhibiting classic signs and symptoms of a stroke. It would be dangerous to have the patient attempt to walk due to the potential for injury and for increasing the extent of the stroke. (EC 433-436 PEC 395-396)

160.

B. Hemorrhagic strokes are commonly associated with hypertension. The severe headache is caused by the increased intracranial pressure associated with rupture of an artery and collection of blood in the skull. (EC 433-436 PEC 405)

161.

B. Emboli can be caused by fat particles from the left side of the heart, carotid arteries, or cerebral circulation. The others would result in a pulmonary embolism. (EC 433-436 PEC 403)

162.

D. A stiff neck is a late sign of stroke caused by hemorrhage. Seizures, headache, and unequal pupils often occur immediately. (EC 433-436 PEC 401-402)

163.

C. Severe intermittent abdominal pain is not a sign or symptom of stroke. Hemiplegia is the medical term used to describe one-sided paralysis. Loss of bowel and bladder control and unequal pupils or vision disturbances are common signs and symptoms. (EC 433-436 PEC 401-402)

164.

B. This patient has signs and symptoms of a stroke. You would not suspect a traumatic brain injury unless the patient has fallen or experienced a traumatic incident recently. This patient awoke with these symptoms, which should cause you to suspect a medical problem rather than a traumatic injury. Hypoglycemia may present with all of the signs and symptoms except unequal pupils. (EC 433-436 PEC 401-402)

ALLERGIES 4.5

165.

B. During an allergic reaction, sympathetic discharge in addition to the hypoxia will result in an increased heart rate. Urticaria is hives and pruritis is itching, the hallmark sign and symptom of allergic reaction. (4-5.1) (EC 447 PEC 425-430)

166.

D. During an allergic reaction, the release of histamine and chemical mediators will cause edema of the airway, increased mucus production, and bronchial smooth muscle constriction. (4-5.4) (EC 445, 447-448 PEC 423-424, 425, 430-431)

167.

A. This patient is exhibiting signs and symptoms of a severe allergic reaction or anaphylaxis. This patient needs aggressive airway management, and ventilatory support is necessary as a primary concern. Contacting ALS is important; however, you must keep airway and ventilation management as a primary concern. (4-5.3) (EC 445, 447-448 PEC 425, 430-431)

168.

C. This patient is exhibiting signs of a mild reaction including the urticaria and pruritis. This patient could advance to a more severe reaction, so constant reassessment of the airway, breathing, and circulation will be necessary during transport. Without respiratory or cardiovascular system involvement, there is no need to administer the epinephrine. Once it is evident that the respiratory system or cardiovascular system is involved, do not delay epinephrine administration. (4-5.2) (EC 448 PEC 430-435)

169.

A. A mild reaction can rapidly deteriorate to severe anaphylaxis involving severe respiratory compromise and cardiovascular collapse. (4-5.7) (EC 445, 447, 448 PEC 423-424, 426, 428)

170.

A. Tachycardia is a common sign even in mild reaction. The tachycardia could be caused by the reaction or by the anxiety that the patient may be experiencing. Likewise, urticaria and flushed skin are found in mild reactions. Hypotension indicates cardiovascular compromise and the immediate need for epinephrine administration. (4-5.1) (EC 447 PEC 425-430)

171.

B. Anaphylactic shock is characterized by cardiovascular collapse, which includes hypoperfusion and subsequent decreased level of consciousness; nasal flaring and tachypnea are signs of respiratory distress. Hemiparesis (weakness to one side of the body) is seen in stroke and head injured patients. (4-5.2) (EC 448 EC 430-435)

172.

C. The high-pitched sounds are stridorous respirations. Stridor indicates obstruction of the upper airway, usually from swelling of the larynx in anaphylaxis. The patient needs rapid and aggressive airway management to include endotracheal intubation. (4-5.3) (EC 445, 447-448 PEC 425, 430-431)

173.

D. Closely assess the airway of the patient with an allergic reaction. Stridor or crowing sounds indicate significant swelling to the upper airway. A swollen tongue and additional signs of anaphylaxis may also be present. (4-5.4) (EC 445, 447-448 PEC 423-424, 425, 430-431)

174.

D. Use of and the administration of the epinephrine auto-injector requires either an off-line or on-line order from medical control. The medication is prescribed to the patient. It is an intramuscular injection. (4-5.6) (EC 448, 451, 452 PEC 432, 434)

175.

A. If the patient is suffering from a mild allergic reaction without respiratory compromise or signs of shock, do not administer epinephrine by auto-injector. Treatment includes high-flow oxygen, placing the patient in a position of comfort, completing your assessment, and transporting the patient. (4-5.7) (EC 445, 447, 448 PEC 423-424, 426, 428)

176.

A. You may need to force air past the swollen laryngeal tissue using the BVM by providing positive pressure ventilation. Delivering ventilation may become difficult due to the high resistance. Deactivating the pop-off valve on the BVM may help deliver adequate ventilation. The airway is compromised due to swelling of laryngeal tissue; thus inserting an airway adjuncts, such as the OPA and NPA, are of little help. (4-5.2) (EC 448 PEC 430-445)

177.

C. The correct administration procedure for a prescribed epinephrine auto-injector is to (1) firmly place the auto-injector against the patient's thigh halfway between the knee and the waist, and (2) hold the injector in place until all of the drug is delivered. The injector will deliver the correct dose automatically if left in place until empty. (4-5.5) (EC 451-453 PEC 434)

178.

C. The possible side effects to the administration of epinephrine are increased heart rate, pale skin, dizziness, chest pain, headache, nausea, vomiting, and anxiousness. You should advise your patient of these possible side effects when administering the drug. (4-5.5) (EC 451-453 PEC 434)

179.

A. There are no contraindications to administration of epinephrine by auto-injector in the severe anaphylactic patient. Never deliver a half dose to any patient, since the auto-injector will automatically deliver the adult a dose of 0.3 mg. Infants and children are prescribed epinephrine auto-injectors that deliver a dose of 0.15 mg. Stridor is an indication that the anaphylactic patient's airway is becoming compromised. Epinephrine by auto-injector is indicated. (4-5.5) (EC 451-453 PEC 434)

POISONING/OVERDOSE 4.6

180.
B. Unequal pupils may indicate a brain injury from a stroke or trauma. Patients with poisoning or an overdose may have dilated or constricted pupils; however, the pupils remain equal. (4-6.2) (EC 459, 461, 465, 466, 468, 471, 472, 474, 476 PEC 443-444, 448, 449-451, 455-459)

181.
D. Many patients that have overdosed on medications or are poisoned can not maintain their airway. Your first concern is to open and maintain the patient's airway. Positioning and the use of airway adjuncts like the nasopharyngeal airway or the oropharyngeal airway may be necessary to maintain an open airway. (4-6.5) (EC 466, 467, 473, 476 PEC 442-459)

182.
B. You must immediately provide positive pressure ventilation to any patient with respirations that become inadequate. (4-6.4) (EC 465, 466, 469, 473, 476-477 PEC 444-447, 448, 450, 451, 453, 454, 455-459)

183.
C. A patient who has overdosed on blood pressure medication is a good candidate for activated charcoal. Activated charcoal can be used up to 4 hours after ingestion of some medications. Activated charcoal is contraindicated in liquid bleach and ammonia. Activated charcoal is an adsorbent that is used in ingested poisonings, not inhalation. (4-6.6) (EC 462-464 PEC 446)

184.
C. Activated charcoal is very porous; thus, it adsorbs the poison and inhibits the absorption into the body. Some poisons have slow absorption rates that allow activated charcoal to be used up to 4 hours after ingestion. (4-6.6) (EC 462-464 PEC 446)

185.
D. The routes of entry into the human body include ingestion, inhalation, injection, and absorption. (4-6.1) (EC 460 PEC 440)

186.
C. The medication is absorbed under the tongue in the very vascular oral mucosa. (4-6.1) (EC 460 PEC 440)

187.
B. An injection is the mode of entry of a substance through a break in the skin. The break can be caused by a stinger, needle, or being bitten. (4-6.1) (EC 460 PEC 440)

188.
C. Dry powders should be brushed off before the area is irrigated. Many chemicals are inactive in the powder form, but are activated, or become more activated, when they come into contact with water, creating a reaction that will increase the heat and extend the burn. (4-6.4) (EC 465, 466, 469, 473, 476-477 PEC 444-447, 448, 450, 451, 453, 454, 455-459)

189.
D. The first priority for the EMT is always scene safety. The scene in this case is obviously unsafe because of the leak. The EMT's job is not to extricate the patient. This job needs to be performed by trained personnel with specialized equipment. (4-6.4) (EC 465, 466, 469, 473, 476-477 PEC 444-447, 448, 450, 451, 453, 454, 455-459)

190.
B. The patient should be placed in the lateral recumbent position to prevent aspiration of secretions, vomitus, blood, and other substances. (4-6.5) (EC 466, 467, 473, 476 PEC 442-459)

191.
C. Whenever you have a question concerning an overdose or toxicology, you should contact the poison control center. It provides the most updated information. (4-6.9) (EC 459, 461, 462, 463, 464, 465, 476 PEC 440, 444, 445, 446, 453)

192.
D. All overdose patients should be transported to be seen by a physician because of the multiple problems that can occur. (4-6.3) (EC 476-477 PEC 444-447, 448, 450, 451, 453, 454, 455-459)

193.
B. Treatment of this patient includes maintaining a patent airway, insertion of a nasopharyngeal airway, and providing oxygen therapy or positive pressure ventilation, depending on the respiratory status. The EMT-B should never give anything by mouth to a patient who has an altered level of consciousness who cannot protect his own airway. This would lead to aspiration of the substance. (4-6.3) (EC 476-477 PEC 444-447, 448, 450, 451, 453, 454, 455-459)

194.

B. Airway control, reassessment if required, and the administration of oxygen are essential treatments for the overdose patient. The administration of activated charcoal may or may not be indicated. Charcoal is contraindicated if the patient has an altered mental status or if the patient has swallowed bleach, ammonia, or hydrochloric acid. (4-6.8) (EC 462-464 PEC 445)

195.

A. Activated charcoal is also known as SuperChar, InstaChar, Actidose, and Liqui-Char, not CharMed. (4-6.6) (EC 462-464 PEC 446)

196.

A. Activated charcoal is only useful for poisonings that occur by ingestion. (4-6.6) (EC 462-464 PEC 446)

197.

C. The contraindications for the use of activated charcoal include the patient who has an altered mental status, has swallowed acids or alkalis (hydrochloric acid, bleach, ammonia, ethanol), or is unable to swallow. (4-6.6) (EC 462-464 PEC 446)

198.

B. Activated charcoal is available as a powder (not recommended for field use) and pre-mixed in water. The bottle contains 12.5 grams of activated charcoal. (4-6.6) (EC 462-464 PEC 446)

199.

A. The usual adult dose is 25 to 50 grams and for a child it is 12.5 to 25 grams. The adult and child dose is 1 gram per kilogram of body weight. (4-6.6) (EC 462-464 PEC 446)

200.

B. Activated charcoal will settle on the bottom of the container. For this reason it should be shaken well or mixed prior to administration. It should never be administered without prior medical direction. Because of its appearance, the patient may be more willing to drink it if he can't see it. Use an opaque container and have the patient drink through a straw. (4-6.6) (EC 462-464 PEC 446)

201.

A. Activated charcoal adsorbs poisons in the stomach and prevents an absorption in the small intestine. Activated charcoal is extremely porous. (4-6.8) (EC 462-464 PEC 445)

202.

C. The most common side effect of activated charcoal is blackened stool. Nausea and vomiting may also occur, especially in a patient who is already nauseated. If the patient vomits after the administration of activated charcoal, contact medical control and request permission to repeat the dose. (4-6.6) (EC 462-464 PEC 446)

203.

D. Early contact is required to provide the most current treatment for the poisoned or overdosed patient. Orders are required to administer activated charcoal. Early contact also allows the receiving facility to prepare for the patient's arrival. (4-6.9) (EC 459, 461, 462, 463, 464, 465, 476 PEC 440, 444, 445, 446, 453)

204.

C. It is important to determine if the patient is suffering from a medical condition or the effects of drugs and/or alcohol. Many medical conditions can mimic the effect of drugs and alcohol. Search the area immediately around the patient for evidence of drug or alcohol use. (4-6.2) (EC 459, 461, 465, 466, 468, 471, 472, 474, 476 PEC 443-444, 448, 449-451, 455-459)

205.

A. Phencyclidine is also known as PCP. PCP patients may become agitated and enraged if this technique is utilized. The "Talk Down Technique" includes making the patient feel welcome, identifying yourself clearly, reassuring the patient, helping the patient verbalize what is taking place, repeating simple concrete statements, and forewarning the patient of actions to be taken. (4-6.3) (EC 476-477 PEC 444-447, 448, 450, 451, 453, 454, 455-459)

ENVIRONMENTAL 4.7

206.

D. The majority of heat lost through the human body is from the head, feet, and hands through radiation. (4-7.1) (EC 483 PEC 495-497)

207.

C. Water conducts heat away from the human body 240 times quicker than any other mechanism. (4-7.1) (EC 483 PEC 495-497)

208.

B. Signs of early hypothermia include shivering, muscle cramps, and rapid heart rate. Bradycardia occurs later in hypothermia with more severe decreases in body core temperature. (4-7.2) (EC 484-489 PEC 497-506, 507)

209.

A. The core body temperature will drop 25 to 30 times faster because the body is in contact with cold water molecules. The body's temperature will cool to that of the temperature of the ambient environment around it, in this case, the water temperature. (4-7.1) (EC 483 PEC 495-497)

210.

D. All the answers are true of the elderly, which places them at a greater risk for heat emergencies. (4-7.4) (EC 491-492 PEC 506, 510-515)

211.

D. This patient is presenting with signs showing that the body's compensatory mechanisms have shut down. This patient can be classified as having heat stroke. The patient needs rapid cooling to prevent cellular breakdown due to the increased body temperature. (4-7.4) (EC 491-492 PEC 506, 510-515)

212.

A. This patient shows all the signs of a possible near drowning or submersion accident. To the patient's benefit, the cool water temperature may have preserved the brain tissues from extensive injury. It is very unlikely that a 16-year-old would suffer a myocardial infarction. (4-7.6) (EC 493 PEC 529, 532, 538-540)

213.

C. All patients that have been involved in a submersion incident or near drowning need to be transported and evaluated in the emergency department. Explain the consequences of pneumonia, pulmonary edema, respiratory failure, and even death to the patient. (4-7.7) (EC 494-495 PEC 528-529, 530-532, 534)

214.

D. Children suffer from environmental emergencies because of their proportionately larger body surface areas, body fat storages, and the inability to dress for the climate. (4-7.1) (EC 483 PEC 495-497)

215.

B. The hypothermic patient should be handled very gently to prevent ventricular fibrillation, which may be caused by rough handling. Don't rub or massage the patient's arms or legs. This may force cold venous blood into the heart, resulting in cardiac arrest. If ventilation is required, avoid hyperventilation; this may cause further cardiac compromise and cool the patient faster if in a cold environment. Only 1 set of 3 defibrillations should be provided if the patient is in cardiac arrest. A cold heart does not respond well to defibrillation or drug therapy. (4-7.5) (EC 491-492 PEC 513-516)

216.

C. If you are unable to obtain a pulse and there are no respirations, but patient movement is detected, delay CPR and the use of the AED. Pulses are very difficult to find in hypothermic patients. You should immediately begin positive pressure ventilation. (4-7.3) (EC 485-490 PEC 504-506, 508-509)

217.

B. The body temperature should be increased slowly. Add heat to the patient gradually and gently. The patient's body temperature should not be increased more than 1 degree F per hour. (4-7.3) (EC 485-490 PEC 504-505, 508-509)

218.

B. Instruct the patient to remain as calm and immobile as possible with just enough effort to remain afloat. Lift the patient from the water in a horizontal or supine position. Remove the wet clothing as quickly and gently as possible to prevent further heat loss and ventricular fibrillation. (4-7.3) (EC 485-490 PEC 504-505, 508-509)

219.

B. Correct management includes the removal of jewelry. Avoid massaging the affected area and the application of salves or ointments. Blisters that are present should be left intact and should not be broken. (4-7.3) (EC 485-490 PEC 504-505, 508-509)

220.

D. Rewarming of localized frozen tissue should generally be avoided unless you have a long or delayed transport. If performed, use water at 100–110 degrees F. Never use dry heat because it is too difficult to control the temperature. Rewarming of tissue is very painful, and medical control will commonly want the patient to have an analgesic. (4-7.3) (EC 485-490 PEC 504-505, 508-509)

221.

C. Remove the stinger by scraping against it with the edge of a credit card or knife. Lower the injection site slightly below the level of the heart. Clean the site with a soap solution or a mild cleansing agent. The application of cold packs may help to reduce swelling at the injection site. Don't use cold on snakebites or marine animal bites. (4-7.3) (EC 485-490 PEC 504-505, 508-509)

222.

D. Begin cooling the patient by moving the patient into the shade or the back of the air-conditioned ambulance. This would be followed by removal of clothing; oxygen administration; and rapid cooling with water, cold packs, or other cooling techniques. (4-7.5) (EC 491-492 PEC 513-516)

223.

A. This patient would require rapid transport. Cooling should be continued en route to the hospital. Maintain an airway and monitor the respirations closely. Provide positive pressure ventilation if necessary. (4-7.5) (EC 491-492 PEC 513-516)

224.

D. The patient is suffering from a heat emergency. This is most likely to occur when the temperature is greater than 90 degrees F with a relative humidity of greater than 75%. (4-7.4) (EC 491-492 PEC 506, 510-515)

225.

B. Family history is not a predisposing factor that increases the risk of hypothermia. A person's age is a major factor in the risk of hypothermia. The young and old are more likely to suffer from hypothermia. Medical conditions such as head injury, spinal cord injury, stroke, diabetes, and a heart condition can increase the likelihood of hypothermia. Alcohol dilates blood vessels and interferes with the normal thermal regulator mechanisms, which can increase the patient's risk of hypothermia. (4-7.2) (EC 484-489 PEC 497-506, 507)

226.

C. Shivering and goose bumps are the body's first reactions to a decrease in body temperature found in the first stage of hypothermia. A decrease in the heart rate and respirations is the fourth stage of hypothermia. The second stage of hypothermia involves a decrease in fine, and then gross, motor function. The fine motor function may be as subtle as a patient's inability to follow simple commands. As the hypothermia continues, the patient may not be able to move the arms or legs. (4-7.2) (EC 484-489 PEC 497-506, 507)

227.

B. This patient should be placed in a supine position with the feet elevated approximately 8 to 12 inches. This will increase the blood flow to the brain. If the patient is responsive and not nauseated, administer a half glass of water every 15 minutes. (4-7.5) (EC 491-492 PEC 513-516)

228.

A. Cold packs should not be applied to the injection site of snakebites or marine animal bites. Cold packs may increase tissue damage at the injection site of a snake bite. Cold packs increase pain considerably at the injection site of marine animal bites. Use heat packs instead of cold packs to treat marine animal stings. (4-7.5) (EC 491-492 PEC 513-516)

229.

B. The stinger should be removed. Leaving the stinger and venom sack in place will result in an increased amount of venom entering the body. Bees, after stinging, will tear their bodies from the stinger and the venom sack. This sack, if not removed, continues to pulsate, pumping venom into the patient. Remove the sack and stinger by scraping a knife or credit card edge against it. Squeezing the sack with tweezers or your fingers while attempting to remove it will force more venom from the sack into the patient. (4-7.8) (EC 500-506 PEC 517-518)

230.

C. This patient is breathing inadequately and should receive immediate ventilatory support by positive pressure ventilation. (4-7.8) (EC 500-506 PEC 517-518)

231.

A. You should immediately obtain an order from medical direction to administer epinephrine by auto-injector. Delaying this action may cause the patient's condition to deteriorate further. Unless you have off-line orders for the administration of epinephrine by auto-injector, you must obtain the order prior to administering the drug. This patient is having a severe allergic reaction (anaphylaxis) and should receive epinephrine as quickly as possible. (4-7.8) (EC 500-506 PEC 517-518)

232.

B. Common side effects of epinephrine are increased heart rate, pale skin, dizziness, chest pain, headache, nausea, vomiting, excitability, and anxiousness. (EC 500-506 PEC 435)

BEHAVIORAL 4.8

233.

B. A person's personality is just one aspect of his or her behavior. Depressions and anxiety are classifications of behaviors. (4-8.1) (EC 512 PEC 545)

234.

C. Society has classified acceptable or "normal" behavior for many situations. Any deviation outside of the norms may be considered abnormal. (4-8.1) (EC 512 PEC 545)

235.

D. There are many different etiologies including oxygen deficits, altered glucose levels, and other deficiencies that could lead to abnormal behavior. Be sure to assess the patient carefully and check for an organic cause for the behavior. (4-8.2) (EC 512-513 PEC 545)

236.

D. Patients that want to hurt themselves often use extreme measures to do so. Others may place themselves in high-risk situations. Report this information to the emergency department staff. (4-8.4) (EC 515-516 PEC 546-547)

237.

C. A leading cause of suicide is depression over the loss of a loved one. (4-8.3) (EC 515-516 PEC 545-547)

238.

B. Approximately 80% of patients that have committed suicide have made a failed previous attempt. This is one reason why all patients who have suicidal tendencies should be transported. (4-8.4) (EC 515-516 PEC 546-547)

239.

C. The EMT-B should be concerned that the patient may have attempted suicide. You should directly ask the patient if he or she was attempting to kill himself or herself. (4-8.4) (EC 515-516 PEC 546-547)

240.

B. Patients who have constructed a plan on how to kill themselves are much more likely to carry out their intentions than are those who have no plan. (4-8.4) (EC 515-516 PEC 546-547)

241.

B. When a patient informs you that he or she has thought of harming himself or herself and has formulated a plan, you should become highly concerned for your safety and that of the patient's, especially when a gun is involved in the plan. Reassess the scene safety and retreat if necessary. (4-8.7) (EC 517 PEC 547)

242.

C. Whenever any scene becomes unsafe you should immediately remove yourself from it. Contact law enforcement to handle the weapon. Once the scene is secure, enter it to manage the patient. (4-8.7) (EC 517 PEC 547)

243.

B. Patients over the age of 40 are more likely to commit suicide. The elderly commonly suffer severe depression and are very likely to commit suicide. Depression in an elderly patient is actually considered a serious emergency. (4-8.4) (EC 515-516 PEC 546-547)

244.

D. When assessing this type of patient, have adequate personnel to help restrain the patient, if necessary. Make sure the scene is free from potential weapons and always have available exit routes. (4-8.6) (EC 514, 515-516, 517 PEC 548-551)

245.

B. Any patient who is a suicide risk should never be left alone. Constant supervision to guarantee your safety and the patient's safety is a priority. (4-8.4) (EC 515-516 PEC 546-547)

246.

B. Many people who are incarcerated for crimes, some very minor, are likely to commit suicide due to the social impact and their reputation. (4-8.4) (EC 515-516 PEC 546-547)

247.

D. All of the factors can cause aggression. Be sure not to rule out an organic cause of aggression. (4-8.6) (EC 514, 515-516, 517 PEC 548-551)

248.

B. The job of the EMT-B is not to be judgmental but rather impartial. You should ask about the patient's intention of killing himself or herself. (4-8.4) (EC 515-516 PEC 546-547)

249.

B. Once a patient is restrained, the restraints should be left on. The patient may be calm one minute and revert back to the aggressive behavior the next. (4-8.7) (EC 517 PEC 547)

ABDOMINAL PAIN

250.

D. Patients that are suffering from acute abdominal pain try to stay completely still and quiet to decrease the pain. Drawing the knees to the chest releases some of the tension on the abdominal muscles and may slightly reduce the pain. (EC 408-410 PEC 482-486)

251.

B. The organs of the right upper quadrant include the liver, gallbladder, and part of the large intestine. The spleen and pancreas are located in the left upper quadrant. (EC 406-407 PEC 479-481)

252.

A. Irritation under the diaphragm can cause referred pain that can present as shoulder pain. (EC 408 PEC 482)

253.

B. The pulsatile mass, tearing pain radiating to the lower back, and the absent femoral pulses are signs indicative of an abdominal aneurysm that is currently rupturing. This is a dire emergency where the treatment is oxygen and rapid transport to an appropriate facility for emergency surgery. (EC 408 PEC 490)

254.

C. Cholecystitis or inflammation of the gallbladder is commonly precipitated by ingesting food high in saturated fat. The green vomitus is likely due to the obstruction of the bile duct. (EC 406-416 PEC 488)

255.

D. Referred pain is pain that is felt in a body part removed from its point of origin. Pain associated with abdominal and other conditions may be referred or felt in other areas of the body. This is associated with nerve tracts and their proximity when entering the spinal cord. (EC 408 PEC 482)

256.

C. Encephalitis involves the head. Causes of abdominal pain include pancretitis, cholecystitis, hernia, ulcer, and abdominal aortic aneurysm. (EC 406-416 PEC 488-490)

257.

C. The correct position for a patient suffering from an acute abdomen with signs of hypoperfusion (shock) is supine with feet elevated. (EC 406-416 PEC 486)

258.

B. When treating a patient for an acute abdomen without signs of hypoperfusion (shock), you should place the patient in the position of most comfort. Typically, patients with an acute abdomen will position themselves bent over at the waist with their knees bent and drawn up towards their chest. Often this position reduces the tension on the abdominal muscles, thus reducing pain. (EC 406-416 PEC 483-486)

259.

B. Never give the acute abdominal patient anything by mouth. These patients need to be prepared to go to surgery if necessary. Food and liquid may cause vomiting after administration of the anesthesia which could lead to aspiration. (EC 406-416 PEC 483-491)

OB-GYN 4.9

260.

C. The uterus is a hollow muscle that houses the fetus until birth. (4-9.1) (EC 526-539 PEC 561-562)

261.

B. The placenta is the organ that allows for nourishment of the fetus. (4-9.1) (EC 526-539 PEC 561-562)

262.

B. Contractions under 2 minutes and lasting 30 to 90 seconds, along with the patient's urgency to move her bowels (caused by the baby placing pressure on the rectum) are all signs that the child is ready to deliver. However, you would always check for crowning to determine the time urgency of the delivery. (4-9.4) (EC 528-529, 530-531 PEC 567-568)

263.

C. The first clamp should be placed approximately 6 inches from the infant's abdomen. (4-9.10) (EC 537-538 PEC 572-573, 578, 579)

264.

D. The birthing process involves many different body fluids so the minimum body substance isolation precautions include mask, gown, gloves, and eye protection. (4-9.7) (EC 531 PEC 569)

265.

B. The second clamp should be placed approximately 3 inches from the first clamp. (4-9.10) (EC 537, 538 PEC 572-573, 578, 579)

266.

D. The inverted pyramid for neonatal resuscitation involves drying, warming, suctioning, stimulating, providing blow by oxygen, positive pressure ventilation, and then CPR. (4-9.13) (EC 536-537 PEC 580-581, 582, 583)

267.

C. If the infant's heart rate drops below 60 bpm with positive pressure ventilation, chest compressions should be initiated. (4-9.13) (EC 536-537 PEC 580-581, 582, 583)

268.

B. Meconium is fecal matter excreted by the infant due to severe distress. Meconium aspiration carries a high mortality rate. The EMT-B must recognize this problem and treat it accordingly. (4-9.16) (EC 528, 545 PEC 575-576)

269.

C. Meconium is the end result of fetal distress caused by decreased oxygen to the fetus or a prolonged labor. (4-9.16) (EC 528, 545 PEC 575, 576)

270.

D. Immediate suctioning of the infant's airway takes precedence over ALL other procedures. (4-9.9) (EC 532, 534 PEC 571-572, 578, 579)

271.

A. The perineum is the area of tissue between the vagina and anus. This area can tear during a rapid delivery or when the infant is large. The perineum is the area where the episiotomy is done to facilitate delivery. (4-9.1) (EC 526-539 PEC 561-562)

272.

B. The foul smell is from the meconium, and the airway needs to be suctioned immediately. (4-9.16) (ECE 528, 545 PEC 575-576)

273.

D. Infants may respond quickly to short periods of ventilation. Once the ventilation is determined to be adequate, stop ventilation and reassess. (4-9.13) (EC 536-537 PEC 580-581, 582, 583)

274.

A. The ratio for infants is 120 compressions to 30 ventilations. The ratio is much higher than the ratio for adults so care must be taken to perform this procedure properly. (4-9.13) (EC 536-537 PEC 580-581, 582, 583)

275.

D. The correct depth is ⅓ the depth of the chest. (4-9.13) (EC 536-537 PEC 580-581, 582-583)

276.

A. Reassess the infant every 30 seconds to see if the infant is responding to the treatment or is getting worse. (4-9.13) (EC 536-537 PEC 580-581, 582, 583)

277.

D. A condition that occurs during the third trimester of pregnancy is called supine hypotensive syndrome. It occurs as a result of the combined weight of the fetus and uterus compressing the inferior vena cava. This pressure obstructs the blood return to the heart via the inferior vena cava while the patient is lying supine, causing hypotension. (4-9.5) (EC 545-548 PEC 565-566, 569-574, 577)

278.

B. Save and transport any passed tissue for examination by hospital personnel. Packing sanitary napkins or pads into the vagina is inappropriate. If a pad becomes soaked with blood it should be replaced. If bleeding is excessive it can become a life-threatening emergency. Carefully evaluate the patient for signs and symptoms of shock. (4-9.5) (EC 545-548 PEC 565-566, 569-574, 577)

279.

D. A miscarriage or spontaneous abortion can occur for many different reasons. Delivery of the fetus occurs before the fetus is viable. Viability is usually considered to begin in the 28th week of pregnancy. Signs and symptoms include cramplike lower abdominal pain, moderate to severe vaginal bleeding, and passage of tissue or blood clots. (4-9.5) (EC 545-548 PEC 565-566, 569-574, 577)

280.

C. BSI precautions are required, including mask, gown, and eye protection. Never hold the mother's legs together to delay delivery. Do not allow the mother to use the bathroom. This is likely a result of the infant's head moving down the birth canal and pressing against the patient's rectum. (4-9.7) (EC 531 PEC 569)

281.

C. Recommended equipment for an obstetric kit includes surgical scissors, hemostats or cord clamps, umbilical tape, bulb syringe, towels, gauze sponges, sterile gloves, infant blanket, individually wrapped sanitary napkins, large plastic bag, and germicidal wipes. A bag-valve-mask is not a part of the OB kit. (4-9.2) (EC 529-530 PEC 569)

282.

B. As soon as the head is delivered, support the head and suction. Suction the mouth first and then the nose. Compress the bulb syringe and suction two or three times to remove fluid and secretions. Insert the tip 1.0 to 1.5 inches into the infant's mouth. Avoid touching the back of the mouth with the tip of the bulb syringe. (4-9.9) (EC 532, 534 PEC 571-572, 578-579)

283.

D. Excessive pressure should be avoided over the fontanel or soft spot. Excessive pressure should not be used for any delivery procedure. (4-9.9) (EC 532, 534 PEC 571-572, 578, 579)

284.

B. The EMT-B should check the position of the umbilical cord and determine if the cord is wrapped around the infant's neck. The creation of a sterile field should have been accomplished prior to the delivery of the head. Avoid deep suctioning of the infant's mouth as this may result in bradycardia. You will have plenty of time after delivery to record the time of birth. (4-9.8) (EC 532, 534 PEC 569-574, 578, 579)

285.

C. Up to 500 cc's is normal. If blood loss is excessive, administer oxygen and provide uterine massage. (4-9.11) (EC 538, 539 PEC 572-573, 578, 579)

286.

D. Massage of the mother's uterus is provided to control excessive bleeding that may occur following delivery. Uterine massage helps to stimulate contractions, which reduces uterine size. This will reduce bleeding. (4-9.11) (EC 538, 539 PEC 572-573, 578, 579)

287.

C. In multiple births (twins, triplets) the infants may share a placenta or have separate ones. (4-9.15) (EC 543 PEC 575)

288.

D. In multiple births, about ⅓ of all the deliveries of the second infant are breech. A breech delivery is one in which the fetal buttocks or the lower extremities are the first to present in the birth canal. (4-9.15) (EC 543 PEC 575)

289.

C. Ensuring the adequacy of the airway, breathing, and circulation always is a priority treatment for all patients. Oxygen administration is the next priority. This is followed by managing bleeding from the vagina. Transport is the last step. (4-9.12) (EC 538, 540 PEC 573, 578, 579)

290.

C. The pregnant trauma patient is able to compensate for blood loss because of an overall increase in body fluid. Late pregnancy patients are at greater risk for injuries to the uterus, liver, spleen or rupture of the mother's diaphragm, even at relatively low speeds. Potential fetal injuries may occur as well. The mother was unrestrained and the potential for injury is present. The best answer presented is to recognize the compensatory capability of the pregnant patient. Encourage the patient to seek med-

ical care and attention. (4-9.5) (EC 545-548 PEC 565-566, 569-574, 577)

291.

D. Determining if any over-the-counter medications are taken is an appropriate question, just not as important as determining the pain characteristics. Evaluation of the quality of the pain will allow you to determine if the patient is experiencing labor pains or pain related to the accident. (4-9.6) (EC 531-532 PEC 569)

292.

C. This patient should be evaluated for signs of crowning. The signs and symptoms presented may indicate immediate delivery. If the patient is crowning, prepare for delivery. (4-9.4) (EC 528-529, 530-531 PEC 567-568)

293.

C. You should suction the mouth and nose of the infant as soon as the head is delivered and prior to delivery of the rest of the body. After the torso is delivered the newborn may breathe deeply due to the chest not being constricted in the birth canal. Suctioning the mouth and nose prior to delivery of the torso will help prevent aspiration of the fluids in the mouth and nose. (4-9.9) (EC 532, 534 PEC 571-572, 578, 579)

294.

B. You should suction the mouth prior to suctioning the nose. Suctioning the mouth first will prevent aspiration of fluid. Placing the bulb syringe into place and then compressing the bulb will force the fluid into the lungs. By advancing the tip of the bulb syringe too deeply into the pharynx, the newborn may become bradycardic. Suction the mouth and nose prior to stimulating the newborn to remove all secretions prior to spontaneous breathing. (4-9.9) (EC 532, 534 PEC 571-572, 578, 579)

295.

D. The pregnant patient who is near full term may experience hypotensive syndrome when lying on her back. To prevent this condition, place the patient supine with her right hip elevated. (4-9.3) (EC 531, 545-548 PEC 563-567)

296.

D. Your first priority is to establish an airway by suctioning and positioning. (4-9.13) (EC 536-537 PEC 580-581, 582, 583)

297.

D. You should avoid applying pressure to the infant's fontanel. The fontanel is the soft area on the infant's head. Gentle pressure can be applied horizontally to prevent an explosive delivery. (4-9.9) (EC 532, 534 PEC 571-572, 578, 579)

298.

A. When the placenta appears, grasp it and gently glide it from the vagina. Under no circumstances should you pull the placenta from the vagina. Do not delay transport while waiting on delivery of the placenta. Transport the placenta to the hospital; do not dispose of it. The physician will need to examine it. (4-9.11) (EC 538, 539 PEC 572-573, 578, 579)

299.

A. The only time it is permissible to place your gloved hand into the mother's vagina is when you encounter a prolapsed cord. A prolapsed cord is a true emergency that can result in injury or death of the infant. When you encounter a prolapsed cord, you should insert your gloved hand into the vagina and gently push the presenting part away from the pulsating cord. (4-9.14) (EC 540-543 PEC 574-575)

300.

A. The patient that presents with a limb presentation should be placed in a supine position with the head lower than the rest of her body with the hips elevated. This position will increase the gravity and slow the progress of the fetus through the birth canal. Administer oxygen and transport immediately. Never push or pull a presenting limb into the vagina. Never try to manipulate the fetus into the correct position by inserting your hand into the vagina. (4-9.14) (EC 540-543 PEC 574-575)

301.

C. The infant born before the 38th week of pregnancy is considered premature. Infants weighing less than 5½ pounds at birth are considered premature. Premature babies appear smaller, skinnier, and will have red and wrinkled skin. Premature babies usually will have a single crease across the soles of their feet. The premature infant will have fine silky hair and very small breast nodules. The premature infant will not have cartilage in the outer ear. (4-9.17) (EC 544 PEC 576)

302.

B. This infant was born before the 38th week of gestation, which makes the infant premature. Premature infants need special care since their lungs and organs are not fully developed. Premature infants must be kept warm by using warmed blankets or a plastic bubble-bag swaddle. Never forcefully direct oxygen into the premature infant's face; hold the end of the oxygen tubing approximately ½ inch above the infant's mouth and nose. You should suction secretions gently, using the bulb syringe. To prevent heat loss, cover the premature infant's head, leaving the face exposed. (4-9.17) (EC 544 PEC 576)

303.

B. Place this patient in a supine position with her hips elevated. This position will help to keep the fetus from putting pressure on the cord. All of the other positions listed may increase pressure on the cord. (4-9.14) (EC 540-543 PEC 574-575)

304.

A. You should place your gloved hand into the vagina and gently push the presenting part of the fetus back and away from the pulsating cord. This is an acceptable time for you to place your gloved hand into the vagina. (4-9.14) (EC 540-543 PEC 574-575)

305.

C. This patient's breathing has become inadequate. You must immediately establish an airway and provide positive pressure ventilation. (4-9.13) (EC 536-537 PEC 580-581, 582, 583)

SEIZURE

306.

B. A seizure is a sudden and temporary alteration caused by the electrical discharge from active foci in the brain. (EC 430-433 PEC 416-419)

307.

D. The sequence of events starts with the aura, next the tonic phase lasting 15 to 20 seconds, then the clonic (tonic-clonic) phase lasting 30 seconds to 5 minutes, and finally the postictal phase, which lasts from 5 to 30 minutes. (EC 430-433 PEC 418)

308.

D. All the conditions can cause irritation to the neurons of the brain, which can trigger a seizure. (EC 430-433 PEC 410-421)

309.

C. Treatment for an actively seizing patient is supportive. Always protect the patient from harm, monitor the airway, suction if necessary. Apply oxygen, assist ventilation if necessary, and transport the patient. Never pry or force anything into the patient's mouth. This can cause further damage. (EC 430-433 PEC 416-419)

310.
C. Status epilepticus is a dire medical emergency. These patients need immediate medical intervention. (EC 430-433 PEC 412)

311.
B. During the tonic phase, the muscles become extremely rigid and the patient may arch his or her back. (EC 430-433 PEC 418)

312.
C. The tonic-clonic phase also referred to as only the clonic phase usually only lasts 30 seconds to 2 minutes. It is this period when the muscles alternate between rigidity and relaxation. (EC 430-433 PEC 418)

313.
A. The nasopharyngeal airway can be inserted in an actively seizing patient to provide a means of airway control without harming the patient. (EC 430-433 PEC 416-419)

314.
D. All of the medications are used to treat seizure disorders. (PEC 414)

315.
C. This condition is status epilepticus. This is a dire medical emergency that requires aggressive airway control and positive pressure ventilation with supplemental oxygen. The patient should be transported rapidly. (EC 430-433 PEC 412)

316.
C. Syncope usually begins in a standing position. The patient remembers feeling faint or lightheaded. The patient will commonly become responsive almost immediately after being placed supine. The seizure patient may remember an aura—an abnormal sound, odor, or visual disturbance—that may precede the seizure. (EC 436-439 PEC 416-417)

317.
C. The aura is a warning that a seizure is about to occur. This stage can present as a sound, twitch, or odor; some patients even experience an unusual taste that precedes the seizure. Some patients experience auras; however, many seizure patients do not. (EC 430-433 PEC 414)

318.
B. The violent and jerky seizure activity caused by alternating relaxation and contraction of muscles is known as the tonic-clonic (convulsion) phase. The aura precedes a seizure and may warn the patient of an upcoming seizure. The tonic phase is after the aura and causes the patient to fall to the ground. The patient's muscles become contracted and tense. The hypertonic phase results in severe muscle rigidity. The postictal phase is the recovery phase. The patient's mental status is altered; however, it progressively improves. (EC 430-433 PC 410-416)

319.
A. The postictal phase is known as the recovery phase. During this phase the patient's mental status may range from complete unresponsiveness to confusion. The patient's mental status improves with time. These patients appear exhausted. (EC 430-433 PEC 410-416)

320.
C. Syncope usually occurs when the patient is standing or the patient stands up from a sitting position. Syncope is caused by a lack of blood flow to the brain. This causes the brain to become deprived of oxygen, rendering the patient unconscious for a brief period. This brief period of unconsciousness is usually corrected once the patient falls to a horizontal position. (EC 436-439 PEC 416)

321.
B. The best position to place a patient who has experienced a syncopal episode is supine with the legs elevated. A supine position will allow more blood to flow to the brain, increasing cerebral oxygenation. The supine position will also allow you to visually inspect the airway and provide oxygen therapy. (EC 436-439 PEC 416)

322.
B. This emergency situation is most likely a syncopal episode. A syncopal episode usually occurs when the patient is in a standing position and usually resolves after the patient is placed in a horizontal position. The skin is usually moist and pale. This also improves when the patient is lying on the floor. (EC 436-439 PEC 416)

323.
D. A condition called Todd's paralysis may occur during the postictal phase following a tonic-clonic seizure. The weakness or paralysis will persist for a brief period of time and resolve itself. (EC 430-433 PEC 410-416)

324.
D. A febrile seizure that lasts longer than 15 minutes would be considered significant. This patient would require aggressive management. (EC 430-433 PEC 420)

325.
B. An aura is a warning symptom of a seizure. Auras may be auditory, visual, or olfactory, or an aura may be pain sensed in any area of the body. The abdominal pain in this patient is most likely an aura. (EC 430-433 PEC 414)

5 Trauma

module objectives

Questions in this module relate to D.O.T.
objectives 5-1.1 to 5-4.44.

1. Your patient has a laceration to the leg; the wound is bleeding heavily in a steady flow that is dark red. You suspect the patient is bleeding from a:
   A. capillary.
   B. artery.
   C. arteriole.
   D. vein.

2. Which of the following **best** describes arterial bleeding?
   A. dark red and flows steadily from wounds
   B. bright red, under high pressure, spurts
   C. oozing flow that usually clots spontaneously
   D. steady flow that is easily controlled due to pressure

3. Your adult patient has lost a large amount of blood and is in shock. He is breathing 20 times a minute with good air exchange. You should manage the patient by:
   A. administering oxygen by nasal cannula at 6 lpm.
   B. administering oxygen by non-rebreather mask at 15 lpm.
   C. administering positive pressure ventilation.
   D. administering oxygen by simple mask at 6 lpm.

4. Your patient is bleeding from a laceration to the lateral forearm. The artery or pressure point that should be utilized to control bleeding is the:
   A. ulna artery.
   B. radial artery.
   C. femoral artery.
   D. brachial artery.

5. A tourniquet should be:
   A. made of a narrow, flat material.
   B. covered with a bandage.
   C. used when direct pressure and pressure points fail.
   D. applied directly over a joint and tight enough to eliminate distal pulses.

6. If bleeding from the lower leg is not controlled with direct pressure, you should attempt to:
   A. utilize a pressure point.
   B. elevate the extremity.
   C. use a tourniquet.
   D. rapidly apply an air splint.

7. Internal bleeding from blunt trauma:
   A. is usually very obvious to identify.
   B. should be suspected with unexplained shock.
   C. never results in severe blood loss.
   D. can be ruled out if the abdomen is rigid.

8. Your patient presents with signs of severe hypoperfusion after falling from a tree. You do not find any signs of external bleeding; your best immediate treatment for this patient is to:
   A. remain on the scene to determine the exact injury site.
   B. provide immediate transport to the hospital.
   C. transport to the hospital only after ALS arrives.
   D. transport to the hospital if the blood pressure decreases.

9. Which of the following early signs would alert you that your 20-year-old patient may have internal bleeding from an assault?

    A. decreased blood pressure
    B. deep bradypneic breathing
    C. capillary refill that is 4 seconds
    D. thready pulse rate of 110

10. Which of the following is **not** a sign or symptom of shock?

    A. nausea and vomiting
    B. restlessness
    C. hot, dry skin
    D. marked thirst

11. The outermost layer of the skin that is composed of dead cells and contains the pigment granules is known as the:

    A. epidermis.
    B. endodermis.
    C. dermis.
    D. subcutaneous layer.

12. You are preparing to treat a patient with a soft tissue injury. Which action should be taken first?

    A. airway control
    B. oxygen administration
    C. BSI precautions
    D. bleeding control

13. A type of soft tissue injury that is caused by scraping, rubbing, or shearing away of the epidermis is called a(n):

    A. abrasion.
    B. puncture.
    C. avulsion.
    D. laceration.

14. Which type of dressing should be used to treat an open chest wound?

    A. water soaked gauze
    B. Vaseline gauze pad
    C. cotton trauma bandage
    D. nonocclusive dressing

15. Your patient has an open chest wound; the best method to secure the occlusive dressing should be:

    A. taping one side.
    B. taping two sides.
    C. taping three sides.
    D. taping all four sides.

16. The treatment for an open abdominal wound with an evisceration should include:

    A. replacing the abdominal organs.
    B. using an absorbent dressing.
    C. keeping the patient's leg flat.
    D. covering the dressing with a bulky material.

17. Your patient has been burned by a grease fire. Large blisters have formed; you recognize this as a:

    A. superficial burn.
    B. full thickness burn.
    C. partial thickness burn.
    D. first degree burn.

18. Your patient is suffering intense pain from a scald burn. The burn includes the epidermis, as well as portions of the dermis. This burn is classified as a:

    A. partial thickness burn.
    B. superficial burn.
    C. full thickness burn.
    D. partial eschar burn.

19. A partial thickness burn involves:

    A. the epidermis only.
    B. the epidermis and dermis.
    C. the dermis and muscle.
    D. the dermis, fat, and muscle.

20. A full thickness burn may appear:
    A. dry, hard, and leathery.
    B. slightly red with blisters.
    C. pink to red.
    D. red with blisters.

21. The classification of a burn that involves the epidermis, dermis and subcutaneous layers of the skin and often results in an eschar is a:
    A. first degree burn.
    B. full thickness burn.
    C. partial thickness burn.
    D. second degree burn.

22. In managing a full thickness burn, special emphasis should be placed upon:
    A. preventing further contamination and injury.
    B. removing clothing that has adhered to the area.
    C. leaving jewelry in the burned areas in place.
    D. calculation of the exact body surface area involved.

23. Which of the following is **inappropriate** treatment for the patient suffering from a full thickness burn?
    A. cover the area with a dry sterile dressing
    B. apply a sterile antiseptic burn ointment
    C. administer oxygen by non-rebreather mask
    D. conserve heat loss by covering the patient

24. Which of the following statements is **incorrect** pertaining to the application of pressure dressings?
    A. If blood soaks through, remove and replace dressing.
    B. Air splints can be used to apply pressure on dressing.
    C. Loss of a distal pulse indicates the dressing is too tight.
    D. The wound is covered with several bulky dressings.

25. Which of the following impaled objects may be removed in the prehospital setting?
    A. screwdriver embedded in the chest
    B. pitchfork impaled through the foot
    C. pencil impaled through the cheek
    D. knife embedded in the upper leg

26. When managing an electrical burn the EMT-B should:
    A. always attempt to remove the patient from the electrical source.
    B. check for a source and ground burn injury.
    C. never attempt CPR unless it is within 4 minutes of contact.
    D. quickly check the pulse, even if the patient is still in contact with the electrical source.

27. Your patient has suffered an electrical burn. Which of the following statements is **incorrect?**
    A. Patients with electrical burns may be treated with the AED and CPR.
    B. Treatment for a source wound is the same as for other thermal burns.
    C. Injury is usually limited to the area around the source and ground wounds.
    D. Patients with burns that appear insignificant are treated as critical injuries.

28. You are treating a patient with a painful swollen and deformed upper arm. You suspect which bone is injured?
    A. scapula
    B. carpals
    C. tibia
    D. humerus

29. A general rule for splinting is to:
    A. check the pulse, motor function, and sensation before splinting.

B. check the pulse and sensation before and after splinting.

C. check the pulse, motor function, and sensation after splinting.

D. check the pulse, motor function, and sensation before and after splinting.

30. Your patient was struck by a car while riding his bicycle; he complains of pain in his right upper arm and lower back. Which of the following treatments should **not** be performed after splinting the arm?

A. elevate the extremity

B. administer oxygen

C. apply cold packs

D. assess motor function

31. Your patient has fallen while skating and complains of pain and swelling to the elbow; you should:

A. immobilize the joint above the elbow joint only.

B. immobilize the joint above and below the elbow.

C. immobilize the bone above the elbow joint only.

D. immobilize the bones above and below the elbow.

32. Your patient has an obviously deformed, painful, and swollen injury to the tibia. The foot is cyanotic and lacks a pulse. The best immediate action for you to take is to:

A. transport immediately without applying a splint, and support the leg manually.

B. apply the splint to the leg in the position found and transport immediately.

C. make one attempt to align the extremity by applying gentle manual traction.

D. make up to three attempts to align the extremity by applying firm traction.

33. Which statement is **false** pertaining to splinting a painful, swollen, or deformed extremity?

A. Motor, sensory, and distal pulses are assessed both prior to and after splinting.

B. Both the above and below joints are immobilized when a long bone is injured.

C. Traction is applied to protruding bones until the bones retract below the skin.

D. A pulseless extremity is not aligned by traction if the injury involves the knee.

34. The nervous system that consists of the brain and spinal cord is known as the:

A. peripheral nervous system

B. central nervous system

C. voluntary nervous system

D. autonomic nervous system

35. The portion of the skeletal system that protects the brain is the:

A. vertebrae.

B. cranium.

C. basilar skull.

D. ischium.

36. Which of the following signs and symptoms of spinal injury is rarely seen?

A. numbness, weakness or tingling in the arms

B. pain without movement

C. obvious deformity of the spine

D. paralysis of the extremities

37. When performing the initial assessment on a patient with a suspected spine injury, you will open and maintain the airway by:

A. performing the cervical traction maneuver.

B. performing the lateral lift maneuver.

C. performing the head-tilt, chin-lift maneuver.

D. performing the jaw-thrust maneuver.

38. Placing a patient with a spinal injury on a long spine board is ideally performed by how many rescuers?
    A. two
    B. three
    C. four
    D. five

39. To size a cervical spine immobilization collar, measure the distance from the top of the shoulder to the:
    A. level of the larynx.
    B. bottom of the chin.
    C. level of C-7.
    D. bottom of the earlobe.

40. You arrive on the scene of an automobile crash and find your patient walking around the scene. The patient complains of neck pain; the correct way to immobilize this patient to minimize movement of the spine is to:
    A. use the standing long board technique.
    B. have the patient sit down on the long board.
    C. use the logrolling technique with a long board.
    D. place the short spinal device on the standing patient.

41. A short spine board is used to immobilize a:
    A. standing patient.
    B. supine patient.
    C. seated patient.
    D. rapid extrication patient.

42. Your patient has been critically injured in a vehicle crash. The patient's injuries are severe and he must be transported immediately. You should extricate the patient, using the:
    A. short spinal extrication device.
    B. rapid extrication technique.
    C. corset-type immobilization device.
    D. standing long board technique.

43. Rapid extrication is indicated in all of the following patient situations **except:**
    A. an unsafe scene.
    B. a stable patient.
    C. a patient blocking access to a critical patient.
    D. an unstable patient.

44. Which of the following cases would require you to remove a helmet?
    A. The patient has an altered mental status.
    B. The patient complains of head pain.
    C. The patient is in cardiac arrest.
    D. The patient complains of neck pain.

45. The two basic types of helmets are the:
    A. sports and motorcycle.
    B. OSHA and sports.
    C. construction and sports.
    D. construction and motorcycle.

46. When you are dealing with an injured football player with a cervical spine injury:
    A. the helmet should never be removed under any circumstances.
    B. the helmet should be left in place unless a critical need requires removal.
    C. the helmet should only be removed by using a special cutting tool.
    D. the helmet should always be removed.

47. It is just after 12 A.M. on a Friday night. You have responded to a motor vehicle accident. The patient is in her mid-20s and is walking about the scene. The patient's car struck a tree and significant damage is noted to the front of the car. The patient appears distraught as you approach. Her right eye is swollen shut and she has a laceration over the left eye. She tells you she had "too much to drink." She is concerned about her car. She complains of neck pain. Given this situation you should:

A. have the patient walk to the ambulance and initiate spinal immobilization.

B. have the patient lie down on the ground and initiate spinal immobilization.

C. secure the patient's cervical spine and initiate a standing takedown.

D. have the patient sit down and initiate seated spinal immobilization techniques.

48. During transport to the hospital she (the patient from #47) begins to complain of a severe headache and dizziness. You should:

A. repeat your assessment of the baseline vitals and level of consciousness.

B. administer oxygen via non-rebreathing mask at 15 lpm.

C. contact medical control and ask for assistance.

D. change your response status from routine to emergency.

49. Her (the patient from #47) level of consciousness declines and she now responds to painful stimuli with flexion (decorticate posturing). You should:

A. consider positive pressure ventilation at 24 breaths per minute.

B. insert an oropharyngeal airway whether a gag reflex exists or not.

C. pull to the side of the road and wait for ALS.

D. continue with your routine response to the hospital and administer oral glucose.

SCENARIO

Questions 50–52 refer to the following scenario:

You and your partner Bill Russell are responding to a burn emergency. Upon arrival you find a 52-year-old patient lying supine on the ground next to a gas grill. Bill makes patient contact and finds the patient awake and responsive with an adequate airway. The patient states he was cleaning his grill with gasoline when it exploded and burned him.

50. The patient has sustained burns that encircle both arms; the burns appear dark brown and involve the subcutaneous layer. You classify this burn as a:

A. superficial thickness burn.

B. half thickness burn.

C. partial thickness burn.

D. full thickness burn.

51. You determine this patient is critically burned using the burn severity classification guidelines. Which guideline was used to determine this patient's classification?

A. superficial burn covering 50% BSA

B. patient's age increased the severity

C. partial thickness burn covering 20% BSA

D. burns encircled both upper extremities

52. You should treat this burn patient by

A. Covering the burns with dry sterile dressing.

B. Continuing to soak the burns while transporting.

C. Administering oxygen by nasal cannula at 6 lpm.

D. Removing adhered clothing by pulling gently.

SCENARIO

Questions 53–55 refer to the following scenario:

You arrive on the scene and find a male patient in his mid-20s who fell from a rocky ledge about 50 feet. Once you gain access to the patient, you find he responds to painful stimuli with flexion of his extremities while arching his back. He is bleeding from his mouth, ears, and nose. His respirations are 35/minute and shallow. His radial pulse is present and bounding.

53. Your first immediate action is to:
    A. suction the mouth and apply a non-rebreather mask at 15 lpm.
    B. move the patient up the embankment to the ambulance.
    C. take a set of vital signs.
    D. suction the airway, insert an oropharyngeal airway, and begin bag-valve-mask ventilation.

54. Which of the signs provides the strongest indication that the patient is suffering from a head injury?
    A. the blood coming from the nose, ears, and mouth
    B. a respiratory rate of 35/minute
    C. flexion of the extremities and arching of the back with painful stimuli
    D. strong radial pulses

55. The best treatment you could provide this patient is to:
    A. administer oral glucose to allow the brain cells to function.
    B. maintain a patent airway and continue to provide effective ventilation.
    C. call for ALS backup to establish IV therapy and fluid resuscitation.
    D. administer oxygen by non-rebreather mask to provide high concentrations of oxygen.

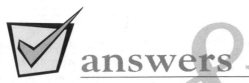

answers & rationales

1.

D. This patient is likely bleeding from veins. Bleeding from veins is dark red, with a steady flow, and can be very heavy. Arterial bleeding usually is bright red, very heavy, and spurts with each contraction of the heart. Capillary bleeding is usually slow or oozing and the color is red; however, the red color is not as bright as arterial bleeding. (5-1.2a) (EC 570 PEC 611)

2.

B. Arterial bleeding is sometimes difficult to control due to the higher pressure. Arterial blood is rich with oxygen, which causes the blood to be bright red. With each contraction of the heart the artery spurts blood from the wound. Dark red with a steady flow describes venous bleeding. Oozing that usually clots spontaneously describes capillary bleeding. (5-1.2b) (EC 570 PEC 611)

3.

B. This patient is in a hypoperfusion state (shock); breathing is adequate at 20 times a minute with good air exchange. This patient should be administered oxygen by non-rebreather mask at 15 lpm. If the patient's breathing becomes inadequate, you must provide immediate positive pressure ventilation with supplemental oxygen. (5-1.5) (EC 572, 580 PEC 608, 611, 620, 622)

4.

D. For bleeding in the upper extremity, the brachial artery or pressure point would be utilized. For bleeding from the lower extremity, the femoral pressure point would be compressed. Use the heel of one hand for the femoral, and the finger tips for the brachial. (5-1.3) (EC 572, 574-578 PEC 611, 613-618)

5.

C. A tourniquet is used only as a last resort to control bleeding. It should be made of a wide, bulky material that will not produce underlying soft tissue injury. The tourniquet should be left uncovered and visible to medical personnel. Avoid placement directly over any joint. The tourniquet should be used after direct pressure and pressure points have failed to control bleeding. (5-1.3) (EC 572, 574-578 PEC 611, 613-618)

6.

B. If direct pressure fails to control bleeding, you should next try direct pressure with elevation of the extremity. Do not elevate the extremity if a fracture is suspected. A tourniquet is reserved for severe uncontrolled bleeding. (5-1.3) (EC 572, 574-578 PEC 611, 613-618)

7.

B. Internal bleeding may not be obvious. Always suspect internal bleeding if the patient presents with unexplained shock. Patients can lose large amounts of blood very rapidly internally. (5-1.6) (EC 579 PEC 619-620)

8.

B. If you suspect the patient is in shock, you should immediately transport to the hospital. Do not delay transport to determine the cause of internal bleeding. You should limit the time on-scene, you should transport and meet ALS on the way to the hospital. Patients that are bleeding internally need immediate transport to the hospital where surgical procedures can be performed and blood can be administered. Do not delay transport. Provide oxygen therapy and positive pressure ventilation if necessary. (5-1.8a) (EC 580 PEC 620)

9.

D. An increased rate, thready, weak pulse is an early sign of possible internal bleeding and shock (hypoperfusion). Decreased blood pressure is a late sign of shock. Bradypneic breathing indicates a slower than normal breathing rate; the patient in shock will usually have a faster than normal breathing rate (tachypnea). A delayed capillary refill in the adult patient is not a reliable sign of hypoperfusion; however, in the child it is a more reliable sign of shock. (5-1.8b) (EC 580 PEC 620)

10.

C. The signs and symptoms of shock include restlessness; anxiety; pale, cool, clammy skin; weak pulse; increased pulse rate; increased respirations; decreasing blood pressure (late); dilated pupils; marked thirst; nausea, vomiting; and pallor. (5-1.9) (EC 582-583 PEC 622)

11.

A. The outermost protective layer of skin, which is composed of dead cells, is the epidermis. The dermis is the layer below the epidermis; this layer contains nerves, blood vessels, and sebaceous glands. The subcutaneous layer contains the fat and soft tissue and is located below the dermis layer. (5-2.2a) (EC 593-594 PEC 634)

12.

C. Because of the obvious hazard of blood and body fluids associated with soft tissue injuries, take body substance isolation precautions prior to patient contact. Be sure to wear gloves, face mask, and eye protection. (5-2.3) (EC 596, 600, 627 PEC 634, 641)

13.

A. An abrasion is caused by scraping of the outermost layer of the skin or epidermis. It is commonly called a "road rash." A puncture is a penetrating injury that results from a sharp, pointed object entering the soft tissue. An avulsion results when a loose flap of skin or soft tissue has been torn loose or pulled completely off. A laceration is a break in the skin of varying depth and may be linear (regular) or stellate (irregular). (5-2.6) (EC 596-600 PEC 636-641)

14.

B. An open wound to the chest is sealed with an occlusive dressing to prevent air from entering the wound. Occlusive dressings are those that do not permit air to pass; these include Vaseline gauze, plastic wrap, and defibrillator pads. The quickest occlusive dressing you can apply is your gloved hand; this will immediately seal the wound until a dressing can be applied. (5-2.8a) (EC 606, 608, 610-611 PEC 642)

15.

C. By securing the occlusive dressing on three sides, trapped air within the chest will be permitted to escape while air outside the chest will not be permitted to enter the chest. Taping on three sides effectively makes the occlusive dressing a one-way (flapper) valve. (5-2.8b) (EC 606, 608, 610-611 PEC 642)

16.

D. The treatment for an open abdominal wound with an evisceration should include NOT touching or replacing the abdominal organs, covering the organs with a sterile (sterile saline/water soaked) dressing. Sterile gauze is recommended. Avoid any dressing that may adhere to the organs such as paper, toilet tissue, or paper towels. Place a bulky dressing on top of the saline/water soaked dressing. This dressing helps to maintain the warmth of the internal organs. The dressing may be held in place by a loose sheet or bandage. Position the patient in a position of comfort, with the hips and knees flexed. (5-2.9) (EC 611-613 PEC 642)

17.

C. Burns are classified as superficial or first degree burn (red skin), partial thickness or second degree (blisters), and full thickness or third degree burn (charring). (5-2.11) (EC 615 PEC 657-659)

18.

A. Burns that involve both the epidermis and portions of the dermis are known as partial thickness burns or second degree burns. These burns can be caused by scalding and are painful. Superficial burns, also called first degree burns, involve only the epidermis and are very painful. Full thickness burns involve all three layers of the skin: epidermis, dermis, and subcutaneous layers. The tough and leathery dead soft tissue formed by this burn is called an eschar. (5-2.11) (EC 615 PEC 657-659)

19.

B. A partial thickness burn or a second degree burn involves the epidermis and dermis. Partial thickness burns cause intense pain from nerve ending damage. (5-2.14) (EC 615 PEC 658)

20.

A. A full thickness burn will appear dry, hard, tough, and leathery. It may appear white and waxy to dark brown or black and charred. The tough and leathery dead soft tissue is called an eschar. (5-2.17) (EC 615, 620 PEC 658-659)

21.

B. The full thickness burn involves the epidermis, dermis, and subcutaneous layers of the skin. This type of burn often results in an eschar, leathery dead soft tissue. The full thickness burn is also known as a third degree burn. (5-2.17) (EC 615, 620 PEC 658-659)

22.

A. Special management of a full thickness burn requires that overall management prevent further contamination and injury to the burn area. Clothing that is adhering to the skin should be left intact. Removal could cause further tissue damage. Remove any jewelry from the hands. This will prevent restrictive blood flow from swelling that may occur. An EXACT calculation of the body surface area (BSA) is not required. (5-2.20) (EC 620-622 PEC 665-666)

23.

B. Never apply any type of ointment or lotion to the burns. Ointments may cause heat retention. Often hospital personnel must then remove the ointment by vigorous cleansing. You should cover the burns with a dry, sterile, particle free burn dressing. Burn patients will often lose too much heat due to damage to their skin, which regulates temperature. Conserve heat loss by covering the patient with blankets. Administer high-flow oxygen by nonrebreather mask if the patient breathing is adequate. If breathing is inadequate, provide positive pressure ventilation. (5-2.20) (EC 620-622 PEC 665-666)

24.

A. If blood soaks through the dressing, do not remove the dressing. This may cause the bleeding to increase. Instead, add additional dressing over the original one and apply pressure. (5-2.23) (EC 625 PEC 645-646)

25.

C. You should never remove an impaled object unless it is impaled through the cheek or it is impaled in the chest and interferes with chest compressions while performing CPR. Removing impaled objects from areas other than the cheek can lead to further injury or even death. Impaled objects should be stabilized in place using bulky dressings and tape. (5-2.26) (EC 602-604 EC 642-644)

26.

B. Never attempt to remove a patient from an electrical source unless trained and equipped to do so. Check for source and ground burn injury. Never touch a patient that is in contact with an electrical source. (5-2.29) (EC 623-624 PEC 669)

27.

C. Injury caused by an electrical burn can be quite extensive and involve many internal organs like the heart, spleen, and lungs. If the source wound is on the left hand and the ground wound is on the feet, right hand, hip, knee, and so on, the path crosses the heart and other vital organs. Many electrical burn patients may need CPR and defibrillation with the AED. Source and ground wounds are treated as other thermal burns. Because of the possible involvement of the heart and other vital organs, you should treat all patients with electrical burns as critical patients. (5-2.29) (EC 623-624 PEC 669)

28.

D. The upper bone of the arm is called the humerus. (5-3.3) (EC 635, 636, 637, 638 PEC 677)

29.

D. Before and after splinting check for pulse, motor function, and sensation in the injured extremity. This should be evaluated every 15 minutes after applying the splint. This ensures that the splint is not impairing circulation. (5-3.6) (EC 645-646 PEC 682, 686)

30.

A. Elevating this patient's extremity is not performed due to possible spinal injury. You should administer oxygen if needed: also, cold packs can decrease pain and edema (swelling). You should assess the patient's motor, sensation, and distal pulse before and after the splint is applied. (5-3.8a) (EC 644 PEC 680-681, 687-698)

31.

D. When a joint is injured, you should immobilize the bones above and below the affected joint. When a bone is injured, you should immobilize the joint above and below the affected bone. (5-3.8b) (EC 644 PEC 680-681, 687-698)

32.

C. If the extremity is cyanotic and pulseless, you may make one attempt to align the extremity by applying gentle traction to the extremity before splinting. If the pain, resistance, or crepitus increase you must stop. Do not try to align a wrist, elbow, knee, hip, or shoulder because of major nerves and blood vessels that lie close to these joints. (5-3.8c)

33.

C. Never intentionally replace a protruding bone into the extremity since further tissue damage may result. You should assess the distal pulse, and motor and sensory function before and after the splint is applied. To effectively immobilize a long bone, you must immobilize the joint above and below the injured bone. Never try to align an injury that involves the wrist, elbow, knee, hip, or shoulder; doing so may cause more injury. (5-3.8d)

34.

B. The nervous system that consists of the brain and the spinal cord is the central nervous system. The peripheral nervous system consists of nerves located outside the brain and spinal cord. The voluntary nervous system influences the activity of the voluntary muscles and moves the body. The autonomic nervous system influences the activity of involuntary muscles and glands and regulates the heart rate and breathing. (5-4.2)

35.

B. The cranium consists of fused bones. This includes the temporal and parietal bones that protect the brain. (5-4.3)

36.

C. A rare sign of spinal injury is an obvious deformity of the spine. This is usually found when palpating the spine. (5-4.6)

37.

D. Patients with possible spine injuries must be managed carefully. Improper handling can cause further injury or death. When you suspect a patient may have a spine injury, you must open and maintain the airway using the jaw-thrust maneuver. Cervical traction is not used in the prehospital setting. This technique can cause further injury including paralysis. Lateral lift or head-tilt maneuvers will compromise the spine and may cause further injury. (5-4.8)

38.

C. Spinal immobilization and placement on a long spine board are ideally performed by four rescuers. One maintains cervical spine stabilization, and three rescuers perform the logroll. A fifth rescuer can be used to place the board under the patient. (5-4.9)

39.

B. Measure the distance from an imaginary line from the top of the shoulder to the bottom of the chin. Use your fingers to measure the distance. (5-4.12)

40.

A. When you encounter a standing patient with a possible spine injury, you must place the patient onto the board, using the standing long board technique. This technique consists of placing the board behind the patient and lowering the patient from the standing position. You must maintain control of the patient's head and cervical spine with manual stabilization and the use of a cervical collar. When lowering the patient, support the patient by placing a rescuer at the side of the board to support the patient under the arms. All of the other techniques will compromise the spine and possibly cause further injury to the patient. (5-4.14)

41.

C. A short spine board or a vest-type device is used to immobilize a patient who is found in a seated position. (5-4.15)

44.

C. If the patient is in cardiac arrest, you must remove the helmet. You should also remove the helmet if the helmet interferes with proper spinal immobilization; the helmet does not fit well and allows excessive movement; the helmet interferes with your ability to adequately manage the airway or breathing; the helmet interferes with your ability to assess or reassess the airway or breathing. (5-4.20)

45.

A. The two basic helmet types are the sports helmet and the motorcycle helmet. (5-4.21)

46.

B. The football helmet should be left in place unless there is a life threat that requires its removal. The player's shoulder pads and helmet create a neutral alignment of the spine. Removal of the helmet causes the head to flex. (5-4.24)

47.

C. The patient is complaining of cervical spine pain and was involved in an incident with a significant mechanism of injury. Immediately provide cervical spine stabilization and initiate a standing takedown. Do not allow the patient to walk, sit down, or lie down.

48.

A. She may be exhibiting early signs and symptoms of a head injury. It is important to provide a trending of her level of consciousness to determine if this is, in fact, occurring. This could also be a normal response to injury. To determine this, trending of the level of consciousness is required.

49.

A. The level of consciousness is continuing to decline. The EMT-B should consider providing positive pressure ventilation at a rate of 24 to 30 per minute. The patient responds to pain, and an oropharyngeal airway is contraindicated. You should change your response to the hospital to emergency as well. The best answer is to consider positive pressure ventilation.

50.

D. Burns that involve all layers of the skin including tissue below the subcutaneous layer are classified as a full thickness burn. Full thickness burns may appear dark brown, black, waxy, dry, hard, leathery, or white. Often the patient with a full thickness burn will experience little pain due to the nerve endings being exposed by the burn injury. (5-2.17)

51.

D. Any burns that encircle a body part, upper extremities, legs, chest, or neck are classified as a critical burn. (5-2.20a)

52.

A. You should apply dry sterile dressings after you remove clothing and initially cool the burn site. Continuing to soak the burn in water may cause hypothermia. Patients that have been burned have lost their temperature regulating capabilities. This patient's breathing is adequate and doesn't warrant positive pressure ventilation; however, oxygen by non-rebreather mask should be administered. Never remove portions of clothing that have adhered to the patient's skin; gently cut the clothing around these areas. (5-2.20b)

53.

D. To establish a patent airway and prevent aspiration of the blood, you should immediately suction the airway. Since the patient is not responding appropriately to painful stimuli, you can insert an oropharyngeal airway. Next, you should begin positive pressure ventilation since the breathing is shallow.

54.

C. Flexion of the extremities and arching of the back on painful stimulation are indications of an injury to the upper brain stem. This is a form of non-purposeful posturing and is also known as decorticate posturing.

55.

B. The best treatment that could be provided to a head injured patient is to establish and maintain a patent airway and provide effective ventilation with supplemental oxygen.

6 Infants and Children

module objectives

Questions in this module relate to D.O.T.
objectives 6-1.1 to 6-1.26.

DIRECTIONS Each of the questions or incomplete statements below is followed by suggested answers or completions. Select the **one answer** that is best in each case.

1. A child up to 12 months of age is referred to as a (an):
   A. preschooler.
   B. toddler.
   C. neonate.
   D. infant.

2. This pediatric age group could be classed as the "do not like" group. These children generally don't like to be touched, separated from parents, or have clothing removed, and they fear needles. Which group is described?
   A. infant
   B. toddler
   C. preschooler
   D. school-age

3. Which pediatric age group uses concrete thinking skills and believes he or she is invincible?
   A. toddler
   B. preschooler
   C. school-age
   D. adolescent

4. Which anatomical or physiological difference in the infant and child patient as compared to the adult is correct?
   A. An infant's rib cage is less pliable resulting in more injury.
   B. Infants have a faster metabolic rate that uses oxygen at a faster rate.
   C. Children's heads are proportionally smaller, leading to more head injuries.
   D. A child's skin surface is small compared to body mass, causing hypothermia.

5. Which statement is **incorrect** relating to anatomical differences between the adult and child/infant?
   A. A child's skin surface area is large when compared to body mass.

   B. Children's heads are proportionally larger than those of adults.
   C. Infants have proportionally larger tongues than those of adults.
   D. Children have a larger circulating blood volume than that of adults.

6. An infant or child responds to illness or injury differently than an adult. Which of the following statements best describes a typical **adult's** response to illness or injury?
   A. While crying, the patient says, "It hurts bad."
   B. "Don't touch me!"
   C. "I want to go home!"
   D. "My left arm hurts just below the elbow."

7. The leading medical cause of cardiac arrest in the infant or child patient is:
   A. cardiovascular disease.
   B. drowning or near drowning.
   C. respiratory failure.
   D. seizures.

8. All of the following are signs of early respiratory distress in the infant or child patient **except:**
   A. intercostal retractions.
   B. nasal flaring.
   C. bradypnea.
   D. increase in respiratory rate.

9. An infant or child patient that presents with agonal respirations, limp muscle tone, unresponsive with a slower than normal heart rates is in:
   A. respiratory arrest.
   B. decompensated respiratory failure.
   C. compensated respiratory failure.
   D. early respiratory failure.

10. Which of the following signs, in addition to the signs of early respiratory distress (compensated respiratory failure), would indicate your infant or child patient is in decompensated respiratory failure?
    A. neck muscle retraction
    B. "See-saw" respirations
    C. decreased muscle tone
    D. nasal flaring on inspiration

11. An alert, crying child presents with stridor, is pink in color, and is displaying retractions of the intercostal muscles. The mother believes that "something is caught in his throat." The potential problem presented is a _____ and requires you to _____.
    A. partial airway obstruction, place the child in a position of comfort and administer oxygen
    B. partial airway obstruction, administer 5 back blows and 5 chest thrusts
    C. complete airway obstruction, administer 5 abdominal thrusts
    D. complete airway obstruction, administer 5 back blows and 5 abdominal thrusts

12. Which treatment is indicated for an 8-month infant with a complete airway obstruction?
    A. head-up position while delivering abdominal thrusts
    B. head-up position while delivering chest thrusts and back blows
    C. head-down position while delivering abdominal thrusts
    D. head-down position while delivering back blows and chest thrust

13. Your partner is preparing to suction your infant patient. You remind your partner to limit suctioning to:
    A. 5–10 seconds.
    B. 10–15 seconds.
    C. 15–20 seconds.
    D. 20–30 seconds.

14. Infants and children require a respiratory tidal volume of _____ ml/kg.
    A. 5–10
    B. 10–15
    C. 15–20
    D. 20–25

15. An unresponsive child with facial trauma requires airway management. Which device or procedure should be avoided?
    A. oropharyngeal airway
    B. nasopharyngeal airway
    C. manual jaw-thrust technique
    D. maintaining the head in a neutral position

16. An early indication of severe hypoperfusion in children is _____ because their _____, which helps to maintain the blood pressure.
    A. common, blood vessels constrict
    B. uncommon, blood vessels constrict
    C. common, blood volume increases
    D. uncommon, respiratory rate increases

17. All of the following are signs of hypoperfusion in the child **except:**
    A. pale, cool skin.
    B. bounding, peripheral pulse.
    C. absence of tears when crying.
    D. decreased urination.

18. The newborn infant should be kept warm and calm following delivery. To what minimum temperature should you heat your ambulance or isollete?
    A. 100 degrees F
    B. 99 degrees F
    C. 98 degrees F
    D. 97 degrees F

19. The least common cause of hypoperfusion in a child is:
    A. cardiac events.
    B. diarrhea.
    C. dehydration.
    D. vomiting.

20. All of the following are signs of adequate perfusion in an infant or child patient **except:**
    A. capillary refill less than 2 seconds.
    B. warm hands and feet.
    C. altered mental status.
    D. normal urinary output.

21. You are treating an 8-year-old patient. Which of the following signs or symptoms would indicate hypoperfusion (shock) in this patient?
    A. peripheral pulse of 80 per minute
    B. bounding peripheral pulse
    C. capillary refill of $<$ 2 seconds
    D. rapid respiratory rate

22. Which of the following is a common cause of seizures in children but not in adults?
    A. epilepsy
    B. hypoglycemia
    C. overdose
    D. fever

23. A seizure in an infant or child that lasts longer than 15 minutes or recurs without a recovery period is called:
    A. grand mal activity.
    B. mega seizure activity.
    C. multi-seizure activity.
    D. status epilepticus.

24. You are treating a child who was an unrestrained front seat passenger in a motor vehicle crash. Your patient is most likely to suffer:
    A. spine and lower extremity injuries.
    B. chest and abdominal injuries.
    C. upper extremity and spine injuries.
    D. head and neck injuries.

25. The leading cause of death of children from 1 to 14 years of age is:
    A. trauma.
    B. cardiovascular disease.
    C. drowning.
    D. asthma.

26. When providing positive pressure ventilation to the injured child, special care must be taken to avoid _____, which can be reduced by using _____ during ventilation.
    A. gastric distention, cricoid pressure
    B. oropharyngeal airway placement, manual airway techniques
    C. head movement, the head-tilt chin-lift
    D. excessive ventilatory pressures, an oropharyngeal airway

27. Which of the following is **not** a general indicator of child abuse?
    A. rapid reporting of injuries
    B. lack of adult supervision
    C. injuries don't match mechanism
    D. a fearful child

28. In most child abuse cases the child suffers from:
    A. physical abuse.
    B. emotional abuse.
    C. sexual abuse.
    D. physical, emotional, and sexual abuse.

29. Which statement is **incorrect** relating to the care of the potential child abuse patient?
    A. Use subjective information in your patient care report.
    B. Don't make accusatory statements to the parents.
    C. Don't allow the child to be alone with the suspected abuser.
    D. Know the abuse reporting law in your community.

30. What action is frequently required following a traumatic child or infant call?
    A. meeting with local law enforcement personnel
    B. extensive cleaning of emergency vehicle
    C. debriefing of parents and friends
    D. CISD assistance

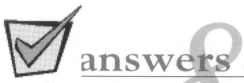

answers & rationales

1.

D. A neonate refers to the first 4 weeks of life, an infant up to 12 months, a toddler from 1 to 3 years and a preschooler from 3 to 6 years of age. (6-1.1) (EC 739-740 PEC 818-820)

2.

B. A toddler, a child from 1 to 3 years of age, creates an assessment challenge for the emergency responder. Remain calm and try to distract the child with a toy or other object during the assessment. (6-1.1) (EC 739-740 PEC 818-820)

3.

D. The 12 to 18-year-olds, or adolescents, believe that nothing bad can happen to them and are able to use abstract and concrete thinking skills. They may take risks that lead to trauma. If injured they fear disfigurement and disability. (6-1.1) (EC 739-740 PEC 818-820)

4.

B. Infants have a faster metabolic rate that uses more oxygen than the adult patient. An infant's rib cage is more pliable, resulting in less rib injury, but in increased injury to the internal organs. Children proportionally have larger heads, predisposing them to head injuries. A child's skin surface area is large compared to its mass, which can increase a child's exposure to a cold environment, causing hypothermia. (6-1.2) (EC 740-743 PEC 820-822)

5.

D. Children have a smaller circulating blood volume than that of adults. Bleeding must be controlled quickly. A seemingly small blood loss in an adult could be life-threatening to the infant or child. (6-1.2) (EC 740-743 PEC 820-822)

6.

D. Children lack the vocabulary and body awareness that adults possess to accurately describe symptoms and assist with care. The adult is able to separate the emotional aspects of illness or injury. The best answer is the most direct answer, "My left arm hurts just below the elbow." (6-1.3) (EC 739-740 PEC 818-820, 822-823)

7.

C. The overriding treatment goal for infants and children is to anticipate and recognize respiratory problems. The leading medical cause of cardiac arrest in the infant or child is respiratory failure. Quickly manage and support respiratory compromise in the infant or child patient. (6-1.4) (EC 766-767 PEC 823-826)

8.

C. Signs of early respiratory distress include intercostal retractions, nasal flaring, increased respiratory rate, and also may include supraclavicular and subcostal retractions, neck muscle retractions, audible breathing sounds including stridor, wheezing and grunting, and "see-saw" respirations. The infant or child progresses from early respiratory distress (compensated respiratory failure) to decompensated respiratory failure to respiratory arrest. An infant or child with bradypnea (slow breathing) is a sign of respiratory distress, not early respiratory failure. (6-1.5) (EC 766-767 PEC 824-825)

9.

A. The signs of respiratory arrest include the signs described in the question stem as well as weak, absent peripheral pulses and hypotension in patients over 3 years of age. Patients presenting with these signs require aggressive ventilatory and airway management. (6-1.5) (EC 766-767 PEC 824-825)

10.

C. In addition to the early signs of respiratory distress (compensated respiratory failure), decreased muscle tone should alert you that your patient is in the advanced stages (decompensated respiratory failure). Neck muscle retraction, "see-saw" respirations, and nasal flaring are all early signs of respiratory distress (compensated respiratory failure). (6-1.5) (EC 766-767 PEC 824-825)

11.

A. This child patient is presenting with a partial airway obstruction. He is moving air and is pink in color. The treatment for a partial airway obstruction with adequate air movement is to place the patient in a position of comfort, administer oxygen, and encourage the patient to remove the obstruction by coughing. (6-1.6) (EC 759-760 PEC 831-834)

12.

D. The management of an infant with a complete airway obstruction includes placing the infant in a head-down position during the back blows and chest thrusts. This position makes use of gravity to help move the obstruction from the infant airway. Abdominal thrusts are contraindicated in infants. (6-1.6) (EC 759-760 PEC 831-834)

13.

A. During suctioning of an infant's or child's airway, oxygen is removed as well as any debris or secretions. For this reason, limit suctions to no longer than 5–10 seconds. (6-1.7) (EC 768-769 PEC 829-835, 837, 838)

14.

A. BVM devices for infants and young children that deliver 500 ml to >50 ml should be used to provide positive pressure ventilation. To estimate the volume needed, remember that infants and children require about 5–10 ml per kg of body weight for each ventilation. (6-1.7) (EC 768-769 PEC 829-835, 837, 838)

15.

B. Avoid the use of a nasopharyngeal airway in adults, infants, and children with possible head trauma and mid-face trauma. Maintaining the head in a neutral position and manual airway control with the jaw-

thrust technique are appropriate management. (6-1.7) (EC 768-769 PEC 829-835, 837, 838)

16.

B. Early signs of severe shock, or hypoperfusion, in children is uncommon because their blood vessels constrict efficiently, which helps to maintain the blood pressure. When the blood pressure does fall, it drops rapidly and quickly. Frequently the child or infant may go into cardiac arrest from this rapid drop. When pediatric patients deteriorate because of hypoperfusion, they deteriorate faster and more severely than adults. (6-1.8) (EC 764-765 PEC 840, 842)

17.

B. The peripheral pulse is absent or weak in the child with hypoperfusion. An altered mental status, delayed capillary refill, and a rapid respiratory rate are also present. (6-1.8) (EC 764-765 PEC 840, 842)

18.

C. Heat the ambulance or isollete to a minimum temperature of 98 degrees F or 36.5 degrees C. Be sure that the baby's head (not face) is covered to prevent heat loss. (6-1.8) (EC 764-765 PEC 840, 842)

19.

A. Cardiac events in children and infants are uncommon. Common causes of hypoperfusion include diarrhea, dehydration, vomiting, trauma, blood loss, infection, and abdominal injuries. (6-1.8) (EC 764-765 PEC 840, 842)

20.

C. Adequate end organ perfusion or tissue perfusion in the infant or child patient is characterized by normal or acceptable findings of capillary refill (2 seconds or less), pulse rate and strength, warmth and color of the hands and feet, urinary output and mental status. Alteration of any one of these factors can be an indication of inadequate perfusion. (6-1.8) (EC 764-765 PEC 840, 842)

21.

D. A rapid respiratory rate may indicate hypoperfusion in the child patient. A bounding peripheral pulse does not indicate hypoperfusion; blood is being pumped adequately to the extremities. A prolonged capillary refill of <2 seconds is normal. (6-1.8) (EC 764-765 PEC 840, 842)

22.
D. Causes of seizure activity in children and adults are similar with one notable exception, fever. Febrile seizures are common in children but occur rarely in adults. (6-1.11) (EC 771 PEC 835)

23.
D. In adults, infants, and children a seizure that lasts longer than 15 minutes or recurs without a recovery period is called status epilepticus. Ensure an airway, be prepared to suction the airway, try to provide positive pressure ventilation, and transport the patient rapidly. (6-1.12) (EC 772 PEC 835)

24.
D. Common injury patterns in children who are unrestrained in a vehicle accident include head and neck injuries. This is due to the head size of children and the likely impact with the dashboard. (6-1.13) (EC 775-777 PEC 846)

25.
A. The leading cause of death in children is trauma. This includes vehicle accidents, bicycle accidents, ATV accidents, falls, recreational activities, and pedestrian accidents. The primary killer of children is the automobile. (6-1.13) (EC 775-777 PEC 846)

26.
A. When providing positive pressure ventilation to the injured infant or child, the rescuer must take special care to avoid high ventilatory pressure which can lead to gastric distention. Gastric distention can be avoided or reduced by using cricoid pressure during ventilation. (6-1.14) (EC 777 PEC 846-848)

27.
A. Rapid reporting of injuries is NOT a general indicator of child abuse. Reports of injuries would be delayed. Additional signs of abuse include multiple abrasions, lacerations, bruises, malnourishment, untreated chronic illness, and injuries on both the front and back or both sides of the child's body. (6-1.15) (EC 778-780 PEC 848-849)

28.
D. A child of abuse will commonly be the victim of a combination of all the forms of abuse listed: physical, emotional, sexual abuse, or neglect. (6-1.15) (EC 778-780 PEC 848-849)

29.
A. Only document objective, not subjective, information. Subjective information such as "The patient was abused" must be avoided. Only document objective information statements or observations made. (6-1.16) (EC 779-782 PEC 851)

30.
D. Critical Incident Stress Debriefing for EMT-Bs is frequently required following a traumatic injury to an infant or child. The stress and anxiety are common and stem from a lack of experience in treating children, the fear of failure, and identifying patients with their own children. (6-1.17) (EC 784 PEC 845, 851-852, 854)

7 Operations

module objectives

Questions in this module relate to D.O.T.
objectives 7-1.1 to 7-3.16.

DIRECTIONS Each of the questions or incomplete statements below is followed by suggested answers or completions. Select the **one answer** that is best in each case.

1. When you are driving to an emergency scene, most state laws allow:
   A. exceeding the speed limit without regard to the safety of others.
   B. proceeding through a traffic light without regard to the safety of others.
   C. parking anywhere at any time without any restriction.
   D. exceeding the speed limit while respecting the safety of others.

2. You are responding to a medical emergency. Which of the following actions is considered unsafe while driving the ambulance?
   A. entering a curve at the outside or high part
   B. accelerating gradually as you leave a curve
   C. driving only as fast as you feel comfortable
   D. braking to the proper speed after entering a curve

3. The use of an escort vehicle is considered dangerous; however, it can be used with extreme caution in which of the following circumstances?
   A. when you are unfamiliar with how to get to the hospital
   B. on emergency response to the hospital
   C. when traffic is congested
   D. when responding through an urban area with intersections

4. Which of the following situations is true pertaining to the use of a police escort?
   A. Use escorts only if you can not quickly travel through high traffic areas.
   B. Use escorts only at traffic intersections, railroad crossings, and bridges.
   C. Use escorts only if you are unfamiliar with how to get to the hospital.
   D. Use escorts to reduce the time it takes you to drive through traffic.

5. You are dispatched to an emergency. Which of the following is considered essential information in order to respond to the call?
   A. gender of the patient
   B. age of the patient
   C. name of the patient
   D. location of the patient

6. You are approaching a railroad crossing with a critical patient, the gate is down, and you see a long train approaching. You determine the train is traveling very slowly; you should:
   A. turn on your lights and siren while waiting for the train to pass.
   B. maintain control of the ambulance and cross the tracks quickly.
   C. wait for the train to pass if there is no immediate alternative route.
   D. signal the train to stop and proceed around the warning gates.

7. Which of the following statements is true regarding ambulance driving techniques?
   A. It is dangerous to brake after entering a curve.
   B. You should accelerate suddenly as you leave a curve.
   C. Stopping distance is shortened when vehicle speed increases.
   D. Brakes in ambulances equipped with antilocking brakes should be pumped.

8. Your patient has vomited on the ambulance floor. Your first action when cleaning the ambulance floor is to:
   A. spread a germicide on top of the vomitus.

B. sweep the vomitus into a bag with a broom.

C. clean up visible vomitus with disposable towels.

D. sterilize the area with a chemical sterilant.

9. Intermediate-level disinfection should be used for surfaces that come into contact with intact skin. Which solution of household bleach and water should be used for intermediate-level disinfecting?

A. 1:1

B. 1:10

C. 1:100

D. 1:1000

10. To clean emergency equipment that comes in contact with a patient's intact skin, such as a stethoscope, you should:

A. immerse in an EPA-registered sterilant for 6 to 10 hours.

B. immerse in an EPA-registered sterilant for 10 to 45 minutes.

C. use low-level disinfection, 1:100 ratio of bleach and water.

D. use intermediate-level disinfection, 1:10 ratio of bleach and water.

11. Which of the following best describes the role of the EMT-B on a scene where a patient is entrapped within a motor vehicle?

A. extrication technician

B. detanglement worker

C. patient care provider

D. scene safety officer

12. After you have determined a vehicle is safe to approach, the most appropriate way to approach your patient trapped in the vehicle is to:

A. approach from the rear of the patient.

B. approach directly facing the patient.

C. approach from the patient's left side.

D. approach from the patient's right side.

13. When preparing to extricate your patient from a motor vehicle, all of the following are acceptable **except to:**

A. inform the patient what you are about to do and what to expect.

B. instruct the patient to focus on an object directly in front of him or her.

C. have the patient lie across the seat for protection prior to extricating.

D. look the patient directly in the eyes while speaking to him or her.

14. You have received dispatch information while responding to a call that informs you that the patient will need to be extricated from a vehicle. Your first action should be:

A. stabilization.

B. gaining access.

C. disentanglement.

D. scene size-up.

15. You are preparing to extricate your patient from a vehicle; you know the access of choice is usually the:

A. door.

B. windshield.

C. side window.

D. removed roof.

16. After gaining safe access to a patient who is entangled in a motor vehicle, your first emergency treatment should be:

A. applying high-flow oxygen.

B. shaking and shouting.

C. extrication of the patient.

D. stabilizing the cervical spine.

17. You have arrived on a motor vehicle crash scene. The police officer states your patient is entangled and access appears to be "complex." You recognize this to be:
    A. access that takes longer than 20 minutes.
    B. access that requires the use of tools.
    C. access that can not be performed by the EMT-B.
    D. access that requires the notification of the police.

18. While waiting for help to arrive on a hazardous material rescue, you should protect bystanders by:
    A. advising them to shut off electronics.
    B. advising them to remain calm.
    C. directing them to keep downhill.
    D. directing them to keep upwind.

19. You are the first to arrive at the scene of a possible hazardous materials spill; your first action should be to:
    A. ensure there are enough additional equipment and personnel.
    B. approach the scene carefully and identify the hazardous material.
    C. protect yourself by donning a hazardous materials protective suit.
    D. secure the scene and prevent the exposure of rescuers and bystanders.

20. The area of a hazardous material scene where contamination is actually present and treatment is limited to life-threatening conditions is known as the:
    A. hot zone.
    B. warm zone.
    C. cold zone.
    D. safe zone.

21. The criteria for a multiple casualty incident (MCI) is best described by:
    A. any event that involves mass transit or a large building where people may be.

B. any event that places excessive demands on EMS personnel and equipment.
C. any event that typically involves more than three emergency vehicles.
D. any event that requires police, fire, and EMS to respond simultaneously.

22. You are the senior EMT-B and have arrived at the scene of a disaster; your responsibility is to assume:
    A. EMS incident manager until relieved.
    B. staging sector command until relieved.
    C. triage sector command until relieved.
    D. supply sector command until relieved.

23. You are the next senior EMT-B who arrives after the first ambulance on the scene of a mass casualty incident (MCI). Your immediate role will be:
    A. EMS incident manager.
    B. treatment sector officer.
    C. primary triage officer.
    D. staging sector officer.

24. To protect yourself at a scene of a hazardous materials incident, you should position yourself and others:
    A. downhill and downwind.
    B. downhill and upwind.
    C. uphill and downwind.
    D. uphill and upwind.

25. You are on the scene of a multiple casualty incident and are assigned as the primary triage sector. You open the airway of an unresponsive victim and find that the patient is not breathing; you should:
    A. move on to the next patient.
    B. provide rescue breaths for 1 minute.
    C. call for assistance and start CPR.
    D. tag the patient "red" for level one.

SCENARIO

Questions 26 and 27 refer to the following scenario:

You and your partner Joshua Adam are cleaning the vehicle as one of your daily chores. The alerting system sounds, "Medic One, respond to a four vehicle crash on I 95, mile marker 147, southbound lane." You and Joshua quickly respond. While en route dispatch advises you of two patients that are critically injured. As you turn onto 20th Street, you notice medic seven just ahead of your unit.

26. Your unit is directly behind unit seven as you both approach a busy intersection. Which of the following practices should you follow?

   A. Use the same siren mode that unit seven is currently using.

   B. Position yourself so motorists can see both units at a glance.

   C. Follow medic seven as closely as possible through the intersection.

   D. Follow medic seven through the intersection without using your siren.

27. You and Joshua Adam have attended to a critically injured trauma patient. You have transported the patient to the hospital and turned the patient over to the hospital staff with a complete oral report. You and Joshua Adam are standing at the rear of the ambulance, looking with disbelief at the incredible mess you both have created while attending to the trauma patient. After you both have picked up all the loose trash and cleaned all the blood from the inside of the ambulance, Joshua Adam states he will clean the laryngoscope blades. Which of the following best describes the correct procedure for cleaning the laryngoscope blades?

   A. Immerse the blades in an EPA-registered sterilant for 10 to 45 minutes.

   B. Immerse the blades in an EPA-registered sterilant for 6 to 10 hours.

   C. Wipe the blades carefully with a 1:10 solution of bleach and water.

   D. Wipe the blades carefully with a 1:100 solution of bleach and water.

SCENARIO

Questions 28–30 refer to the following scenario:

You and your partner Russ are reviewing your department's protocol when the alerting system sounds: "Medic One, respond to an automobile crash with injuries at 1729 17th Avenue." You both quickly move to the ambulance. While you are en route to the accident scene, dispatch advises you that a bystander stated there are nine persons injured, some of whom may be critical. You advise dispatch to activate the multiple casualty incident plan.

28. What criteria did you use to determine that the multiple casualty incident plan would need to be implemented?

   A. This event will likely take longer than 2 hours to complete.

   B. This event and location will limit the number of rescuers on the scene.

   C. This event will require an emergency response from EMS, fire, and police.

   D. This event will place excessive demand on personnel and equipment.

29. Your unit is the first to arrive on the crash scene and you are the most senior EMT-B; your initial role would be:

   A. primary triage manager.

   B. primary incident manager.

   C. primary treatment manager.

   D. primary staging manager.

30. Your partner Russ is assigned to the triage sector. Triage is best described as a:

   A. system ensuring that ambulances are accessible and transportation occurs with direction of EMS incident manager.

   B. system responsible for distributing the medical material and equipment necessary to render care.

   C. system that monitors, inventories, and directs available emergency ambulances to the treatment sector.

   D. system used for sorting patients to determine the order in which they will receive care and transport.

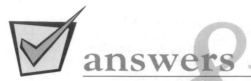

answers & rationales

1.

D. When operating an ambulance, you must always respect the safety and well-being of others. This is called due regard for the safety of others. This due regard must be respected when traveling through a traffic light, parking, or exceeding the speed limit. (7-1.3) (EC 816-820 PEC 882-883, 885)

2.

D. Braking to the proper speed after entering a curve is considered dangerous. You should decelerate to a safe speed prior to entering the curve. (7-1.4a) (EC 816 PEC 884-885, 899-901)

3.

A. The only acceptable use of an escort vehicle is when the driver of the ambulance is unfamiliar with how to get to the scene or the hospital. When using an escort, extreme caution must be exercised. (7.14b) (EC 816 PEC 884-885, 899-901)

4.

C. You should only use a police escort if you are uncertain with how to reach a patient or with how to go to the hospital. (7-1.5) (EC 819 PEC 884-885)

5.

D. The location of the patient is considered essential information needed to respond to a call. Neither the gender nor the age is essential information; however, it is often included as additional information. The name of the patient should not be given over the radio and may be considered a breech of patient confidentiality. (7-1.7) (EC 815-816 PEC 887-888)

6.

C. Never proceed through a crossing gate at a railroad crossing! Simply be calm and monitor your patient. If there is no immediate alternative route, wait for the train to pass. Turning on your lights and siren while waiting for the train to pass will likely upset the patient and others. (7-1.8a) (EC 819-820 PEC 884-885, 899-901)

7.

A. After entering a curve, it is dangerous to apply the brakes. Anticipate the curve and apply the brakes prior to entering the curve; accelerate gradually and carefully as you leave the curve. Stopping distances increase as the speed of the vehicle increases. Ambulances equipped with antilocking brakes should not be pumped; apply the brakes firmly and steadily. (7-1.8b) (EC 819-820 PEC 884-885, 899-901)

8.

C. When cleaning any body fluid or substances that have spilled, you should first protect yourself by wearing gloves, a mask, and eyewear. The visible spill should first be cleaned by using disposable towels to pick up the majority of the spill. After the spill has been picked up and disposed of properly, you will need to clean the surface with a germicide or mixture of bleach and water. Never try to pick up a spill with a broom, this will only create a larger spill and may cause further contamination. (7-1.13a) (EC 831 PEC 894-896)

9.

B. A ratio of 1:10 or 1 part household bleach and 10 parts water is the correct mixture to use for an intermediate-level disinfection. A 1:1 mixture is too strong; a 1:100 ratio is too weak for an intermediate-level disinfection. A mixture of 1:100 is used for a low-level disinfection such as routine cleaning of the ambulance. A 1:1000 mixture is too weak. (7-1.13b) (EC 831 PEC 894-896)

10.

D. When cleaning equipment that comes in contact with the patient's intact skin, use a 1:10 ratio of bleach and water. A ratio of 1:100 is used for routine housekeeping on surfaces such as floors. Equipment that comes in contact with a patient's mucous membranes should be soaked for 10 to 45 minutes in an EPA-registered sterilant. Immersion in an EPA-registered sterilant for 6 to 10 hours is used on equipment that is used invasively, primarily in the hospital. (7-1.14) (EC 831 PEC 894-896)

11.

C. Your primary role as an EMT-B on a crash scene is as a patient care provider. Although you will work closely with the detanglement team and help to ensure minimal risk to the patient's condition, you will provide emergency care to the patient. (7-2.2) (EC 842-860 PEC 910-912)

12.

B. When approaching a patient inside a vehicle, you should approach directly facing the patient. Approaching the patient from his or her front will help to keep the patient's attention forward, thus keeping the patient from turning his or her head. When you have made direct eye contact with your patient, instruct the patient not to move his or her head. Approaching from the right, left, and behind may cause the patient to move his or her head, possibly further injuring the patient. (7-2.4a) (EC 842-860 PEC 910)

13.

C. Having the patient lie across the seat may further injure the patient. You must maintain in-line spinal stabilization during extrication. It is important to explain to your patient what to expect; this will lessen the patient's apprehension during the extrication process. Having the patient focus on an object directly in front of him or her will help to keep the head and spine in-line and not moving. When speaking to your patient, look the patient directly in the eyes; this will help keep the patient from moving his or her head unnecessarily. (7-2.4b) (EC 842-860 PEC 910)

14.

D. You first must size up the scene; this will help you organize your resources and prepare for the extrication. A good scene size-up can help reduce injury to the rescuers and patient. (7-2.4c) (EC 842-860 PEC 910)

15.

A. The door is usually the best access when extricating a patient from a motor vehicle because of its large opening. In addition, it is fairly easy to open. The windshield can be a difficult choice through which to gain access. The side window is usually too small and may cause the spine to be manipulated. The removal of the roof opens the vehicle considerably and can make extrication much easier. Roof removal usually requires special training and equipment and can be costly to the vehicle owner. (7-2.4d) (EC 842-860 PEC 910)

16.

D. After gaining safe access to your patient, you will stabilize the cervical spine with manual in-line stabilization. Provide the same care as you would on other trauma patients. Apply high-flow oxygen after securing the cervical spine manually. Shaking and shouting to establish responsiveness may cause injury to an unsecured cervical spine. (7-2.5) (EC 846-847 PEC 911-912)

17.

B. Complex access requires the use of tools or specialized equipment. Access that does not require tools or specialized equipment is known as "simple access." (7-2.7) (EC 857 PEC 909)

18.

D. While waiting for help to arrive on a hazardous materials incident, you should protect yourself and bystanders by remaining upwind, uphill, and away from the scene. Turning off electronics will not protect you from hazardous materials. (7-3.2) (EC 868-877 PEC 926-927)

19.

D. As the first responding EMT-B on the scene of a hazardous material incident, you should first secure the scene. Securing the scene will limit the exposure of other rescuers and bystanders. (7-3.4) (EC 868-872 PEC 926-927)

20.

A. The hot zone is where contamination is actually present. Treatment in this area is provided by trained personnel wearing protective equipment. Treatment is limited to life-threatening conditions. The warm zone is the area outside the hot zone where patients and personnel must remain until they are fully decontaminated. The cold or safe zone is outside the warm zone. This area is where personnel can remove protective clothing; all life-threatening conditions should have been attended to before the patient reaches this zone. (7-3.5) (EC 868-872 PEC 926)

21.

B. A MCI is typically defined as any event that places excessive demands on personnel and equipment. This demand is specific for your individual system. Often an incident involving mass transit or a large building may turn into a MCI; however, the incident must meet the above criteria. A rural system may be taxed by a response of three emergency vehicles; another system may not be taxed by the same response. Often many systems routinely require police, fire, and EMS to respond simultaneously. (7-3.7) (EC 877 PEC 937)

22.

A. The senior EMT-B who arrives at the scene of a disaster first assumes EMS incident manager until relieved by the pre-designated officer. When the EMT-B is relieved by the pre-designated officer, he or she may be reassigned as a sector officer. (7-3.10) (EC 877-889 PEC 948)

23.

C. Your immediate role as the next senior EMT-B on a MCI is as the primary triage officer. You will remain at this post until relieved by the EMS incident commander. (7-3.11) (EC 878-880 PEC 938-939)

24.

D. To protect yourself and others from possible exposure of a hazardous materials incident, you should position yourself and others uphill and upwind. Positioning in this manner limits exposure for the following reasons: many chemicals being carried with the wind, liquids flowing downhill, and some gasses being heavier than air. (7-3.12) (EC 872-877 PEC 926-932)

25.

A. It may be difficult to do, but you must move on to the next patient if you find that there is no breathing or no pulse. Remember you must move on; attending to this patient would take too many of your much needed resources. (7-3.13) (EC 877-888 PEC 936, 938-939)

26.

B. You should position your vehicle at a safe distance behind medic seven but close enough so that motorists can see both units at a glance. Do not follow too closely; reaction time decreases and motorists may think there is only one emergency vehicle and proceed, striking your vehicle. Always use all your lights and siren when approaching and proceeding through an intersection. When following another emergency vehicle, use a different siren mode than the other vehicle. (7-1.5) (EC 819 PEC 884-885)

27.

A. Equipment that comes in contact with mucous membranes like laryngoscope blades should be cleaned by soaking the blades in an EPA-registered sterilant for 10 to 45 minutes. Soaking equipment in an EPA-registered sterilant for 6 to 10 hours is usually performed by hospitals on their invasive equipment. Simply wiping the blades with a 1:100 or 1:10 bleach and water solution will not disinfect them adequately. (7-1.14) (EC 831 PEC 894-896)

28.

D. This event will likely place an excessive demand on your personnel and equipment resources. It is far better to activate the MCI plan and have too many rescuers and equipment en route to the scene than to have too little responding. (7-3.7) (EC 877 PEC 937)

29.

B. If you are the most senior EMT-B to arrive on the scene of a multiple casualty incident, your initial role will be that of the EMS incident manager. You will remain the EMS incident manager until relieved by the pre-designated officer if there is one. (7-3.10) (EC 877-889 PEC 948)

30.

D. Triage is a system that sorts patients to determine the order that they will receive care and transportation to the hospital. Triage usually divides patients into groups that are high priority, second priority and lowest priority. (7-3.13) (EC 877-888 PEC 936, 938-939)

8 Advanced Airway

module objectives

Questions in this module relate to D.O.T. objectives 8-1.1 to 8-1.35.

DIRECTIONS Each of the questions or incomplete statements below is followed by suggested answers or completions. Select the **one answer** that is best in each case.

1. The depression that is located between the base of the tongue and the epiglottis is known as the:
   A. vallecula.
   B. glottic opening.
   C. vocal cords.
   D. larynx.

2. The space between the true vocal cords where the endotracheal tube is placed is known as the:
   A. glottic opening.
   B. vallecula.
   C. larynx.
   D. epiglottis.

3. The narrowest portion of the infant's airway is at the level of the:
   A. true vocal cords.
   B. laryngopharynx.
   C. cuneiform cartilage.
   D. cricoid cartilage.

4. Because the head is proportionately larger in children, padding should not be placed under the head of a child younger than:
   A. 9 years of age.
   B. 11 years of age.
   C. 13 years of age.
   D. 15 years of age.

5. Which statement is true regarding airway compromise in children?
   A. Because the tongue is larger in a child, it is the most common cause of airway obstruction.
   B. Most airway obstruction in the child patient is caused by a foreign body lodged in the carina.
   C. Because a child's head is smaller, it is less likely to flex the neck forward, thus compromising the airway.

   D. The trachea is firmer and less flexible, which likely will cause an airway compromise.

6. You are treating a responsive trauma patient. Which of the following will help maintain an open airway?
   A. oropharyngeal airway
   B. head-tilt, chin-lift
   C. head-tilt, extension technique
   D. nasopharyngeal airway

7. Insertion of a nasogastric (NG) tube is indicated in which of the following?
   A. 4-year-old involved in a bicycle accident who has sustained significant facial trauma
   B. 2-year-old for whom you can not provide effective ventilation due to gastric distention
   C. 1-year-old who complains of a painful throat and has a seal-like bark when he coughs
   D. 3-year-old who may have ingested a caustic chemical substance like drain cleaner

8. The procedure where pressure is applied on the cricoid cartilage, closing off the esophagus and reducing the chance of aspiration is called:
   A. Trendelenburg position.
   B. McIntosh pressure.
   C. Buck's extension.
   D. Sellick's maneuver.

9. In which of the following patients would endotracheal intubation be contraindicated?
   A. 54-year-old without a gag reflex who can not protect his or her own airway
   B. 34-year-old unresponsive patient who will not tolerate an oropharyngeal airway

C. 18-year-old patient with mouth trauma for whom you are unable to get a good seal with the mask

D. 73-year-old cardiac arrest patient with a history of cardiomegaly

10. Because of anatomical differences, which laryngoscope blade is preferred for intubating infants and children?

A. curved

B. McIntosh

C. convex

D. Miller

11. Which laryngoscope blade lifts the epiglottis indirectly by pressing on the glossoepiglottic ligament?

A. Miller

B. Wisconsin

C. Flagg

D. McIntosh

12. The straight laryngoscope blade exposes the vocal cords and the glottic opening by:

A. indirectly lifting the epiglottis.

B. fitting into the vallecula.

C. directly lifting the epiglottis.

D. pressing the glossoepiglottic ligament.

13. Select the **untrue** statement pertaining to the use of a malleable stylet when performing an endotracheal intubation.

A. The stylet provides stiffness to alter the shape of the tube.

B. The stylet should be lubricated with a water soluble lubricant.

C. The stylet should extend past the Murphy eye 1 to 2 cm.

D. The stylet must be recessed ½ inch from the distal end.

14. In the emergency setting, which size endotracheal tube will fit either the adult male or female?

A. 6.5 mm i.d.

B. 7.0 mm i.d.

C. 7.5 mm i.d.

D. 8.0 mm i.d.

15. You have responded to a 2-year-old who is in cardiac arrest. Which formula is used to estimate the correct size endotracheal tube for this child?

A. tube size = (age in months + 16) ÷ 2

B. tube size = (4 ÷ age in years) + 4

C. tube size = (age in months × 4) ÷ 16

D. tube size = (16 + age in years) ÷ 4

16. Common complications of endotracheal intubation of the adult patient include all of the following **except:**

A. tachycardia.

B. arrhythmia.

C. hypotension.

D. hypovolemia.

17. An alternative method for estimating the size of the endotracheal tube needed for a child is to:

A. choose a tube with the same outside diameter as the patient's little finger.

B. select a tube with an inside diameter the same as the patient's fingernail.

C. measure from the tip of the patient's nose to the angle of the lower jaw.

D. choose a tube that is slightly larger than the patient's glottic opening.

18. You are preparing to intubate your adult patient. You should ventilate the patient at a rate of:

A. 12 breaths per minute for 4 to 6 minutes.

B. 20 breaths per minute for 2 to 4 minutes.

C. 24 breaths per minute for 1 to 2 minutes.

D. 28 breaths per minute for 1 to 3 minutes.

19. When preparing to intubate a nontraumatic patient, all of the following are appropriate techniques to maximize visualization of the vocal cords **except:**
    A. placing a folded towel under the patient's shoulder blades.
    B. positioning the patient's head in a sniffing position.
    C. positioning the head backward while lifting the chin forward.
    D. placing the patient's head so that it hangs over the edge of the bed.

20. Of the following, the correct sequence for inserting the laryngoscope is to:
    A. hold the laryngoscope in the left hand, insert into the right corner of the mouth, sweep the tongue to the left.
    B. hold the laryngoscope in the right hand, insert into the right corner of the mouth, sweep the tongue to the left.
    C. hold the laryngoscope in the left hand, insert into the left corner of the mouth, sweep the tongue to the left.
    D. hold the laryngoscope in the left hand, insert into the left corner of the mouth, sweep the tongue to the right.

21. You know you have successfully intubated your patient when:
    A. the distal cuff inflates and secures the tube in place.
    B. you visualize the tube pass through the glottic opening.
    C. you place the tube through the oval esophageal opening.
    D. you hear air rush into the patient's mouth and nose.

22. After you witness the endotracheal tube pass through the vocal cords, you hear lung sounds only on the right chest. You should:
    A. deflate the cuff and extubate the patient; then try again.
    B. deflate the cuff and withdraw the tube slightly; then reinflate.
    C. gently advance the tube forward and add air to the cuff.
    D. ask the patient if his right lung has been surgically removed.

23. Your partner has intubated a patient; after assessing for proper placement, you are unsure if the endotracheal tube has been properly placed. You should:
    A. leave the tube in place and reassess.
    B. deflate the cuff and pull back gently.
    C. perform a rapid medical assessment.
    D. immediately remove the tube.

24. You are attempting to intubate an infant when the heart rate falls below 80 beats per minute, you should:
    A. continue the intubation attempt and start CPR immediately.
    B. stop the intubation attempt and hyperventilate with a BVM.
    C. continue the intubation attempt and insert an oropharyngeal airway.
    D. stop the intubation attempt and perform a finger sweep.

25. The best indicator of proper endotracheal tube placement in infants and children is:
    A. auscultating bilateral breath sounds anteriorly.
    B. watching the diaphragm move by observing the abdomen.
    C. observing changes in the pulse oximeter device.
    D. observing the symmetrical rise and fall of the chest.

26. Insertion of an oropharyngeal airway after intubating a child is recommended because:
    A. the OPA acts as a bite block.
    B. the OPA keeps the tongue forward.
    C. the OPA helps to secure the tube.
    D. the OPA will keep the airway open.

27. You have successfully intubated your infant patient when you notice inadequate lung expansion. Which of the following can be the cause of the inadequate lung expansion?

    A. the tube is too small for this patient.

    B. the tube has become blocked by secretions.

    C. there is a leak in the bag-valve-mask.

    D. all of the above.

28. Confirming correct endotracheal tube placement is accomplished by:

    A. auscultating over the epigastrium.

    B. watching for chest rise and fall.

    C. auscultating breath sounds.

    D. all of the above.

29. You suspect your partner has intubated the esophagus; you should:

    A. extubate and hyperventilate with a BVM.

    B. extubate and reattempt to intubate the patient.

    C. leave the tube in place and intubate around the tube.

    D. leave the tube in place and hyperventilate with a BVM.

30. After you have successfully intubated your child patient, which of the following will help limit the possibility of a dislodged tube?

    A. inflating the cuff with 10 cc of air

    B. inserting an oropharyngeal airway

    C. immobilizing the patient's head

    D. deactivating the pop-off valve

SCENARIO

Questions 31–34 refer to the following scenario:

You and your partner Mim are taking a well deserved break at the station when the station alerting system sounds: "Medic One, respond to a respiratory call at 455 Nell Avenue." You put down your coffee and pick up your run report computer and walk briskly to the ambulance. After assuring that the scene is safe, you enter the patient's house. You are led by the husband to a back bedroom where you find the patient, a 68-year-old female, lying on the floor unresponsive to any stimulus and breathing 6 times a minute. Mim, being the most senior and experienced EMT-B, asks you to insert an airway adjunct and hyperventilate the patient with the BVM. Mim decides to intubate this patient with an endotracheal tube.

31. Why did Mim decide to intubate this patient rather than to ventilate with the BVM and airway adjunct?

    A. The patient is unresponsive to any type of stimulus.

    B. The bag-valve-mask is contraindicated in this patient.

    C. An airway adjunct will not be tolerated in this patient.

    D. The patient's age dictates the endotracheal tube is needed.

32. Mim chooses to use the McIntosh (curved) blade to intubate her patient. Which best describes the correct sequence and technique for using the McIntosh blade?

    A. Enter the mouth on the left side, sweep the tongue to the right, and lift the epiglottis directly.

    B. Enter the mouth on the right side, sweep the tongue to the left, and lift the epiglottis directly.

    C. Enter the mouth on the right side, sweep the tongue to the left, and lift the epiglottis indirectly.

    D. Enter the mouth on the left side, sweep the tongue to the right, and lift the tongue indirectly.

33. Mim observes the tube pass through the vocal cords and glottic opening. She securely holds the tube in place and inflates the cuff by injecting air. How much air should be injected?

    A. 1 to 3 cc

    B. 5 to 10 cc

    C. 15 to 20 cc

    D. 20 to 30 cc

34. Immediately after passing the endotracheal tube, you should first assess for tube placement by:
    A. auscultating over the 2nd intercostal space on the midclavicular line.
    B. auscultating over the epigastrium.
    C. watching for an increase on the pulse oximeter.
    D. inspecting for rise and fall of the abdomen.

35. The average sized endotracheal tube used in the adult male patient is _____ mm.
    A. 6.0
    B. 7.0
    C. 7.5
    D. 8.0

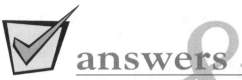

answers & rationales

1.

A. The depressed space between the epiglottis and the base of the tongue is the vallecula. The McIntosh (curved) laryngoscope blade fits into the vallecula to indirectly lift the epiglottis during endotracheal intubation. (8-1.1a) (EC 930-933 PEC 971-973)

2.

A. The area between the true vocal cords is known as the glottic opening. You must actually see the endotracheal tube pass through the glottic opening to be certain that the tube is placed correctly. (8-1.1b) (EC 930-933 PEC 971-973)

3.

D. The narrowest portion of the infant's and child's airway is the cricoid cartilage. It is important to remember this because the endotracheal tube may pass easily through the vocal cords but be too large to pass the cricoid ring. (8-1.2a) (EC 930-933 PEC 973)

4.

A. The head of a child under the age of 9 years is proportionately larger. Placing a pad under the head may occlude the airway by flexing the head and neck forward. (8-1.2b) (EC 930-933 PEC 973)

5.

A. The tongue is larger in the child and is the most common cause of airway obstruction. Most often a foreign body will lodge at the level of the cricoid cartilage since this is the narrowest portion of the pediatric airway anatomy. Proportionately the child's head is larger and can easily flex the neck forward, compromising the airway. The trachea is not as firm and more flexible than that of the adult, which can cause an airway compromise. (8-1.3) (EC 930-933 PEC 971-973)

6.

D. The nasopharyngeal airway will help to maintain an adequate airway in the trauma patient. The oropharyngeal airway is contraindicated in the responsive patient. A and C Movement of the patient's head, is contraindicated in the trauma patient. (8-1.4) (EC 933 PEC 974)

7.

B. If you are unable to effectively ventilate your pediatric patient because of gastric distention, you should relieve the pressure by inserting a nasogastric tube. The use of a nasogastric tube is contraindicated in the patient with facial trauma. (8-1.6) (EC 948 PEC 970-973)

8.

D. Sellick's maneuver is a procedure that applies pressure to the cricoid cartilage by pressing backwards on the Adam's apple. Applying pressure to the cricoid cartilage closes off the esophagus, thus reducing the chance of aspiration. The Trendelenburg position is also known as the shock position; feet are elevated slightly above the head while in the supine position. Buck's extension refers to Gurdon Buck, an early American surgeon who invented a device made of weight and pulley for applying extension to a limb. (8-1.7) (EC 942-943 PEC 979)

9.

B. If the patient will not tolerate an oropharyngeal airway, he or she is not likely to accept endotracheal intubation. A patient without a gag reflex who can not protect his or her own airway should be intubated. Patients who have mouth trauma and for whom you are unable to maintain an adequate mask seal should be intubated. A patient in cardiac arrest should be intubated. Cardiomegaly describes the patient's history of hypertrophy (increased size) of the heart. (8-1.8) (EC 930-933, 938, 945 PEC 975)

10.

D. The Miller blade is preferred when intubating infants and children. The Miller blade provides better displacement of the tongue and allows for better visualization of the glottic opening. (8-1.9) (EC 935-938 PEC 975-979)

11.

D. The curved or McIntosh laryngoscope blade lifts the epiglottis indirectly. The tip of the McIntosh blade is inserted into the vallecula where it presses the glossoepiglottic ligament, causing the epiglottis to be lifted. The other distracters are all straight blades that lift the epiglottis directly. (8-1.10) (EC 935-936, 942 PEC 976)

12.

C. The straight blade (Miller, Wisconsin, or Flagg) lifts the epiglottis directly by placing the tip under the epiglottis and lifting. All other distracters describe the curved or McIntosh blade. (8-1.11) (EC 935-936, 942 PEC 976)

13.

C. The Murphy eye is located at the distal end of the tube, and the stylet should not extend past this area. Extending the stylet beyond the Murphy eye may injure the patient. (8-1.12) (EC 937-938 PEC 978)

14.

C. The 7.5 mm i.d. endotracheal tube will usually fit both the adult male and female in the emergency setting. (8-1.13) (EC 936-937 PEC 977-978)

15.

D. The following is the correct formula to estimate the endotracheal tube size for a child over the age of 1 year: tube size = (16 + age in years) ÷ 4. An example for a 4-year-old child is thus: 16 + 4 = 20; 20 divided by 4 is 5. The patient should receive a 5.0 mm i.d. endotracheal tube. (8-1.14) (EC 945-946 PEC 988)

16.

C. Hypotension is rarely seen when intubating the adult patient; however, this is a common complication when intubating infants and children. Tachycardia and arrhythmia are common complications when intubating the adult patient. (8-1.16) (EC 945-946 PEC 988-989)

17.

A. To estimate the correct endotracheal tube size for a child, select a tube with the same outside diameter as the child's little finger. Never choose a tube larger than the glottic opening. (8-1.17a) (EC 938, 942-944 PEC 979-985)

18.

C. The adult patient needing intubated should be hyperventilated at a rate of 24 breaths per minute for 1 to 2 minutes. (8-1.17a) (EC 938, 942-944 PEC 979-985)

19.

D. Never place the patient's head in a position that does not allow for support; this may cause serious injury. All of the others are appropriate techniques for the nontraumatic patient. (8-1.17b) (EC 938, 942-944 PEC 979-985)

20.

A. The correct sequence for inserting the laryngoscope, which will help to maximize visualization of the vocal cords and the glottic opening, is to hold the scope in the left hand, insert into the right corner of the mouth, sweep the tongue to the left. (8-1.17a) (EC 938, 942-944 PEC 979-985)

21.

B. When you visualize the endotracheal tube pass directly through the glottic opening, you can be sure the tube has been correctly placed. Beware, just because the tube has been placed correctly does not mean that it can not become dislodged and then intubate the esophagus. The purpose of the distal cuff is to seal the airway, not to secure the tube in place. If the tube is placed and left in the esophagus, this is a grave mistake and will cause the patient to die. If the patient is properly intubated and the cuff inflated, you should not hear air escaping. (8-1.17d) (EC 938, 942-944 PEC 979-985)

22.

B. After the tube has passed through the glottic opening, if lung sounds are only heard on the right side of the chest the tube is likely in the right mainstem bronchus. You should carefully deflate the cuff and gently withdraw the tube 1 to 2 cm. Next, reinflate the cuff and recheck the lung sounds. A lobectomy (surgical removal of lung) on the right side of the chest will cause the absence of lung sounds. (8-1.17e) (EC 938, 942-944 PEC 979-985)

23.

D. If at any time you are unsure if the endotracheal tube has been properly placed, you should immediately remove the tube. It is far better to remove the tube and ventilate with a BVM than to leave the tube in place. Leaving the tube in the esophagus will cause the death of the patient and may subject you to litigation. (8-1.17f) (EC 938, 942-944 PEC 979-985)

24.

B. If the heart rate falls below 80 beats per minute in the infant, this is an ominous sign of hypoxia. You should immediately stop the intubation attempt and hyperventilate the patient with the BVM with supplemental oxygen. (8-1.18a) (EC 945-947 PEC 989-993)

25.

D. The best indicator of proper tube placement in the infant or child patient is watching the symmetrical (both sides) rise and fall of the chest. Lung sounds can be deceiving in the infant and child. Pulse oximeter may not have immediate changes in these patients. The abdomen moving is not a good indication of proper tube placement. (8-1.8b) (EC 945-947 PEC 989-993)

26.

A. The OPA will act as a bite block and prevent the patient from biting the soft tube and obstructing the airflow. There is no reason to keep the tongue forward; the tube is a direct airway. The OPA does not secure the tube. There is no need to keep the airway open because the endotracheal tube is a direct airway. (8-1.18c) (EC 945-947 PEC 989-993)

27.

D. After you watch the endotracheal tube pass directly through the vocal cords and you are sure the tube is properly placed, you notice poor tidal volume. You should assess the patient and equipment. Is the tube too small for this patient? Does the BVM have a leak or a pop-off valve? Is the EMT delivering a great enough tidal volume? Has the tube become blocked? (8-1.18d) (EC 945-947 PEC 989-993)

28.

D. All of these are used to confirm correct placement of the endotracheal tube. (8-1.19) (EC 943-944, 947 PEC 983-985, 989-990)

29.

A. If you suspect the endotracheal tube has been placed into the esophagus, you must immediately extubate (remove) the tube and hyperventilate the patient. You must not attempt to reintubate the patient until the patient has been hyperventilated. The first tube being in the esophagus does not ensure the next will be placed into the trachea. The esophagus is elastic and can easily accommodate two tubes. Intubating the esophagus and leaving the tube in place are lethal mistakes and will cause your patient to die. Trying to ventilate a patient with a BVM around a tube will prevent a good mask seal. (8-1.20) (EC 934, 943-944, 947 PEC 983, 985-986)

30.

C. Immobilizing the child's or infant's head will reduce movement, which can help limit the possibility of a dislodged tube. Inflating the cuff only seals the tube; it does not help to secure the tube. Inserting an OPA can act as a bite block but will not help secure the tube. When you are ventilating a patient, the pop-off valve should always be deactivated. (8-1.21) (EC 938, 944, 947 PEC 985, 990)

31.

A. Mim is correct in choosing to intubate this patient because the patient is deeply unresponsive and does not respond to any stimulus. By intubating this patient, you establish a secure airway that the patient can not protect on her own. By using the BVM and an airway adjunct, there is a risk of vomiting and aspiration into the lungs. The BVM and airway adjunct are not contraindicated in this type of patient; however, if permitted by your medical direction, the best choice is orotracheal intubation. (8-1.8) (EC 930-933, 938, 945 PEC 975)

32.

C. The correct technique for using the curved McIntosh blade to intubate a patient is to enter the mouth from the right side, sweep the tongue to the left, and lift the epiglottis indirectly by inserting the tip of the blade into the vallecula. (8-1.10) (EC 935-936, 942 PEC 976)

33.

B. The distal cuff should be inflated with 5 to 10 cc of air. Overfilling the cuff could cause injury to the trachea. Underfilling the cuff could cause air to escape around the tube, causing inadequate air exchange. Moreover, an underfilled cuff may not prevent secretions from entering the airway. (8-1.18) (EC 945-947 PEC 989-993)

34.

B. Immediately after passing the endotracheal tube, you should listen over the epigastrium for sounds in the stomach. This would indicate the tube is in the esophagus. If so, you would immediately remove the tube. After the epigastrium, you would auscultate the chest at the 2nd intercostal space midclavicular and then 4th intercostal space midaxillary. At the same time, you would inspect the chest for adequate rise and fall. (EC 930-959 PEC 971-1006)

35.

D. The average sized endotracheal tube used in the adult male patient is 8.0 mm. An adult female typically takes a 7.5 mm sized tube. (EC 930-959 PEC 971-1006)

EXAM

1. An example of an unsafe on-scene activity is:
   A. wearing reflective clothing at night.
   B. using latex gloves.
   C. wearing protective clothing.
   D. entering a crime scene quickly.

2. Which of the following is a behavioral response to stress?
   A. depression
   B. overeating
   C. defensiveness
   D. mood swings

3. The single most important way to prevent the spread of infection is by:
   A. wearing latex gloves.
   B. wearing a disposable face mask.
   C. using antiseptic wipes.
   D. vigorous handwashing.

4. You are responding to a possible crime scene; the patient is reported to be bleeding heavily. You should:
   A. make patient contact and immediately begin your treatment.
   B. get access to the residence and speak to the patient from a distance.
   C. wait for police to secure the scene before entering the scene.
   D. position your vehicle on-scene and wait for police to arrive.

5. Most states require EMT-Bs to report certain conditions. Which of the following is **not** one of these conditions that requires reporting to proper authorities?
   A. abuse
   B. crime
   C. asthmatic attack
   D. drug related injury

6. The term that means "on both sides" is:
   A. unilateral.
   B. lateral.
   C. bilateral.
   D. proximal.

7. The shoulder joint that allows for the widest range of motion is what type of joint?
   A. gliding
   B. pivot
   C. ball and socket
   D. hinged

8. Which of the following patients is breathing adequately?
   A. 6-month-old breathing with abdominal muscles at 20 times a minute
   B. 42-year-old breathing irregularly from sighs at 20 times a minute
   C. 8-year-old breathing with accessory muscles at 30 times a minute
   D. 60-year-old breathing with unequal chest expansion at 22 times a minute

9. You are treating an 8-year-old patient who was kicked in the head by a horse; you should open the airway by:
   A. jaw-thrust maneuver.
   B. head-tilt, chin-lift.
   C. in-line traction maneuver.
   D. head-tilt, flex maneuver.

10. Stimulation of the back of the throat while suctioning a patient may result in:
    A. tachypnea.
    B. bronchospasm.
    C. bradypnea.
    D. bradycardia.

11. When you are preparing to suction the nasopharynx with a French catheter, the length is determined by:
    A. measuring from the tip of the patient's nose to the angle of the jaw.
    B. measuring from the corner of the patient's mouth to the tip of the ear.
    C. measuring from the tip of the patient's nose to the tip of the ear.

D. measuring from the corner of the patient's mouth to the angle of the jaw.

12. After inserting an oropharyngeal airway (OPA), the patient begins to gag; you should:
A. insert a nasopharyngeal airway in addition to the oropharyngeal airway.
B. immediately remove the oropharyngeal airway and prepare to suction.
C. reassure the patient that the oropharyngeal airway is necessary.
D. do nothing; the gagging will subside within a few minutes.

13. You have determined that the number of patients has exceeded your ability to effectively handle a scene. You have summoned additional resources; your next action should be to:
A. move all patients to the transport area.
B. immediately begin treating the patients.
C. perform a focused history on the patients.
D. triage and prioritize the patients.

14. Which of the following best describes a deeply unresponsive patient?
A. may have an intact gag reflex
B. responds to tactile stimulation
C. may cough when an airway adjunct is placed
D. does not respond to pain

15. Which upper respiratory sound may indicate a liquid substance in the airway?
A. crowing
B. snoring
C. gurgling
D. stridor

16. While assessing a patient, you find that the patient's skin is pale, cool and moist; you suspect:
A. hyperthermia.
B. hypoperfusion.
C. vasogenic shock.

D. dehydration.

17. All of the following are examples of life threats that should be managed in the initial assessment **except:**
A. inadequate breathing.
B. open chest injury.
C. closed humerus fracture.
D. major bleeding.

18. When performing a rapid trauma assessment, you are most concerned with:
A. assessing the specific injury site.
B. obtaining accurate vital signs.
C. obtaining the SAMPLE history.
D. identifying life-threatening injuries.

19. A rapid trauma assessment is performed:
A. while en route to the hospital on an unstable patient following vital sign assessment.
B. on the stable trauma patient after the ongoing assessment.
C. prior to movement of the patient from the scene.
D. just before arrival at the hospital on the unstable patient.

20. A major decision point for determining the sequence of assessment steps in the medical patient is:
A. the patient's blood pressure.
B. the patient's level of consciousness.
C. the patient's respiratory status.
D. the patient's pulse rate.

21. During the SAMPLE history for a responsive medical patient, the OPQRST question you used to have the patient rate his or her pain on a scale of 1 to 10 is known as:
A. radiation.
B. quality.
C. severity.
D. provocation.

22. You are assessing a patient who complains of pelvis pain after a fall from a ladder. Choose the correct answer for assessing this injury.
    A. Do not palpate the pelvis; visually inspect it.
    B. Rock the pelvis, checking for instability.
    C. Compress inward and downward.
    D. Apply firm pressure to the pubic bone.

23. Mucous that is coughed up is referred to as a:
    A. mucous cough.
    B. rhonchi cough.
    C. productive cough.
    D. hacking cough.

24. Palpation of the pelvic area in a trauma patient should be:
    A. omitted in the patient with pelvic pain.
    B. performed in the patient with pelvic pain.
    C. performed always with suspected injury.
    D. omitted if the patient is unresponsive.

25. The dorsalis pedis pulse is located:
    A. behind the inner ankle bone.
    B. at the bend of the elbow.
    C. behind the knee.
    D. on the top surface of the foot.

26. The first step in the ongoing assessment is to:
    A. check your interventions.
    B. repeat the focused assessment for other injuries or complaints.
    C. reassess and record vital signs.
    D. repeat the initial assessment.

27. You note a change in the patient's mental status during transport. You should immediately:
    A. take a complete set of vital signs.
    B. assess effectiveness of emergency care.
    C. increase the oxygenation of the patient.
    D. repeat the initial assessment.

28. Which of the following signs found during the ongoing assessment of an adult would indicate the patient's condition is improving?
    A. The patient's breathing was bradypneic and is now tachypneic.
    B. The patient's skin color changes from cyanotic to blue-gray.
    C. The patient begins to use accessory muscles to breathe.
    D. The patient's heart rate increases from 40 beats a minute to 100.

29. Components of the ongoing assessment—the initial assessment and baseline vital signs—should be repeated every _____ minutes in the unstable patient.
    A. 2
    B. 3
    C. 4
    D. 5

30. When you are dealing with a patient who seems hostile or aggressive, it may be necessary to assert your authority. Which position is likely to convey authority?
    A. Keep your eye level below the patient's.
    B. Keep your eye level above the patient's.
    C. Communicate without making eye contact.
    D. Communicate while staring at the patient.

31. After you have made numerous attempts to persuade a patient to be treated and transported, the patient refuses both. The patient refuses to sign the refusal-of-care form; you should:
    A. force the patient to sign the form by refusing to leave until it is signed.
    B. have a family member sign the form verifying that the patient refused to sign.
    C. leave the scene without the signature and advise dispatch of the situation.
    D. sign the patient's name for the patient and document the unusual circumstances.

32. Which of the following is **not** a sign of breathing difficulty?
    A. restlessness and agitation
    B. acute abdominal pain
    C. accessory muscle use
    D. incomprehensible speech

33. When providing emergency care for the adult patient with breathing difficulty, you should:
    A. take time to determine the exact cause of the patient's distress.
    B. expose and inspect the chest in the trauma patient.
    C. provide positive pressure ventilation only if you are certain of the need.
    D. consider the patient a low treatment priority.

34. On auscultation of the patient with breathing difficulty, you note diminished wheezing.
    A. This is always indicative of patient improvement.
    B. This is seldom indicative of patient improvement.
    C. This never indicates patient improvement.
    D. This commonly indicates patient improvement but may indicate patient decline.

35. Increased oxygenation should have what effect on a breathing patient's mental status.
    A. It generally has little effect.
    B. It generally causes an improvement.
    C. It generally causes a worsening.
    D. It generally has no effect.

36. During your initial assessment of a patient complaining of difficulty breathing, you find the pulse is 140 beats a minute and the patient's neck is cyanotic. The correct sequence for appropriate immediate treatment is to:
    A. provide positive pressure ventilation, transport expeditiously, and continue assessment.
    B. apply high-flow oxygen, continue the assessment, and transport to the hospital.
    C. complete the physical assessment, apply positive pressure ventilation, and transport.
    D. continue assessment, apply high-flow oxygen, call for ALS backup, and transport.

37. You are treating a patient who is complaining of shortness of breath. The patient has minimal rise and fall of the chest. Little air flow is felt from the patient's mouth and nose. Your emergency treatment should be to:
    A. provide positive pressure ventilation.
    B. provide oxygen by non-rebreather mask.
    C. provide oxygen by nasal cannula at 6 lpm.
    D. provide no oxygen therapy at this time.

38. Which of the following is **incorrect** pertaining to assisting a patient with the use of the metered-dose inhaler (MDI)?
    A. Shake the canister for at least 30 seconds.
    B. Instruct the patient to breathe slowly and deeply.
    C. Instruct the patient to breathe through the nose.
    D. Depress the canister as the patient begins to inhale.

39. Exposure to cool night air will frequently reduce a child's distress associated with:
    A. epiglottis.
    B. croup.
    C. asthma.
    D. pulmonary embolism.

40. A common cause of mechanical AED failure is:
    A. cable breakage.
    B. 80 cycle interference.
    C. battery failure.
    D. cold temperature.

41. In providing treatment for a cardiac arrest patient, which of the following actions should be performed first?
    A. placement of a oropharyngeal airway.
    B. setting up an oxygen delivery device.
    C. obtaining a patient history.
    D. providing care with the AED.

42. Which of the following patients should **not** receive a dose of nitroglycerin?
    A. 52-year-old who has taken four nitroglycerin tablets before your arrival
    B. 77-year-old with a blood pressure of 110/64, pulse 90 beats each minute
    C. 62-year-old who continues to complain of chest pain after taking two nitro
    D. 88-year-old who has taken one nitro and now complains of a headache

43. Which of the following is **not** a common side effect of nitroglycerin spray?
    A. severe headache
    B. heart rate increase
    C. hypertension
    D. heart rate decrease

44. Nitroglycerin spray is administered sublingualy. To achieve the same dose as one nitroglycerin tablet, you would need to depress the container how many times?
    A. Depress the container once, delivering one short spray.
    B. Depress the container twice, delivering two short sprays.
    C. Depress the container three times, delivering one continuous spray.
    D. Depress and hold the container down, delivering one continuous extended spray.

45. The number one killer in America today is:
    A. automobile accidents.
    B. falls.
    C. cancer.
    D. heart disease.

46. A patient experiencing a heart attack without chest pain is said to be having:
    A. silent heart attack.
    B. phantom heart attack.
    C. quiet heart attack.
    D. minor heart attack.

47. You are preparing to administer a defibrillation shock using an AED; you notice the patient has a nitroglycerin patch on; you should:
    A. place the adhesive defibrillation pad over the nitroglycerin patch and shock.
    B. not remove the patch, place the defibrillation pad next to the patch, and shock.
    C. remove the patch and wipe the area after you deliver three stacked shocks.
    D. remove the patch and wipe the area with a cloth before defibrillating.

48. The two basic categories of external defibrillators are the:
    A. automatic and semi-automatic.
    B. automatic and implantable.
    C. automatic and manual.
    D. manual and implantable.

49. You have successfully defibrillated your pulseless patient. The patient has a strong radial pulse; however, the breathing is shallow and slow; you should:
    A. wait a few minutes for the respiratory drive to return.
    B. provide oxygen by nasal cannula at 6 liters per minute.
    C. administer oxygen by non-rebreather mask at 15 lpm.
    D. control the breathing with positive pressure ventilation.

50. Which of the following is a true statement pertaining to nitroglycerin?
    A. Nitroglycerin administration may cause a slight increase in the patient's pulse rate.
    B. Nitroglycerin administration may result in an increase in the patient's blood pressure.
    C. Nitroglycerin administration may result in sudden and intense diarrhea and nausea.
    D. Nitroglycerin administration may increase the workload of the heart.

51. The most common cause of an automated external defibrillator (AED) failure is:
    A. battery failure.
    B. lack of training.
    C. cable failure.
    D. outdated pads.

52. The condition in which there is a lack of insulin and a high level of sugar in the blood is called:
    A. hypoglycemia.
    B. insulin shock.
    C. hypoinsulin.
    D. hyperglycemia.

53. In which position should you place a patient with an altered mental status who has a history of diabetes that is controlled by medication?
    A. supine or prone
    B. semi-Fowler
    C. Trendelenburg
    D. on the patient's side

54. Which symptom is a late sign of neurological deficit that has resulted from a nontraumatic brain injury?
    A. double vision
    B. stiff neck
    C. headache
    D. garbled speech

55. The stage of a seizure known as the recovery phase in which the patient's mental status progressively improves over time is known as the:
    A. aura period.
    B. tonic phase.
    C. clonic phase.
    D. postictal state.

56. The stage of a generalized seizure during which the muscles become rigid is known as the:
    A. aura phase.
    B. tonic phase.
    C. clonic phase.
    D. postictal phase.

57. The symptoms associated with a transient ischemic attack generally subside within _____ minutes.
    A. 10
    B. 20
    C. 30
    D. 40

58. A major contributing factor to a stroke is:
    A. recent exercise.
    B. fever.
    C. high blood pressure.
    D. seizure.

59. A condition in which the patient has a sudden and temporary loss of consciousness is called:
    A. neuropoxia.
    B. syncope.
    C. postictal.
    D. eclampsia.

60. Which pair of signs and symptoms is the most likely indicator of anaphylaxis?
    A. headache and restlessness
    B. respiratory distress and shock
    C. runny or watery eyes
    D. general weakness and abdominal cramping

61. You have just administered epinephrine by auto-injector to a patient having an anaphylactic reaction to a bee sting. The drug effect is immediate. How long would you expect the duration of its effectiveness?
    A. 10 to 20 minutes
    B. 30 to 40 minutes
    C. 50 to 60 minutes
    D. 2 to 3 hours

62. A 65-year-old patient is suffering from a mild allergic reaction. There are no signs of respiratory compromise or shock; you should:
    A. inject ½ the adult dose of epinephrine via the auto-injector.
    B. administer ¼ the adult dose of epinephrine via the auto-injector.
    C. not administer the epinephrine at any dose unless directed by medical control.
    D. give a full adult dose of epinephrine via the auto-injector.

63. A substance that triggers an allergic reaction is called:
    A. an allergen.
    B. an allergic substance.
    C. an access particle.
    D. an antibody.

64. Activated charcoal is the medication of choice for ingested poisonings because:
    A. it inhibits poisons from being absorbed into the body.
    B. it neutralizes poisons while in the stomach and GI tract.
    C. it prevents poisons from entering the cells by neutralization.
    D. it acts as an antidote to most household and commercial poisons.

65. In which position should the patient complaining of an acute abdomen with signs of hypoperfusion be placed?
    A. left lateral recumbent
    B. supine with feet elevated
    C. semi-Fowler with knees bent
    D. position of comfort for the patient

66. Which of the following persons would likely tolerate a cold environment best and have a reduced risk of hypothermia?
    A. a 3-year-old who is wet from a rain shower
    B. a 20-year-old who has been drinking alcohol
    C. a 34-year-old walking briskly in a stiff wind
    D. a 50-year-old who takes blood pressure medication

67. You are treating a patient who has been bitten by a rattlesnake. Which of the following treatments is correct?
    A. Wash the area around the bite with mild soap and water.
    B. Elevate the injection site above the level of the patient's heart.
    C. Make two small lacerations over the bite and evacuate the wound.
    D. Place a tourniquet superior and inferior to the bite injection site.

68. Choose the phrase that best describes reasonable force.
    A. Use of moderate force to control a dangerous patient whom you have determined a risk
    B. The amount of force needed to overpower and restrain an unruly patient who may injure others
    C. The use of physical and tactile force to subdue a patient and prevent injury to all concerned
    D. Minimal amount of force required to keep the patient from injuring self or others

69. Which position will help reduce the risk of supine hypotension syndrome in the patient who is near full term of her pregnancy?
    A. prone position
    B. shock position
    C. supine position
    D. sitting position

70. Which statement pertaining to the normal delivery of an infant is correct?
    A. The placenta most often is delivered 1 to 2 hours after birth.
    B. Gentle pressure should be applied to the fontanel during delivery.
    C. Bleeding after delivery may be up to 1000 cc and is well tolerated.
    D. The placenta must be transported to the hospital for examination.

71. Your patient has just delivered her baby in your ambulance. Which of the following is correct pertaining to treatment of this patient?
    A. Gentle pressure should be applied to cord to aid delivery of placenta.
    B. The placenta usually delivers on its own within 10 to 20 minutes. Transport without delay.
    C. Delay transport until the placenta is completely delivered.
    D. Apply direct pressure over the vaginal area with a nonocclusive dressing and transport immediately.

72. You and your partner have just helped deliver a baby. The umbilical cord should be cut:
    A. as soon after delivery as possible.
    B. after the cord pulsations cease.
    C. before cord pulsations cease.
    D. after the single clamp has been placed.

73. During delivery the gloved fingertips are positioned on the bony part of the infant's head to:
    A. delay delivery until arrival at the hospital.

B. prevent an explosive delivery of the head.
    C. slow delivery until arrival at the hospital.
    D. monitor the infant's pulse rate during labor.

74. Your patient has a deep laceration to the upper arm; bright red blood is spurting from the wound. Which vessel is likely severed?
    A. brachial artery
    B. femoral artery
    C. cephalic vein
    D. peroneal vein

75. Your patient has been involved in an industrial accident; he is bleeding dark red blood profusely from the leg. You should first control this patient's bleeding:
    A. during the focused history and physical.
    B. during the detailed physical exam.
    C. during the initial assessment of the patient.
    D. before assuring an airway and breathing.

76. Your patient has sustained a large hematoma from an accident on the playground; which order is correct for treating a closed soft tissue injury?
    A. assure airway and breathing, splint injuries, BSI precautions, treat shock
    B. assure airway and breathing, BSI precautions, splint injuries, treat shock
    C. BSI precautions, assure airway and breathing, treat shock, splint injuries
    D. BSI precautions, treat shock, assure airway and breathing, splint injuries

77. While removing a burn patient's clothing, you find that a portion of the shirt has adhered to the patient's back; you should:
    A. gently remove clothing from the adhered area by pulling.
    B. cut the shirt around the adhered portion.
    C. apply a burn ointment to the adhered area.
    D. soak the adhered area with water, and them remove adhered clothing.

78. Which of the following is **inappropriate** treatment for a patient suffering from burns?
    A. Cover the patient to prevent body heat loss.
    B. Separate burned fingers with dry dressings.
    C. Stop the burning process by applying water.
    D. Attempt to drain blisters by direct pressure.

79. Which of the following is correct pertaining to the use of a bandage?
    A. A bandage holds a dressing in place.
    B. A bandage should be sterile or free from any organisms.
    C. A bandage should be removed if bleeding is not controlled.
    D. A bandage covers an open wound and prevents infection.

80. Blood has soaked through the pressure dressing you applied to your patient's injury; your next immediate action should be to:
    A. apply a loose tourniquet until you can feel a pulse.
    B. apply a tight tourniquet because the bleeding is uncontrollable.
    C. remove the original dressings and then apply new ones.
    D. apply additional dressings over the original ones.

81. Leaving the fingertips or toes exposed after bandaging an extremity:
    A. provides for patient comfort through temperature control.
    B. eliminates the potential for circulatory obstruction.
    C. allows for rapid removal of bandages if required.
    D. allows for the assessment of circulation.

82. Your patient has a knife embedded in the right side of his chest. Your immediate emergency medical care for this injury should be to:
    A. expose the wound area.
    B. control wound bleeding.
    C. gently remove the object.
    D. manually secure the object.

83. The anterior bone of the lower leg is called the:
    A. fibula.
    B. ulna.
    C. tibia.
    D. femur.

84. Which of the following is an appropriate treatment for a patient with an isolated fracture?
    A. Make three attempts to align a fracture if the distal pulses are absent.
    B. Pad the splint to prevent pressure and discomfort to the patient.
    C. To prevent loss of any jewelry around the injury site, leave it in place.
    D. To reduce infection, you should return protruding bones back beneath the skin.

85. When assessing your patient for a potential spine injury, which of the following is inappropriate:
    A. ask the patient to move to determine the specific area of injury.
    B. realize that impaired breathing is not a sign of potential injury.
    C. know that soft tissue injuries of the head and neck are not reliable indicators of injury.
    D. assess the motor and sensory functions.

86. You and your partner have responded to a motorcycle crash. The patient was wearing a helmet. You should leave the helmet in place if:
    A. it interferes with your ability to assess the airway and breathing.

B. it interferes with your ability to manage the airway and breathing.

C. it does not fit well and allows excessive movement of the head.

D. you can properly immobilize the spine with the helmet in place.

87. When providing care for chemical burns to the eye, you should:

A. delay flushing of the eyes until transport has begun.

B. flush alkali burns with vinegar for at least 10 minutes.

C. flush the eyes immediately and continue during transport.

D. be certain to never remove hard or soft contact lenses.

88. Which of the following signs and symptoms indicates a pediatric patient is in decompensated respiratory failure?

A. cyanosis

B. nasal flaring

C. subcostal retractions

D. increased respiratory rate

89. Which of the following signs or symptoms is the best indication of hypoperfusion (shock) in the pediatric patient?

A. noisy respiration

B. weak or absent peripheral pulse

C. pink, warm, and dry skin

D. capillary refill less than 2 seconds

90. When a caregiver fails to provide sufficient attention or respect to an individual, this is called:

A. abuse.

B. neglect.

C. molestation.

D. violation.

91. When you are navigating a curve while driving the ambulance, which action could be considered dangerous?

A. entering the curve on the outside

B. braking prior to entering the curve

C. decelerating before entering the curve

D. accelerating while in the curve

92. To protect yourself and the patient during the extrication process from debris such as glass and metal, you should:

A. direct the hydraulic spreader operator to be careful.

B. quickly perform a rapid extrication procedure.

C. cover the patient and yourself with a tarpaulin.

D. remove your heavy coat and cover the patient.

93. Which of the following best describes simple access to a patient?

A. access that takes less than 20 minutes

B. access that does not require the use of tools

C. access that requires special training

D. access gained by using a manually forced tool

94. You are approaching a motor vehicle crash site and notice a truck overturned with a plume of yellow gas surrounding the site; your first action should be to:

A. cordon off the area and evacuate all bystanders from the area.

B. approach the site slowly in an attempt to identify the cargo.

C. approach the site quickly and remove any injured patients.

D. assist bystanders to an area downhill and down wind of the site.

95. You are the first to arrive on a scene of a mass casualty incident (MCI). What is your initial role as the first EMT-B on-scene?

A. EMS treatment manager

B. EMS incident manager

C. EMS triage officer

D. EMS staging sector

96. You are at the scene of a MCI and have been assigned to the triage sector. Your patient has sustained a large burn without airway problems; you would prioritize this patient as:
    A. red—high priority
    B. yellow—second priority
    C. green—low priority
    D. black—lowest priority

97. Placement of a nasogastric tube is indicated for a child patient when:
    A. an endotracheal tube can be placed within 30 seconds.
    B. the responsive patient is developing gastric distention.
    C. effective ventilations are prevented due to gastric distention.
    D. the responsive patient is at risk of vomiting.

98. Which of the following is **not** a piece of equipment required for endotracheal intubation?
    A. endotracheal tube mask
    B. laryngoscope and blades
    C. suction unit
    D. stylet

99. During endotracheal intubation, the stylet is used to:
    A. facilitate suctioning of the endotracheal tube.
    B. secure the endotracheal tube in place.
    C. alter the shape of the endotracheal tube and provide stiffness.
    D. remove an improperly positioned endotracheal tube

100. All of the following are common complications that can occur with endotracheal intubation **except:**

A. hypoxia.
B. left mainstem intubation.
C. trauma to the lips, tongue, or teeth.
D. bradycardia.

101. Stimulation of the epiglottis or vocal cords during intubation attempts may result in:
    A. acute laryngospasm.
    B. endotracheal swelling.
    C. aspiration due to vomiting.
    D. loss of tube sterility.

102. During intubation attempts in the infant or child patient, the presence of bradycardia may indicate:
    A. a need for nasogastric tube placement.
    B. correct tube placement.
    C. hypoxia.
    D. gastric distention.

103. Placement of an endotracheal tube by using the fingers of one hand is called:
    A. digital intubation.
    B. manual intubation.
    C. fingertip intubation.
    D. oral intubation.

SCENARIO

Questions 104 and 105 refer to the following scenario:

You arrive on the scene and find a 32-year-old male patient who the police claim was stabbed in the chest following an altercation in a parking lot. Upon your arrival at the scene, the police are present and have the perpetrator in custody. You find the patient lying supine and fully clothed. His face and neck are cyanotic. He moans when you apply painful stimuli. The first responders on the scene indicate that his airway is clear, and he is breathing at 42 beats per minute with shallow breaths. His radial pulse is rapid. His skin is warm and dry to the touch, and his capillary refill is less than two seconds. His nail beds are cyanotic.

104. What should be your next immediate action?

    A. Apply a non-rebreather mask at 15 lpm and prepare the patient for transport.

    B. Obtain a set of vital signs.

    C. Attempt to get a SAMPLE history from the patient.

    D. Expose the chest and occlude the open wound with your hand.

105. The skin signs in this patient indicate:

    A. severe bleeding and hypovolemic shock.

    B. hypoxia and inadequate oxygen exchange.

    C. a head injury.

    D. inadequate perfusion and adequate ventilation.

1.

D. An example of an unsafe on-scene activity is entering a crime scene too quickly, before the situation has been controlled by law enforcement.

2.

B. People react to stress differently. Behavioral reactions include overeating, increased alcohol and drug use, teeth grinding, hyperactivity, or the lack of energy. Choices A, C, and D are all psychological reactions to stress. In addition to behavioral and psychological reactions, some people react socially (increased interpersonal conflicts) or cognitively, which includes confusion and loss of objectivity.

3.

D. The single most important way to prevent the spread of infection is by handwashing. Contaminants can be removed from the hands by 10 to 15 seconds of vigorous scrubbing with plain soap.

4.

C. As an EMT-B you will be called to crime scenes or dangerous situations. Never enter a possibly dangerous scene; always position your vehicle away from the scene and wait for the police to stabilize the situation. Parking in view of the scene may endanger the EMS crew, as well as escalate the anger of the people on the scene due to your not making patient contact. If you enter a scene and it then becomes hostile, quickly leave the scene and wait for the police to arrive and secure it.

5.

C. Most states require EMT-Bs to report elder or child abuse or neglect, crimes, and drug related injuries. Some states may require reporting of infectious disease exposure, use of patient restraints, mentally incompetent or intoxicated patients, attempted suicides, and dog bites.

6.

C. The term that means "on both sides" is bilateral. Lateral is toward the side or away from the midline. Unilateral means on one side. Proximal means near the point of reference.

7.

C. The ball and socket joint permits the widest range of motion of all the joints. These joints permit flexion, extension, adduction, abduction and rotation. Examples of a ball and socket joint are the hip and the shoulder. The pivot joint permits a turning motion; examples are head and neck and wrist. Gliding joints permit the sliding of one bone against another, such as those joints located in the hands and feet. Hinged joints permit flexion and extension; examples are those found in the elbow, fingers, and knee.

8.

B. Breathing may be slightly irregular when the patient sighs; this is a normal event that allows for deeper breaths to occur. The adult patient should be breathing between 12 to 20 times a minute. It is normal for a 6-month-old to breathe with the use of abdominal muscles; however, the rate should be between 25 and 50 times a minute. A patient breathing with the use of accessory muscles is in respiratory distress. Use of accessory muscles is an attempt to force more air into the lungs to relieve the shortness of breath. Unequal chest expansion is a sign of distress and may be caused by injury.

9.

A. Using the jaw-thrust maneuver will open the airway without compromising the spine. Use the jaw-thrust maneuver whenever you suspect the possibility of a spinal injury. The head-tilt, chin-lift maneuver will compromise the spine when opening the airway. This is a general distracter; however, you should never pull traction on the spine because this may lead to further injury. Tilting the head of a possibly spine injured patient may injure the patient further. Open the airway by using the jaw-thrust maneuver.

10.

D. Stimulating the back of the throat while suctioning may result in bradycardia, a slowing of the heart. There are sensitive nerves in this area and if stimulated they may cause a decrease in the heart rate, further complicating the patient's condition. Bronchospasm refers to the constriction of the bronchi. Tachypnea is a fast breathing rate. Bradypnea is a slow breathing rate.

11.

C. The correct way to measure the length of catheter needed to suction the nasopharynx is from the tip of the patient's nose to the tip of the ear. Choices B, and D are both correct ways to measure the proper length of an oropharyngeal airway (OPA).

12.

B. After inserting an OPA if the patient begins to gag or vomit, you must immediately remove the airway and prepare to suction. The OPA must only be used in the completely unresponsive patient. If the patient gags, remove the OPA prepare to suction and insert a nasopharyngeal airway.

13.

D. You should first triage and prioritize the patients. This will help to organize the emergency care they receive. The critically injured patient should be treated before patients with minor injuries. Triaging will help to organize the whole scene. Treating and transporting patients in an organized manner will reduce on-scene time and increase the survival of the patients.

14.

D. An unresponsive patient does not respond to any stimuli. The patient does not cough or gag when an airway adjunct is placed into the throat.

15.

C. Liquid substances in the upper airway result in gurgling sounds. Crowing and stridor are produced on inspiration and are associated with upper airway swelling or muscle spasm. Snoring is caused by a partial airway obstruction of the tongue or epiglottis.

16.

B. The patient who presents with pale, cool, and moist skin is likely in a state of decreased perfusion (hypoperfusion). This hypoperfusion state should clue you to look for the onset of shock. Hyperthermia, an elevated body core temperature, usually presents with hot, red skin. Vasogenic shock, a state of shock that causes the vascular to dilate, usually presents with red skin.

17.

C. Life threats that require immediate treatment during the initial assessment include airway control, breathing inadequacy, injuries to the chest, and major bleeding. Fracture management is a secondary injury and is not considered as a life threat.

18.

D. When performing the rapid trauma assessment, which is based on the mechanism of injury, you are most concerned with identifying life-threatening injuries. Assessing the specific injury site is done when performing the focused trauma assessment.

19.

C. The rapid trauma assessment is performed rapidly prior to movement or immobilization of the patient and before leaving the scene. The detailed physical exam is performed while transporting the patient. If other injuries are suspected when evaluating a stable trauma patient, always perform a rapid trauma assessment. This determines if other life-threatening injuries are present.

20.

B. The patient's level of consciousness is a major determining factor in the sequence of the history and physical exam of the medical patient. If the patient is responsive you obtain the history and perform a focused medical assessment. If the patient is unresponsive you perform the rapid medical assessment followed by the history.

21.

C. Severity questions relate to how bad the pain is. Many patients can rate the pain on a scale from 1 to 10 with 10 being the worst. This method will help you when you reevaluate the patient. If the pain was originally a 4 and is now a 8, the pain has become worse.

22.

A. If a **patient complains of pelvis pain or there is obvious injury to the pelvis,** do not palpate the pelvis. Palpating or manipulating the pelvis may cause further injury and severe pain. If the **patient does not complain of pelvis pain or is unresponsive,** palpate by placing both hands on the anterior lateral wings of the pelvis. When palpating the pelvis, you should use gentle inward and downward compression. Do not rock the pelvis or apply too much pressure.

23.

C. A productive cough is one that produces mucous. Make note of the color, consistency, and amount.

24.

A. Palpation of the pelvic region is omitted in a patient who is complaining of pelvic pain. It should be performed in the patient who denies pain or is unresponsive.

25.

D. The dorsalis pedis pulse is located on the top surface of the foot. The posterior tibial pulse is located behind the inner ankle bone. The brachial pulse is located at the bend of the elbow. The popliteal is located behind the knee.

26.

D. The first step in the ongoing assessment is to repeat the initial assessment. This is followed by reassessing and recording vital signs, repeating the focused assessment, and rechecking your interventions.

27.

D. If the patient's condition has worsened, you should first perform an ongoing assessment, which begins with a repeat of the initial assessment.

28.

D. The patient's heart rate was too slow (bradycardia) and is now 100 beats each minute, which is normal in the adult patient. It is not a sign of improvement when the patient who was breathing too slowly (bradypnea) is now breathing too fast (tachypnea). The patient's skin color is a good indication of the effectiveness of oxygenation of the patient. Skin color that changes from cyanotic to blue-gray is inadequate; both are signs of inadequate oxygenation and poor perfusion of the tissue. When a patient begins to use accessory muscles to breathe the patient is deteriorating and needs to be ventilated with positive pressure ventilation.

29.

D. The initial assessment and the baseline vital signs should be repeated every 5 minutes in the critical patient. Repeat every 15 minutes in the stable patient.

30.

B. Keeping your eye level above a patient's who is hostile or aggressive will help to assert your authority. This simple positioning can make a great deal of difference in the difficult patient. Positioning yourself below the patient's eye level may convey a submissive position. You should avoid staring at a patient; make eye contact just as you would in a normal conversation. Some patients are on the edge of aggression, and using the correct body language can make a difference in the patients' demeanor.

31.

B. If the patient will not sign the refusal-of-care form, have a family member, police officer, or bystander sign, stating that the patient refused to sign. The family member or police officer is witnessing that the patient refused to sign the document; they are not signing the refusal for the patient. They are witnesses for your protection; the patient may state later that he or she wanted to be treated and did not sign the report.

32.

B. Abdominal pain is not a sign of respiratory distress. Restlessness and agitation are signs that the brain is not getting enough oxygen. Accessory muscle use is a sign of inadequate breathing; the intercostal muscles and the diaphragm are used to try to force more air into the lungs. Incomprehensible or mumbled speech may indicate the brain is not receiving enough oxygen.

33.

B. It is not important to determine the cause of a patient's breathing difficulty, except for the trauma patient. Expose and inspect the trauma patient's chest and treat accordingly. The EMT-B should provide positive pressure ventilation whenever in doubt as to the patient's ventilatory status. Patients with breathing difficulty are considered priority patients.

34.

D. Diminished wheezing is frequently, although not always, an indication of patient improvement. Decreased wheezing may indicate severe bronchospasm with less air movement.

35.

B. Improvement in oxygenation will frequently improve cerebral oxygenation. Improved cerebral oxygenation will result in improvement in the patient's mental status.

36.

A. This patient has late signs of respiratory distress. Cyanosis and tachycardia are ominous signs of severe respiratory distress. This patient must be immediately ventilated with positive pressure ventilations. This patient is a priority patient and should be transported immediately. Continue your assessment while en route to the hospital. You should also consider ALS backup with priority patients.

37.

A. You should provide positive pressure ventilation immediately. The patient is making efforts to breathe; however, breathing is not effective. Never withhold oxygen from a patient who complains of breathing difficulty. Oxygen by nasal cannula or non-rebreather mask is not sufficient for this patient; ventilate this patient.

38.

C. Do not instruct the patient to breathe through the nose. Breathing through the nose will seriously decrease the amount of medication delivered to the patient. The patient should also be instructed to hold his or her breath for as long as possible after administration.

39.

B. Croup, a childhood condition, is characterized by a high pitched sound from swelling of the larynx. Exposing the child to the cool night air will frequently diminish the signs and symptoms.

40.

C. The most common cause of mechanical failure is related to batteries. Ensure that the batteries are properly maintained to prevent this type of equipment failure.

41.

D. When caring for adult victims of cardiac arrest, defibrillation with the AED should come first over the other actions listed. Delay in rapidly defibrillating the patient can reduce the patient's chances for surviving the cardiac arrest.

42.

A. When the patient has taken more than three nitroglycerin tablets prior to your arrival, refrain from administering any additional doses. If the systolic blood pressure is below 100 mmHg, do not administer nitroglycerin. Patients with head injuries should not receive nitro. Headaches are a common side effect of nitroglycerin.

43.

C. Hypertension is not a common side effect when administering nitroglycerin. Because nitroglycerin is a potent vasodilator, you would expect a drop in the patient's blood pressure. Changes in the heart rate, and severe headache are common side effects.

44.

A. To deliver nitroglycerin spray, depress the container once, delivering one short spray. The nitroglycerin spray container is metered and will deliver only the correct dose each time it is depressed.

45.

D. Diseases of the heart and blood vessels are the number one killer of people in America today.

46.

A. Approximately 20% of heart attacks are painless or silent. There is no pain associated with a silent heart attack. You must rely on other signs and symptoms of a heart attack to help you determine the patient is having a silent heart attack.

47.

D. You should remove nitroglycerin patches and wipe the area with a cloth before defibrillating the patient. If the nitroglycerin patch is not removed, the current from the defibrillator may melt the plastic, causing a fire.

48.

C. External defibrillators are categorized into two main types. A manual defibrillator requires extensive skills to operate. The second type is the automatic. There are two types of automatic defibrillators, the automatic and semi-automatic. The implantable defibrillator is categorized as an internal defibrillator.

49.

D. This patient's breathing is shallow and slow (bradypnea). This inadequate breathing must be assisted by positive pressure ventilation immediately. If the patient is breathing adequately, you should administer oxygen by non-rebreather mask at 15 lpm.

50.

A. Nitroglycerin causes coronary artery vasodilation. Blood vessels in other parts of the body dilate also. The body may compensate for this by increasing the pulse rate slightly. The patient's blood pressure will most likely decrease. Nitroglycerin decreases the workload of the heart.

51.

A. Poor maintenance is the most common cause of AED failure. Battery failure causes most failures. Batteries must be maintained on a regular basis. At the beginning of every shift the AED and batteries should be checked and maintained in good order.

52.

D. A high level of sugar in the blood is called hyperglycemia. A low blood sugar level in the blood is called hypoglycemia. When insulin production is insufficient, the sugar can not leave the blood and enter the body cells. This causes an increase in the blood sugar level.

53.

D. The diabetic patient who has an altered mental status should be placed on his or her side. This position will help to protect the airway if the patient's vomit. All of the other positions may cause secretions to be aspirated into the airway due to the patient's inability to protect his or her airway.

54.

B. A stiff neck is a late sign of neurological deficit that has resulted from a nontraumatic brain injury. There are many different signs and symptoms of neurological deficit, depending on the location of the brain injury.

55.

D. The stage of a seizure that is known as the recovery phase is the postictal state. During this period of time the patient's mental status progressively im-

proves. The patient may present with a severe headache or temporary hemiparesis.

56.

B. The aura is the first phase and involves some type of sensory perception by the patient. The second phase occurs when the patient's muscles contract and tense and the patient exhibits extreme muscular rigidity with arching of the back. This is called the tonic phase. This is followed by the occurrence of convulsions, or the clonic phase. The last phase is the postictal state, or the recovery period. This lasts from 10 to 30 minutes.

57.

A. A transient ischemic attack generally subsides within 5 to 10 minutes. The signs and symptoms are identical to the presentation of a stroke patient. The patient recovers without any neurological deficit.

58.

C. Strokes most often affect elderly patients with a history of hardening of the arteries (atherosclerosis) or hypertension (high blood pressure). More than half the stroke patients die, and many others suffer from permanent neurological damage.

59.

B. Syncope occurs when there is a temporary lack of blood and oxygen flow to the brain that occurs over a short time period. It commonly occurs when the patient is standing. When the patient assumes a supine position, the patient improves rapidly.

60.

B. In anaphylaxis the two primary body systems affected are the respiratory and circulatory systems. This results from bronchoconstriction and peripheral vasodilatation that are associated with the reaction.

61.

A. Epinephrine works almost immediately; however, the effectiveness duration is short, approximately 10 to 20 minutes. Because of the short effectiveness time, you should transport immediately and consider ALS backup.

62.

C. Do not administer epinephrine to the patient who is suffering a mild reaction unless you are directed to do so by medical control. This patient is an elderly patient who may suffer serious side effects from the administration of epinephrine. The adverse side effects do not outweigh the benefits for this patient's current condition as described.

63.

A. An allergen is a substance that enters the body by ingestion, injection, inhalation, or contact and triggers an allergic reaction.

64.

A. Activated charcoal is the medication of choice to use for ingested poisonings. Activated charcoal works by absorbing the poison and thus inhibiting absorption into the body.

65.

B. The acute abdomen patient that is in shock (hypoperfusion) should be placed in a supine position with the patient's feet elevated. This position will help to increase perfusion to the brain and other vital organs.

66.

C. The 34-year-old is middle aged and tolerates cold better than the young and old. This patient is walking briskly, which increases body temperature through muscle contractions. Certain medications and alcohol will decrease a person's ability to tolerate a cold environment. A person who is wet will lose more heat than a dry person.

67.

A. You should wash the bite area with a mild soap and water, being careful not to aggressively scrub the area. The injection site should be placed slightly lower than the level of the patient's heart. Never lacerate the injection site to try to evacuate the poison; this may further complicate the patient's recovery and does not remove toxins. Tourniquets should not be used in a snake bite injury. Some protocols may use restricting bands; consult your local medical direction.

68.

D. Simply stated, reasonable force is the minimum amount of force required to keep a patient from injuring self or others.

69.

D. To prevent supine hypotension syndrome in the patient who is near full term of her pregnancy, place her in a sitting position. If the patient must lie flat, place her on her left side. If placed in the supine position, the weight of the uterus and fetus presses on the inferior vena cava and causes inadequate blood return to the heart, causing poor cardiac output.

70.

D. The placenta must be transported to the hospital for examination by a physician. The physician will then determine if the delivery was complete. Normal blood loss after delivery is up to 500 cc and is well tolerated. The placenta usually delivers within 10 minutes of the fetus and almost always within 20 minutes. Do not apply pressure to the infant's fontanel, this is the soft depressed area of the infant's head.

71.

B. The placenta usually delivers within 10 to 20 minutes following delivery. Do not delay transport while waiting for the delivery of the placenta. The placenta, enclosed in a plastic bag, should be transported with the patient. This will allow a physician to examine it to confirm that the placenta delivery was complete.

72.

B. The umbilical cord should be cut after the pulsations that are present in the cord cease. Two clamps are positioned on the cord prior to cutting the cord.

73.

B. The fingertips of the gloved hand are positioned on the bony part of the infant's head to prevent an explosive delivery. A rapid or explosive delivery can result in tearing of the birth canal.

74.

A. The brachial artery is located in the upper arm; arterial bleeding is bright red and spurts with each heart contraction. The femoral artery is located in the upper leg. The cephalic vein is located in the upper arm; however, bleeding from a vein is dark red and steady. The peroneal vein is located in the lower leg.

75.

C. Severe bleeding that is life-threatening should be controlled during the initial assessment. Control severe bleeding after you secure the airway, breathing, and circulation. Often, bleeding control can be accomplished simultaneously with airway and breathing management.

76.

C. When treating a closed soft tissue injury like a large hematoma, you must first take BSI precautions. Next, assure the patient has an open airway and that the patient is breathing adequately. If the patient is not breathing adequately or has a closed airway, stop and correct the airway or breathing problem. After assuring the airway is adequate, quickly treat for shock. After treating for shock, you should next splint any painful, swollen, or deformed extremities.

77.

B. You should cut the shirt away from the adhered portion. Never remove adhered clothing. This can cause extreme pain and further damage the burn site. Never apply ointments of any kind to burns; most often these ointments must be removed at the hospital.

78.

D. Never attempt to break or drain blisters from a burn; doing so will likely introduce contaminants and increase the possibility of infection.

79.

A. A bandage holds a dressing in place. A dressing $(2 \times 2, 4 \times 4)$ should be sterile and is placed directly on the wound. Common bandages include self-adhering, gauze rolls, and triangular bandages.

80.

D. When blood soaks through the original dressings, you should apply additional dressings over the original ones. Removing the original dressings will aggravate the wound and increase the bleeding. Tourniquets should only be applied as an absolute last resort. A loose tourniquet will act as a restricting band and cause the pressure in the blood vessel to increase, thus increasing the bleeding.

81.

D. Leaving the fingertips or toes exposed after bandaging allows for the assessment of circulation. This enables examination of skin color and temperature. Bandages must not impair circulation distal to an injury.

82.

D. Your first action should be to manually secure the object; this will reduce the likelihood of the object causing further injury or becoming dislodged. Never remove any object that is embedded in the chest. Next, expose the wound site. After exposing the wound site, you should control the bleeding from around the object. Last, use a bulky dressing to help stabilize the object.

83.

C. The anterior bone of the lower leg is called the tibia. The posterior bone is called the fibula.

84.

B. Limit your alignment attempt to one if the distal pulse is absent in an extremity. Splints should be appropriately padded to prevent pressure. Any jewelry around the injury site should be removed. **Never** intentionally return broken bone ends to beneath the skin.

85.

A. The EMT-B should never ask the patient to move in an attempt to determine the anatomical location of a potential spinal injury. This may cause irreversible spinal cord injury. Impaired breathing may result from damage at the level of the cervical spine. Soft tissue injury of the head and neck are frequent indications of possible spinal injury.

86.

D. A helmet should be removed if it interferes with the assessment or management of the airway or breathing. If the helmet does not fit well and excessive head movement occurs within the helmet, it should be removed. It should be left in place if you can properly immobilize the head, and the helmet does not allow for head movement.

87.

C. The EMT-B must quickly and continuously provide irrigation of the patient's eyes when dealing with eye burns. Do not use any irrigant other than saline or water. Continue flushing the eyes during transport. Remove contact lenses. This prevents the trapping of chemical agents under the lens.

88.

A. Cyanosis (blue color) indicates that your pediatric patient is in decompensated respiratory failure, and positive pressure ventilation must be performed. All other distracters are early signs of respiratory distress in the pediatric patient.

89.

B. Absent or weak peripheral pulses indicate poor circulation, which indicates hypoperfusion (shock). Other signs are rapid respiratory rate; pale, cool, and clammy skin; decreased mental status; and prolonged capillary refill in the patient under 6 years of age.

90.

B. Physical abuse occurs when improper or excessive action is taken so as to injure or cause harm. Neglect is when the caregiver provides insufficient respect or attention to an individual for whom the caregiver is responsible. This may apply to elderly patients or children.

91.

D. It is dangerous to accelerate while navigating a curve. You should carefully and gradually accelerate after exiting the curve. You should brake or decelerate prior to entering the curve; you should only drive as fast as feels comfortable. You should enter a curve on the outside or highest part.

92.

C. To protect yourself and the patient from debris, cover up using a tarpaulin or heavy blanket. Even the most careful spreader operator can not keep debris from becoming projectiles. A rapid extrication should be performed if the patient's condition requires it or there is a real threat to the well-being of the rescue personnel. Giving your protective clothing to the patient will not protect you.

93.

B. Simple access is best described as access that does not require the use of tools or specialized equipment.

94.

A. Your immediate role as the EMT-B who responds to a possible hazardous material spill is to cordon off the area and evacuate all bystanders. Do not approach the site even if there are patients visible. Move bystanders uphill and upwind. Do not approach the site to try to identify the type of cargo being transported.

95.

B. Your initial role as the first EMT-B on the scene of a MCI is the EMS incident manager. You will remain the EMS incident manager until you are relieved by the designated EMS incident manager.

96.

B. A patient with burns without airway problems should be tagged yellow—second priority. Red is the highest priority: airway problems, severe bleeding, and shock. Green is a low priority: minor burns, minor injuries, and walking wounded. Black is the lowest priority: obviously dead patients.

97.

C. A nasogastric tube is indicated in the infant or child patient when you are unable to provide positive pressure ventilation due to gastric distention. It is also indicated when an unresponsive patient is at risk of vomiting or developing gastric distention.

98.

A. Ventilation of a patient with an endotracheal tube in place does not require the use of a mask. The endotracheal tube provides a direct route to the patient's lungs for ventilation. In addition to the equipment listed, the following is needed to intubate a patient: endotracheal tube, water-soluble lubricant, 10 cc syringe, endotracheal tube securing device, towels or padding, and a stethoscope.

99.

C. The stylet is used to alter the shape of the endotracheal tube and to make the tube stiffer. Be sure the stylet does not extend beyond the end of the endotracheal tube. This could cause damage to the soft tissues of the airway.

100.

B. The right mainstem bronchus, not the left mainstem, is more likely to be intubated. In addition to the complications listed, others include bradycardia, hypertension, vomiting, and laryngospasm.

101.

A. Touching or stimulating the patient's vocal cords or epiglottis may result in laryngospasm of the vocal cords. The vocal cords will close completely and not allow air to pass through. The cords will eventually relax and allow air to pass through. Positive pressure ventilation will be necessary if the cords do not relax immediately.

102.

C. Bradycardia in the infant or child is an early sign of hypoxia. If the heart rate drops below 80 beats per minute in the infant or 60 in the child patient, stop the intubation attempt and hyperventilate the patient. Then reattempt the intubation.

103.

A. The technique is called digital intubation. Oral intubation is placement of an endotracheal tube through the mouth. Technically, it is a digital intubation that is placed orally.

104.

D. The open wound to the chest is an immediate life threat. You must expose the chest, occlude the open wound with your gloved hand and then with an occlusive dressing. You must inspect the entire thorax, looking for other possible stab wounds. Once you have done that, begin positive pressure ventilation. The patient's breathing is shallow at 42/minute. Be careful to assess the patient frequently since positive pressure ventilation in a patient with a pneumothorax could worsen the pneumothorax and potentially create a tension pneumothorax. You would then proceed with the rapid trauma assessment.

105.

B. The cyanosis to the face, neck, and nail beds is an indication of poor ventilation and inadequate oxygen exchange. The patient is hypoxic. If there were shock or inadequate tissue perfusion, you would expect to see pale, cool, clammy skin. Skin signs do not provide an indication of head injury.

Appendix D.O.T. Objectives

MODULE 1 PREPARATORY

LESSON 1-1 INTRODUCTION TO EMERGENCY MEDICAL CARE

Cognitive Objectives

At the completion of this lesson, the EMT-Basic student will be able to:

1-1.1   Define Emergency Medical Services (EMS) systems.(C-1)

1-1.2   Differentiate the roles and responsibilities of the EMT-Basic from other prehospital care providers.(C-3)

1-1.3   Describe the roles and responsibilities related to personal safety.(C-1)

1-1.4   Discuss the roles and responsibilities of the EMT-Basic towards the safety of the crew, the patient, and the bystanders.(C-1)

1-1.5   Define quality improvement and discuss the EMT-Basic's role in the process.(C-1)

1-1.6   Define medical direction and discuss the EMT-Basic's role in the process.(C-1)

1-1.7   State the specific statutes and regulations in your state regarding the EMS system.(C-1)

Affective Objectives

At the completion of this lesson, the EMT-Basic student will be able to:

1-1.8   Assess areas of personal attitude and conduct of the EMT Basic.(A-3)

1-1.9   Characterize the various methods used to access the EMS system in your community.(A-3)

Psychomotor Objectives

No psychomotor objectives identified.

LESSON 1-2 WELL-BEING OF THE EMT-BASIC

Cognitive Objectives

At the completion of this lesson, the EMT-Basic student will be able to:

1-2.1   List possible emotional reactions that the EMT-Basic may experience when faced with trauma, illness, death, and dying.(C-1)

1-2.2   Discuss the possible reactions that a family member may exhibit when confronted with death and dying.(C-1)

1-2.3   State the steps in the EMT-Basic's approach to the family confronted with death and dying.(C-1)

1-2.4   State the possible reactions that the family members of the EMT-Basic may exhibit due to his or her outside involvement in EMS.(C-1)

1-2.5   Recognize the signs and symptoms of critical incident stress.(C-1)

1-2.6   State possible steps that the EMT-Basic may take to help reduce/alleviate stress.(C-1)

1-2.7   Explain the need to determine scene safety.(C-2)

1-2.8   Discuss the importance of body substance isolation (BSI).(C-1)

1-2.9   Describe the steps the EMT-Basic should take for personal protection from airborne and bloodborne pathogens.(C-1)

1-2.10 List the personal protective equipment necessary for each of the following situations:(C-1)
- Hazardous materials
- Rescue operations

- Violent scenes
- Crime scenes
- Exposure to bloodborne pathogens
- Exposure to airborne pathogens

Affective Objectives

At the completion of this lesson, the EMT-Basic student will be able to:

1-2.11 Explain the rationale for serving as an advocate for the use of appropriate protective equipment.(A-3)

Psychomotor Objectives

1-2.12 Given a scenario with potential infectious exposure, the EMT Basic will use appropriate personal protective equipment. At the completion of the scenario, the EMT-Basic will properly remove and discard the protective garments.(P-1,2)

1-2.13 Given the above scenario, the EMT-Basic will complete disinfection/cleaning and all reporting documentation.(P-1,2)

LESSON 1-3 MEDICAL/LEGAL AND ETHICAL ISSUES

Cognitive Objectives

At the completion of this lesson, the EMT-Basic student will be able to:

1-3.1 Define the EMT-Basic scope of practice.(C-1)

1-3.2 Discuss the importance of Do Not Resuscitate (DNR) advance directives and local or state provisions regarding EMS application.(C-1)

1-3.3 Define consent and discuss the methods of obtaining consent.(C-1)

1-3.4 Differentiate between expressed and implied consent.(C-3)

1-3.5 Explain the role of consent of minors in providing care.(C-1)

1-3.6 Discuss the implications for the EMT-Basic in patient refusal of transport.(C-1)

1-3.7 Discuss the issues of abandonment, negligence, and battery and their implications to the EMT-Basic.(C-1)

1-3.8 State the conditions necessary for the EMT-Basic to have a duty to act.(C-1)

1-3.9 Explain the importance, necessity, and legality of patient confidentiality.(C-1)

1-3.10 Discuss the considerations of the EMT-Basic in issues of organ retrieval.(C-1)

1-3.11 Differentiate the actions that an EMT-Basic should take to assist in the preservation of a crime scene.(C-3)

1-3.12 State the conditions that require an EMT-Basic to notify local law enforcement officials.(C-1)

Affective Objectives

At the completion of this lesson, the EMT-Basic student will be able to:

1-3.13 Explain the role of EMS and the EMT-Basic regarding patients with DNR orders.(A-3)

1-3.14 Explain the rationale for the needs, benefits, and usage of advance directives.(A-3)

1-3.15 Explain the rationale for the concept of varying degrees of DNR.(A-3)

Psychomotor Objectives

No psychomotor objectives identified.

LESSON 1-4 THE HUMAN BODY

Cognitive Objectives

At the completion of this lesson, the EMT-Basic student will be able to:

1-4.1 Identify the following topographic terms: medial, lateral, proximal, distal, superior, inferior, anterior, posterior, midline, right and left, mid-clavicular, bilateral, and mid-axillary.(C-1)

1-4.2 Describe the anatomy and function of the following major body systems: respiratory, circulatory, musculoskeletal, nervous, and endocrine.(C-1)

Affective Objectives

No affective objectives identified.

Psychomotor Objectives

No psychomotor objectives identified.

LESSON 1-5 BASELINE VITAL SIGNS AND SAMPLE HISTORY

Cognitive Objectives

At the completion of this lesson, the EMT-Basic student will be able to:

1-5.1 Identify the components of the extended vital signs.(C-1)

1-5.2 Describe the methods to obtain a breathing rate.(C-1)

1-5.3 Identify the attributes that should be obtained when assessing breathing.(C-1)

1-5.4 Differentiate between shallow, labored, and noisy breathing.(C-3)

1-5.5 Describe the methods to obtain a pulse rate.(C-1)

1-5.6 Identify the information obtained when assessing a patient's pulse.(C-1)

1-5.7 Differentiate between a strong, weak, regular, and irregular pulse.(C-3)

1-5.8 Describe the methods to assess the skin color, temperature, condition, and capillary refill in infants and children.(C-1)

1-5.9 Identify the normal and abnormal skin colors.(C-1)

1-5.10 Differentiate between pale, blue, red, and yellow skin color.(C-3)

1-5.11 Identify the normal and abnormal skin temperature.(C-1)

1-5.12 Differentiate between hot, cool, and cold skin temperature.(C-3)

1-5.13 Identify normal and abnormal skin conditions.(C-1)

1-5.14 Identify normal and abnormal capillary refill in infants and children.(C-1)

1-5.15 Describe the methods to assess the pupils.(C-1)

1-5.16 Identify normal and abnormal pupil size.(C-1)

1-5.17 Differentiate between dilated (big) and constricted (small) pupil size.(C-3)

1-5.18 Differentiate between reactive and non-reactive pupils and equal and unequal pupils.(C-3)

1-5.19 Describe the methods to assess blood pressure.(C-1)

1-5.20 Define systolic pressure.(C-1)

1-5.21 Define diastolic pressure.(C-1)

1-5.22 Explain the difference between auscultation and palpation for obtaining a blood pressure.(C-1)

1-5.23 Identify the components of the SAMPLE history.(C-1)

1-5.24 Differentiate between a sign and a symptom.(C-3)

1-5.25 State the importance of accurately reporting and recording the baseline vital signs.(C-1)

1-5.26 Discuss the need to search for additional medical identification.(C-1)

Affective Objectives

At the completion of this lesson, the EMT-Basic student will be able to:

1-5.27 Explain the value of performing the baseline vital signs.(A-2)

1-5.28 Recognize and respond to the feelings patients experience during assessment.(A-1)

1-5.29 Defend the need for obtaining and recording an accurate set of vital signs.(A-3)

1-5.30 Explain the rationale of recording additional sets of vital signs.(A-1)

1-5.31 Explain the importance of obtaining a SAMPLE history.(A-1)

Psychomotor Objectives

At the completion of this lesson, the EMT-Basic student will be able to:

1-5.32 Demonstrate the skills involved in assessment of breathing.(P-1,2)

1-5.33 Demonstrate the skills associated with obtaining a pulse.(P-1,2)

1-5.34 Demonstrate the skills associated with assessing the skin color, temperature, condition, and capillary refill in infants and children.(P-1,2)

1-5.35 Demonstrate the skills associated with assessing the pupils.(P-1,2)

1-5.36 Demonstrate the skills associated with obtaining blood pressure.(P-1,2)

1-5.37 Demonstrate the skills that should be used to obtain information from the patient, family, or bystanders at the scene.(P-1,2)

LESSON 1-6 LIFTING AND MOVING PATIENTS

Cognitive Objectives

At the completion of this lesson, the EMT-Basic student will be able to:

1-6.1 Define body mechanics.(C-1)

1-6.2 Discuss the guidelines and safety precautions that need to be followed when lifting a patient.(C-1)

1-6.3   Describe the safe lifting of cots and stretchers.(C-1)

1-6.4   Describe the guidelines and safety precautions for carrying patients and/or equipment.(C-1)

1-6.5   Discuss one-handed carrying techniques.(C-1)

1-6.6   Describe correct and safe carrying procedures on stairs.(C-1)

1-6.7   State the guidelines for reaching and their application.(C-1)

1-6.8   Describe correct reaching for logrolls. (C-1)

1-6.9   State the guidelines for pushing and pulling.(C-1)

1-6.10   Discuss the general considerations of moving patients.(C-1)

1-6.11   State three situations that may require the use of an emergency move.(C-1)

1-6.12   Identify the following patient carrying devices:
- Wheeled ambulance stretcher
- Portable ambulance stretcher
- Stair chair
- Scoop stretcher
- Long spine board
- Basket stretcher
- Flexible stretcher (C-1)

Affective Objectives

At the completion of this lesson, the EMT-Basic student will be able to:

1-6.13   Explain the rationale for properly lifting and moving patients.(A-3)

Psychomotor Objectives

1-6.14   Working with a partner, prepare each of the following devices for use, transfer a patient to the device, properly position the patient on the device, move the device to the ambulance, and load the patient into the ambulance:
- Wheeled ambulance stretcher
- Portable ambulance stretcher
- Stair chair
- Scoop stretcher
- Long spine board

- Basket stretcher
- Flexible stretcher (P-1,2)

1-6.15   Working with a partner, the EMT-Basic will demonstrate techniques for the transfer of a patient from an ambulance stretcher to a hospital stretcher.(P-1,2)

MODULE 2   AIRWAY

LESSON 2-1   AIRWAY

Cognitive Objectives

At the completion of this lesson, the EMT-Basic student will be able to:

2-1.1   Name and label the major structures of the respiratory system on a diagram.(C-1)

2-1.2   List the signs of adequate breathing.(C-1)

2-1.3   List the signs of inadequate breathing.(C-1)

2-1.4   Describe the steps in performing the head-tilt, chin-lift maneuver.(C-1)

2-1.5   Relate mechanism of injury to opening the airway.(C-3)

2-1.6   Describe the steps in performing the jaw-thrust maneuver.(C-1)

2-1.7   State the importance of having a suction unit ready for immediate use when providing emergency care.(C-1)

2-1.8   Describe the techniques of suctioning.(C-1)

2-1.9   Describe how to artificially ventilate a patient with a pocket mask.(C-1)

2-1.10   Describe the steps in performing the skill of artificially ventilating a patient with a bag-valve-mask while using the jaw-thrust.(C-1)

2-1.11   List the parts of a bag-valve-mask system.(C-1)

2-1.12   Describe the steps in performing the skill of artificially ventilating a patient with a bag-valve-mask for one and two rescuers.(C-1)

2-1.13   Describe the signs of adequate artificial ventilation using the bag-valve-mask.(C-1)

2-1.14   Describe the signs of inadequate artificial ventilation using the bag-valve-mask.(C-1)

2-1.15   Describe the steps in artificially ventilating a patient with a flow restricted, oxygen-powered ventilation device.(C-1)

2-1.16 List the steps in performing the actions taken when providing mouth-to-mouth and mouth-to-stoma artificial ventilation.(C-1)

2-1.17 Describe how to measure and insert an oropharyngeal (oral) airway.(C-1)

2-1.18 Describe how to measure and insert a nasopharyngeal (nasal) airway.(C-1)

2-1.19 Define the components of an oxygen delivery system.(C-1)

2-1.20 Identify a non-rebreather face mask and state the oxygen flow requirements needed for its use.(C-1)

2-1.21 Describe the indications for using a nasal cannula versus a non-rebreather face mask.(C-1)

2-1.22 Identify a nasal cannula and state the flow requirements needed for its use.(C-1)

Affective Objectives

At the completion of this lesson, the EMT-Basic student will be able to:

2-1.23 Explain the rationale for basic life support, artificial ventilation, and airway protective skills taking priority over most other basic life support skills.(A-3)

2-1.24 Explain the rationale for providing adequate oxygenation through high inspired oxygen concentrations to patients who, in the past, may have received low concentrations.(A-3)

Psychomotor Objectives

At the completion of this lesson, the EMT-Basic student will be able to:

2-1.25 Demonstrate the steps in performing the head-tilt, chin-lift.(P-1,2)

2-1.26 Demonstrate the steps in performing the jaw-thrust.(P-1,2)

2-1.27 Demonstrate the techniques of suctioning.(P-1,2)

2-1.28 Demonstrate the steps in providing mouth-to-mouth artificial ventilation with body substance isolation (barrier shields).(P-1,2)

2-1.29 Demonstrate how to use a pocket mask to artificially ventilate a patient.(P-1,2)

2-1.30 Demonstrate the assembly of a bag-valve-mask unit.(P-1,2)

2-1.31 Demonstrate the steps in performing the skill of artificially ventilating a patient with a bag-valve-mask for one and two rescuers.(P-1,2)

2-1.32 Demonstrate the steps in performing the skill of artificially ventilating a patient with a bag-valve-mask while using the jaw-thrust.(P-1,2)

2-1.33 Demonstrate artificial ventilation of a patient with a flow restricted, oxygen-powered ventilation device.(P-1,2)

2-1.34 Demonstrate how to artificially ventilate a patient with a stoma.(P-1,2)

2-1.35 Demonstrate how to insert an oropharyngeal (oral) airway.(P-1,2)

2-1.36 Demonstrate how to insert a nasopharyngeal (nasal) airway.(P-1,2)

2-1.37 Demonstrate the correct operation of oxygen tanks and regulators.(P-1,2)

2-1.38 Demonstrate the use of a non-rebreather face mask and state the oxygen flow requirements needed for its use.(P-1,2)

2-1.39 Demonstrate the use of a nasal cannula and state the flow requirements needed for its use.(P-1,2)

2-1.40 Demonstrate how to artificially ventilate the infant and child patient.(P-1,2)

2-1.41 Demonstrate oxygen administration for the infant and child patient.(P-1,2)

MODULE 3 PATIENT ASSESSMENT

LESSON 3-1 SCENE SIZE-UP
Cognitive Objectives

At the completion of this lesson, the EMT-Basic student will be able to:

3-1.1 Recognize hazards/potential hazards.(C-1)

3-1.2 Describe common hazards and a medical patient found at the scene of a trauma.(C-1)

3-1.3 Determine if the scene is safe to enter.(C-2)

3-1.4 Discuss common mechanisms of injury/nature of illness.(C-1)

3-1.5 Discuss the reason for identifying the total number of patients at the scene.(C-1)

3-1.6 Explain the reason for identifying the need for additional help or assistance.(C-1)

Affective Objectives

At the completion of this lesson, the EMT-Basic student will be able to:

3-1.7 Explain the rationale for crew members to evaluate scene safety prior to entering.(A-2)

3-1.8 Serve as a model for others explaining how patient situations affect your evaluation of mechanism of injury or illness.(A-2)

Psychomotor Objectives

At the completion of this lesson, the EMT-Basic student will be able to:

3-1.9 Observe various scenarios and identify potential hazards.(P-1)

LESSON 3-2 INITIAL ASSESSMENT

Cognitive Objectives

At the completion of this lesson, the EMT-Basic student will be able to:

3-2.1 Summarize the reasons for forming a general impression of the patient.(C-1)

3-2.2 Discuss methods of assessing altered mental status.(C-1)

3-2.3 Differentiate between assessing the altered mental status in the adult, child, and infant patient.(C-3)

3-2.4 Discuss methods of assessing the airway in the adult, child, and infant patient.(C-1)

3-2.5 State reasons for management of the cervical spine once the patient has been determined to be a trauma patient.(C-1)

3-2.6 Describe methods used for assessing if a patient is breathing.(C-1)

3-2.7 State what care should be provided to the adult, child, and infant patient with adequate breathing.(C-1)

3-2.8 State what care should be provided to the adult, child, and infant patient without adequate breathing.(C-1)

3-2.9 Differentiate between a patient with adequate and inadequate breathing.(C-3)

3-2.10 Distinguish between methods of assessing breathing in the adult, child, and infant patient.(C-3)

3-2.11 Compare the methods of providing airway care to the adult, child, and infant patient.(C-3)

3-2.12 Describe the methods used to obtain a pulse.(C-1)

3-2.13 Differentiate between obtaining a pulse in an adult, child, and infant patient.(C-3)

3-2.14 Discuss the need for assessing the patient for external bleeding.(C-1)

3-2.15 Describe normal and abnormal findings when assessing skin color.(C-1)

3-2.16 Describe normal and abnormal findings when assessing skin temperature.(C-1)

3-2.17 Describe normal and abnormal findings when assessing skin condition.(C-1)

3-2.18 Describe normal and abnormal findings when assessing skin capillary refill in the infant and child patient.(C-1)

3-2.19 Explain the reason for prioritizing a patient for care and transport.(C-1)

Affective Objectives

At the completion of this lesson, the EMT-Basic student will be able to:

3-2.20 Explain the importance of forming a general impression of the patient.(A-1)

3-2.21 Explain the value of performing an initial assessment.(A-2)

Psychomotor Objectives

At the completion of this lesson, the EMT-Basic student will be able to:

3-2.22 Demonstrate the techniques for assessing mental status.(P-1,2)

3-2.23 Demonstrate the techniques for assessing the airway.(P-1,2)

3-2.24 Demonstrate the techniques for assessing if the patient is breathing.(P-1,2)

3-2.25 Demonstrate the techniques for assessing if the patient has a pulse.(P-1,2)

3-2.26 Demonstrate the techniques for assessing the patient for external bleeding.(P-1,2)

3-2.27 Demonstrate the techniques for assessing the patient's skin color, temperature, condition, and capillary refill (infants and children only).(P-1,2)

3-2.28 Demonstrate the ability to prioritize patients.(P-1,2)

LESSON 3-3 FOCUSED HISTORY AND PHYSICAL EXAM - TRAUMA PATIENTS

Cognitive Objectives

At the completion of this lesson, the EMT-Basic student will be able to:

3-3.1 Discuss the reasons for reconsideration concerning the mechanism of injury.(C-1)

3-3.2 State the reasons for performing a rapid trauma assessment.(C-1)

3-3.3 Recite examples and explain why patients should receive a rapid trauma assessment.(C-1)

3-3.4 Describe the areas included in the rapid trauma assessment and discuss what should be evaluated.(C-1)

3 3.5 Differentiate when the rapid assessment may be altered in order to provide patient care.(C-3)

3-3.6 Discuss the reasons for performing a focused history and physical exam.(C-1)

Affective Objectives

At the completion of this lesson, the EMT-Basic student will be able to:

3-3.7 Recognize and respect the feelings that patients might experience during assessment.(A-1)

Psychomotor Objectives

At the completion of this lesson, the EMT-Basic student will be able to:

3-3.8 Demonstrate the rapid trauma assessment that should be used to assess a patient based on mechanism of injury.(P-1,2)

LESSON 3-4 FOCUSED HISTORY AND PHYSICAL EXAM - MEDICAL PATIENTS

Cognitive Objectives

At the completion of this lesson, the EMT-Basic student will be able to:

3-4.1 Describe the unique needs for assessing an individual with a specific chief complaint with no known prior history.(C-1)

3-4.2 Differentiate between the history and physical exam that are performed for responsive patients with no known prior history and patients who are responsive with a known prior history.(C-3)

3-4.3 Describe the unique needs for assessing an individual who is unresponsive or has an altered mental status.(C-1)

3-4.4 Differentiate between the assessment that is performed for a patient who is unresponsive or has an altered mental status and other medical patients requiring assessment.(C-3)

Affective Objectives

At the completion of this lesson, the EMT-Basic student will be able to:

3-4.5 Attend to the feelings that these patients might be experiencing.(A-1)

Psychomotor Objectives

At the completion of this lesson, the EMT-Basic student will be able to:

3-4.6 Demonstrate the patient care skills that should be used to assist with a patient who is responsive with no known history.(P-1,2)

3-4.7 Demonstrate the patient care skills that should be used to assist with a patient who is unresponsive or has an altered mental status.(P-1,2)

LESSON 3-5 DETAILED PHYSICAL EXAM

Cognitive Objectives

At the completion of this lesson, the EMT-Basic student will be able to:

3-5.1 Discuss the components of the detailed physical exam.(C-1)

3-5.2 State the areas of the body that are evaluated during the detailed physical exam.(C-1)

3-5.3 Explain what additional care should be provided while performing the detailed physical exam.(C-1)

3-5.4 Distinguish between the detailed physical exam that is performed on a trauma patient and that of the medical patient.(C-3)

Affective Objectives

At the completion of this lesson, the EMT-Basic student will be able to:

3-5.5 Explain the rationale for the feelings that these patients might be experiencing.(A-3)

Psychomotor Objectives

At the completion of this lesson, the EMT-Basic student will be able to:

3-5.6　Demonstrate the skills involved in performing the detailed physical exam.(P-1,2)

LESSON 3-6　ONGOING ASSESSMENT
Cognitive Objectives

At the completion of this lesson, the EMT-Basic student will be able to:

3-6.1　Discuss the reasons for repeating the initial assessment as part of the ongoing assessment.(C-1)

3-6.2　Describe the components of the ongoing assessment.(C-1)

3-6.3　Describe trending of assessment components.(C-1)

Affective Objectives

At the completion of this lesson, the EMT-Basic student will be able to:

3-6.4　Explain the value of performing an ongoing assessment.(A-2)

3-6.5　Recognize and respect the feelings that patients might experience during assessment.(A-1)

3-6.6　Explain the value of trending assessment components to other health professionals who assume care of the patient.(A-2)

Psychomotor Objectives

At the completion of this lesson, the EMT-Basic student will be able to:

3-6.7　Demonstrate the skills involved in performing the ongoing assessment.(P-1,2)

LESSON 3-7　COMMUNICATIONS
Cognitive Objectives

At the completion of this lesson, the EMT-Basic student will be able to:

3-7.1　List the proper methods of initiating and terminating a radio call.(C-1)

3-7.2　State the proper sequence for delivery of patient information.(C-1)

3-7.3　Explain the importance of effective communication of patient information in the oral report.(C-1)

3-7.4　Identify the essential components of the oral report.(C-1)

3-7.5　Describe the attributes for increasing effectiveness and efficiency of oral communications.(C-1)

3-7.6　State legal aspects to consider in oral communication.(C-1)

3-7.7　Discuss the communication skills that should be used to interact with the patient.(C-1)

3-7.8　Discuss the communication skills that should be used to interact with the family, bystanders, and individuals from other agencies while providing patient care and the difference between skills used to interact with the patient and those used to interact with others.(C-1)

3-7.9　List the correct radio procedures in the following phases of a typical call:(C-1)
- To the scene
- At the scene
- To the facility
- At the facility
- To the station
- At the station

Affective Objectives

At the completion of this lesson, the EMT-Basic student will be able to:

3-7.10　Explain the rationale for providing efficient and effective radio communications and patient reports.(A-3)

Psychomotor Objectives

At the completion of this lesson, the EMT-Basic student will be able to:

3-7.11　Perform a simulated, organized, concise radio transmission.(P-2)

3-7.12　Perform an organized, concise patient report that would be given to the staff at a receiving facility.(P-2)

3-7.13　Perform a brief, organized report that would be given to an ALS provider arriving at an incident scene at which the EMT-Basic was already providing care.(P-2)

LESSON 3-8 DOCUMENTATION
Cognitive Objectives
At the completion of this lesson, the EMT-Basic student will be able to:

3-8.1   Explain the components of the written report and list the information that should be included on the written report.(C-1)

3-8.2   Identify the various sections of the written report.(C-1)

3-8.3   Describe what information is required in each section of the prehospital care report and how it should be entered.(C-1)

3-8.4   Define the special considerations concerning patient refusal.(C-1)

3-8.5   Describe the legal implications associated with the written report.(C-1)

3-8.6   Discuss all state and/or local record and reporting requirements.(C-1)

Affective Objectives
At the completion of this lesson, the EMT-Basic student will be able to:

3-8.7   Explain the rationale for patient care documentation.(A-3)

3-8.8   Explain the rationale for the EMS system gathering data.(A-3)

3-8.9   Explain the rationale for using medical terminology correctly.(A-3)

3-8.10 Explain the rationale for using an accurate and synchronous clock so that information can be used in trending.(A-3)

Psychomotor Objectives
At the completion of this lesson, the EMT-Basic student will be able to:

3-8.11 Complete a prehospital care report.(P-2)

MODULE 4 MEDICAL/BEHAVIORAL/OBSTETRICS

LESSON 4-1 GENERAL PHARMACOLOGY
Cognitive Objectives
At the completion of this lesson, the EMT-Basic student will be able to:

4-1.1   Identify which medications will be carried on the unit.(C-1)

4-1.2   State the medications carried on the unit by the generic name.(C-1)

4-1.3   Identify the medications that the EMT-Basic may assist the patient with administering.(C-1)

4-1.4   State the medications by the generic name that the EMT-Basic can assist the patient with administering.(C-1)

4-1.5   Discuss the forms in which the medications may be found.(C-1)

Affective Objectives
At the completion of this lesson, the EMT-Basic student will be able to:

4-1.6   Explain the rationale for the administration of medications.(A-3)

Psychomotor Objectives
At the completion of this lesson, the EMT-Basic student will be able to:

4-1.7   Demonstrate general steps for assisting patient with self-administration of medications.(P-2)

4-1.8   Read the labels and inspect each type of medication.(P-2)

LESSON 4-2 RESPIRATORY
Cognitive Objectives
At the completion of this lesson, the EMT-Basic student will be able to:

4-2.1   List the structure and function of the respiratory system.(C-1)

4-2.2   State the signs and symptoms of a patient with breathing difficulty.(C-1)

4-2.3   Describe the emergency medical care of the patient with breathing difficulty.(C-1)

4-2.4   Recognize the need for medical direction to assist in the emergency medical care of the patient with breathing difficulty.(C-3)

4-2.5   Describe the emergency medical care of the patient with breathing distress.(C-1)

4-2.6   Establish the relationship between airway management and the patient with breathing difficulty.(C-3)

4-2.7   List signs of adequate air exchange.(C-1)

4-2.8   State the generic name, medication forms, dose, administration, action, indications, and contraindications for the prescribed inhaler.(C-1)

4-2.9 Distinguish between the emergency medical care of the infant, child, and adult patient with breathing difficulty.(C-3)

4-2.10 Differentiate between upper airway obstruction and lower airway disease in the infant and child patient.(C-3)

Affective Objectives

At the completion of this lesson, the EMT-Basic student will be able to:

4-2.11 Defend EMT-Basic treatment regimens for various respiratory emergencies.(A-1)

4-2.12 Explain the rationale for administering an inhaler.(A-3)

Psychomotor Objectives

At the completion of this lesson, the EMT-Basic student will be able to:

4-2.13 Demonstrate the emergency medical care for breathing difficulty.(P-1,2)

4-2.14 Perform the steps in facilitating the use of an inhaler.(P-2)

LESSON 4-3 CARDIOVASCULAR
Cognitive Objectives

At the completion of this lesson, the EMT-Basic student will be able to:

4-3.1 Describe the structure and function of the cardiovascular system.(C-1)

4-3.2 Describe the emergency medical care of the patient experiencing chest pain/discomfort.(C-1)

4-3.3 List the indications for automated external defibrillation (AED).(C-1)

4-3.4 List the contraindications for automated external defibrillation.(C-1)

4-3.5 Define the role of the EMT-Basic in the emergency cardiac care system.(C-1)

4-3.6 Explain the impact of age and weight on defibrillation.(C-1)

4-3.7 Discuss the position of comfort for patients with various cardiac emergencies.(C-1)

4-3.8 Establish the relationship between airway management and the patient with cardiovascular compromise.(C-3)

4-3.9 Predict the relationship between the patient experiencing cardiovascular compromise and basic life support.(C-2)

4-3.10 Discuss the fundamentals of early defibrillation.(C-1)

4-3.11 Explain the rationale for early defibrillation.(C-1)

4-3.12 Explain why not all chest pain patients result in cardiac arrest and do not need to be attached to an automated external defibrillator.(C-1)

4-3.13 Explain the importance of prehospital ACLS intervention if it is available.(C-1)

4-3.14 Explain the importance of urgent transport to a facility with Advanced Cardiac Life Support if it is not available in the prehospital setting.(C-1)

4-3.15 Discuss the various types of automated external defibrillators.(C-1)

4-3.16 Differentiate between the fully automated and the semi-automated defibrillator.(C-3)

4-3.17 Discuss the procedures that must be taken into consideration for standard operations of the various types of automated external defibrillators.(C-1)

4-3.18 State the reasons for assuring that the patient is pulseless and apneic when the EMT-Basic is using the automated external defibrillator.(C-1)

4-3.19 Discuss the circumstances that may result in inappropriate shocks.(C-1)

4-3.20 Explain the considerations for interruption of CPR when using the automated external defibrillator.(C-1)

4-3.21 Discuss the advantages and disadvantages of automated external defibrillators.(C-1)

4-3.22 Summarize the speed of operation of automated external defibrillation.(C-1)

4-3.23 Discuss the use of remote defibrillation through adhesive pads.(C-1)

4-3.24 Discuss the special considerations for rhythm monitoring.(C-1)

4-3.25 List the steps in the operation of the automated external defibrillator.(C-1)

4-3.26 Discuss the standard of care that should be used to provide care to a patient with persistent ventricular fibrillation and no available ACLS.(C-1)

4-3.27 Discuss the standard of care that should be used to provide care to a patient with recurrent ventricular fibrillation and no available ACLS.(C-1)

4-3.28 Differentiate between the single rescuer and multi-rescuer care with an automated external defibrillator.(C-3)

4-3.29 Explain the reason for pulses not being checked between shocks with an automated external defibrillator.(C-1)

4-3.30 Discuss the importance of coordinating ACLS trained providers with personnel using automated external defibrillators.(C-1)

4-3.31 Discuss the importance of post-resuscitation care.(C-1)

4-3.32 List the components of post-resuscitation care.(C-1)

4-3.33 Explain the importance of frequent practice with the automated external defibrillator.(C-1)

4-3.34 Discuss the need to complete the Automated Defibrillator: Operator's Shift Checklist.(C-1)

4-3.35 Discuss the role of the American Heart Association (AHA) in the use of automated external defibrillation.(C-1)

4-3.36 Explain the role medical direction plays in the use of automated external defibrillation.(C-1)

4-3.37 State the reasons why a case review should be completed following the use of the automated external defibrillator.(C-1)

4-3.38 Discuss the components that should be included in a case review.(C-1)

4-3.39 Discuss the goal of quality improvement in automated external defibrillation.(C-1)

4-3.40 Recognize the need for medical direction of protocols to assist in the emergency medical care of the patient with chest pain.(C-3)

4-3.41 List the indications for the use of nitroglycerin.(C-1)

4-3.42 State the contraindications and side effects for the use of nitroglycerin.(C-1)

4-3.43 Define the function of all controls on an automated external defibrillator, and describe event documentation and battery defibrillator maintenance.(C-1)

Affective Objectives

At the completion of this lesson, the EMT-Basic student will be able to:

4-3.44 Defend the reasons for obtaining initial training in automated external defibrillation and the importance of continuing education.(A-3)

4-3.45 Defend the reasons for maintenance of automated external defibrillators.(A-3)

4-3.46 Explain the rationale for administering nitroglycerin to a patient with chest pain or discomfort.(A-3)

Psychomotor Objectives

At the completion of this lesson, the EMT-Basic student will be able to:

4-3.47 Demonstrate the assessment and emergency medical care of a patient experiencing chest pain/discomfort.(P-1,2)

4-3.48 Demonstrate the application and operation of the automated external defibrillator.(P-1,2)

4-3.49 Demonstrate the maintenance of an automated external defibrillator.(P-1,2)

4-3.50 Demonstrate the assessment and documentation of patient response to the automated external defibrillator.(P-1,2)

4-3.51 Demonstrate the skills necessary to complete the Automated Defibrillator: Operator's Shift Checklist.(P-1,2)

4-3.52 Perform the steps in facilitating the use of nitroglycerin for chest pain or discomfort.(P-2)

4-3.53 Demonstrate the assessment and documentation of patient response to nitroglycerin.(P-1,2)

4-3.54 Practice completing a prehospital care report for patients with cardiac emergencies.(P-2)

LESSON 4-4 DIABETES/AMS
Cognitive Objectives

At the completion of this lesson, the EMT-Basic student will be able to:

4-4.1 Identify the patient taking diabetic medications with altered mental status and the implications of a diabetes history.(C-1)

4-4.2   State the steps in the emergency medical care of the patient taking diabetic medicine with an altered mental status and a history of diabetes.(C-1)

4-4.3   Establish the relationship between airway management and the patient with altered mental status.(C-3)

4-4.4   State the generic and trade names, medication forms, dose, administration, action, and contraindications for oral glucose.(C-1)

4-4.5   Evaluate the need for medical direction in the emergency medical care of the diabetic patient.(C-3)

Affective Objectives

4-4.6   Explain the rationale for administering oral glucose.(A-3)

Psychomotor Objectives

4-4.7   Demonstrate the steps in the emergency medical care for the patient taking diabetic medicine with an altered mental status and a history of diabetes.(P-1,2)

4-4.8   Demonstrate the steps in the administration of oral glucose.(P-1,2)

4-4.9   Demonstrate the assessment and documentation of patient response to oral glucose.(P-1,2)

4-4.10 Demonstrate how to complete a prehospital care report for patients with diabetic emergencies.(P-2)

Lesson 4-5 Allergies
Cognitive Objectives

At the completion of this lesson, the EMT-Basic student will be able to:

4-5.1   Recognize the patient experiencing an allergic reaction.(C-1)

4-5.2   Describe the emergency medical care of the patient with an allergic reaction.(C-1)

4-5.3   Establish the relationship between the patient with an allergic reaction and airway management.(C-3)

4-5.4   Describe the mechanisms of allergic response and the implications for airway management.(C-1)

4-5.5   State the generic and trade names, medication forms, dose, administration, action, and contraindications for the epinephrine auto-injector.(C-1)

4-5.6   Evaluate the need for medical direction in the emergency medical care of the patient with an allergic reaction.(C-3)

4-5.7   Differentiate between the general category of those patients having an allergic reaction and those patients having an allergic reaction and requiring immediate medical care, including immediate use of the epinephrine auto-injector.(C-3)

Affective Objectives

4-5.8   Explain the rationale for administering epinephrine using an auto-injector.(A-3)

Psychomotor Objectives

4-5.9   Demonstrate the emergency medical care of the patient experiencing an allergic reaction.(P-1,2)

4-5.10 Demonstrate the use of the epinephrine auto-injector.(P-1,2)

4-5.11 Demonstrate the assessment and documentation of patient response to an epinephrine injection.(P-1,2)

4-5.12 Demonstrate proper disposal of equipment.(P-1,2)

4-5.13 Demonstrate completing a prehospital care report for patients with allergic emergencies.(P-2)

Lesson 4-6 Poisoning/Overdose
Cognitive Objectives

At the completion of this lesson, the EMT-Basic student will be able to:

4-6.1   List various ways that poisons enter the body.(C-1)

4-6.2   List signs/symptoms associated with poisoning.(C-1)

4-6.3   Discuss the emergency medical care for the patient with possible overdose.(C-1)

4-6.4   Describe the steps in the emergency medical care for the patient with suspected poisoning.(C-1)

4-6.5 Establish the relationship between the patient suffering from poisoning or overdose and airway management.(C-3)

4-6.6 State the generic and trade names, indications, contraindications, medication form, dose, administration, actions, side effects and reassessment strategies for activated charcoal.(C-1)

4-6.7 Recognize the need for medical direction in caring for the patient with poisoning or overdose.(C-3)

Affective Objectives

At the completion of this lesson, the EMT-Basic student will be able to:

4-6.8 Explain the rationale for administering activated charcoal.(A-3)

4-6.9 Explain the rationale for contacting medical direction early in the prehospital management of the poisoning or overdose patient.(A-3)

Psychomotor Objectives

At the completion of this lesson, the EMT-Basic student will be able to:

4-6.10 Demonstrate the steps in the emergency medical care for the patient with possible overdose.(P-1,2)

4-6.11 Demonstrate the steps in the emergency medical care for the patient with suspected poisoning.(P-1,2)

4-6.12 Perform the necessary steps required to provide a patient with activated charcoal.(P-2)

4-6.13 Demonstrate the assessment and documentation of patient response.(P-1,2)

4-6.14 Demonstrate proper disposal of equipment used in the administration of activated charcoal.(P-1,2)

4-6.15 Demonstrate completing a prehospital care report for patients with a poisoning/overdose emergency.(P-1,2)

LESSON 4-7 ENVIRONMENTAL
Cognitive Objectives

At the completion of this lesson, the EMT-Basic student will be able to:

4-7.1 Describe the various ways that the body loses heat.(C-1)

4-7.2 List the signs and symptoms of exposure to cold.(C-1)

4-7.3 Explain the steps in providing emergency medical care to a patient exposed to cold.(C-1)

4-7.4 List the signs and symptoms of exposure to heat.(C-1)

4-7.5 Explain the steps in providing emergency care to a patient exposed to heat.(C-1)

4-7.6 Recognize the signs and symptoms of water-related emergencies.(C-1)

4-7.7 Describe the complications of near drowning.(C-1)

4-7.8 Discuss the emergency medical care of bites and stings.(C-1)

Affective Objectives

No affective objectives identified.

Psychomotor Objectives

4-7.9 Demonstrate the assessment and emergency medical care of a patient with exposure to cold.(P-1,2)

4-7.10 Demonstrate the assessment and emergency medical care of a patient with exposure to heat.(P-1,2)

4-7.11 Demonstrate the assessment and emergency medical care of a near drowning patient.(P-1,2)

4-7.12 Demonstrate completing a prehospital care report for patients with environmental emergencies.(P-2)

LESSON 4-8 BEHAVIORAL
Cognitive Objectives

At the completion of this lesson, the EMT-Basic student will be able to:

4-8.1 Define behavioral emergencies.(C-1)

4-8.2 Discuss the general factors that may cause an alteration in a patient's behavior.(C-1)

4-8.3 State the various reasons for psychological crises.(C-1)

4-8.4 Discuss the characteristics of an individual's behavior that suggest the patient is at risk for suicide.(C-1)

4-8.5 Discuss special medical/legal considerations for managing behavioral emergencies.(C-1)

4-8.6   Discuss the special considerations for assessing a patient with behavioral problems.(C-1)

4-8.7   Discuss the general principles of an individual's behavior that suggest he or she is at risk for violence.(C-1)

4-8.8   Discuss methods to calm behavioral emergency patients.(C-1)

Affective Objectives

At the completion of this lesson, the EMT-Basic student will be able to:

4-8.9   Explain the rationale for learning how to modify your behavior toward the patient with a behavioral emergency.(A-3)

Psychomotor Objectives

At the completion of this lesson, the EMT-Basic student will be able to:

4-8.10   Demonstrate the assessment and emergency medical care of the patient experiencing a behavioral emergency.(P-1,2)

4-8.11   Demonstrate various techniques to safely restrain a patient with a behavioral problem.(P-1,2)

LESSON 4-9   OB-GYN

Cognitive Objectives

At the completion of this lesson, the EMT-Basic student will be able to:

4-9.1   Identify the following structures: uterus, vagina, fetus, placenta, umbilical cord, amniotic sac, perineum.(C-1)

4-9.2   Identify and explain the use of the contents of an obstetrics kit.(C-1)

4-9.3   Identify predelivery emergencies.(C-1)

4-9.4   State indications of an imminent delivery.(C-1)

4-9.5   Differentiate the emergency medical care provided to a patient with predelivery emergencies from a normal delivery.(C-3)

4-9.6   State the steps in the predelivery preparation of the mother.(C-1)

4-9.7   Establish the relationship between body substance isolation and childbirth.(C-3)

4-9.8   State the steps to assist in the delivery.(C-1)

4-9.9   Describe care of the baby as the head appears.(C-1)

4-9.10   Describe how and when to cut the umbilical cord.(C-1)

4-9.11   Discuss the steps in the delivery of the placenta.(C-1)

4-9.12   List the steps in the emergency medical care of the mother post-delivery.(C-3)

4-9.13   Summarize neonatal resuscitation procedures.(C-1)

4-9.14   Describe the procedures for the following abnormal deliveries: breech birth, prolapsed cord, limb presentation.(C-1)

4-9.15   Differentiate the special considerations for multiple births.(C-3)

4-9.16   Describe special considerations of meconium.(C-1)

4-9.17   Describe special considerations of a premature baby.(C-1)

4-9.18   Discuss the emergency medical care of a patient with a gynecological emergency.(C-1)

Affective Objectives

At the completion of this lesson, the EMT-Basic student will be able to:

4-9.19   Explain the rationale for understanding the implications of treating two patients (mother and baby).(A-3)

Psychomotor Objectives

At the completion of this lesson, the EMT-Basic student will be able to:

4-9.20   Demonstrate the steps to assist in the normal cephalic delivery.(P-1,2)

4-9.21   Demonstrate necessary care procedures of the fetus as the head appears.(P-1,2)

4-9.22   Demonstrate infant neonatal procedures.(P-1,2)

4-9.23   Demonstrate post-delivery care of infant.(P-1,2)

4-9.24   Demonstrate how and when to cut the umbilical cord.(P-1,2)

4-9.25   Attend to the steps in the delivery of the placenta.(P-1,2)

4-9.26   Demonstrate the post-delivery care of the mother.(P-1,2)

4-9.27 Demonstrate the procedures for the following abnormal deliveries: vaginal bleeding, breech birth, prolapsed cord, limb presentation.(P-1,2)

4-9.28 Demonstrate the steps in the emergency medical care of the mother with excessive bleeding.(P-1,2)

4-9.29 Demonstrate completing a prehospital care report for patients with obstetrical/gynecological emergencies.(P-2)

MODULE 5   TRAUMA

LESSON 5-1 BLEEDING AND SHOCK
Cognitive Objectives

At the completion of this lesson, the EMT-Basic student will be able to:

5-1.1 List the structure and function of the circulatory system.(C-1)

5-1.2 Differentiate between arterial, venous, and capillary bleeding.(C-3)

5-1.3 State methods of emergency medical care for external bleeding.(C-1)

5-1.4 Establish the relationship between body substance isolation and bleeding.(C-3)

5-1.5 Establish the relationship between airway management and the trauma patient.(C-3)

5-1.6 Establish the relationship between mechanism of injury and internal bleeding.(C-3)

5-1.7 List the signs of internal bleeding.(C-1)

5-1.8 List the steps in the emergency medical care of the patient with signs and symptoms of internal bleeding.(C-1)

5-1.9 List signs and symptoms of shock (hypoperfusion).(C-1)

5-1.10 State the steps in the emergency medical care of the patient with signs and symptoms of shock (hypoperfusion).(C-1)

Affective Objectives

At the completion of this lesson, the EMT-Basic student will be able to:

5-1.11 Explain the sense of urgency to transport patients who are bleeding and show signs of shock (hypoperfusion).(A-1)

Psychomotor Objectives

At the completion of this lesson, the EMT-Basic student will be able to:

5-1.12 Demonstrate direct pressure as a method of emergency medical care for external bleeding.(P-1,2)

5-1.13 Demonstrate the use of diffuse pressure as a method of emergency medical care for external bleeding.(P-1,2)

5-1.14 Demonstrate the use of pressure points and tourniquets as a method of emergency medical care for external bleeding.(P-1,2)

5-1.15 Demonstrate the care of the patient exhibiting signs and symptoms of internal bleeding.(P-1,2)

5-1.16 Demonstrate the care of the patient exhibiting signs and symptoms of shock (hypoperfusion).(P-1,2)

5-1.17 Demonstrate completing a prehospital care report for the patient with bleeding and/or shock (hypoperfusion).(P-2)

LESSON 5-2 SOFT TISSUE INJURIES
Cognitive Objectives

At the completion of this lesson, the EMT-Basic student will be able to:

5-2.1 State the major functions of the skin.(C-1)

5-2.2 List the layers of the skin.(C-1)

5-2.3 Establish the relationship between body substance isolation (BSI) and soft tissue injuries.(C-3)

5-2.4 List the types of closed soft tissue injuries.(C-1)

5-2.5 Describe the emergency medical care of the patient with a closed soft tissue injury.(C-1)

5-2.6 State the types of open soft tissue injuries.(C-1)

5-2.7 Describe the emergency medical care of the patient with an open soft tissue injury.(C-1)

5-2.8 Discuss the emergency medical care considerations for a patient with a penetrating chest injury.(C-1)

5-2.9 State the emergency medical care considerations for a patient with an open wound to the abdomen.(C-1)

5-2.10 Differentiate the care of an open wound to the chest from an open wound to the abdomen.(C-3)

5-2.11 List the classifications of burns.(C-1)

5-2.12 Define superficial burn.(C-1)

5-2.13 List the characteristics of a superficial burn.(C-1)

5-2.14 Define a partial thickness burn.(C-1)

5-2.15 List the characteristics of a partial thickness burn.(C-1)

5-2.16 Define a full thickness burn.(C-1)

5-2.17 List the characteristics of a full thickness burn.(C-1)

5-2.18 Describe the emergency medical care of the patient with a superficial burn.(C-1)

5-2.19 Describe the emergency medical care of the patient with a partial thickness burn.(C-1)

5-2.20 Describe the emergency medical care of the patient with a full thickness burn.(C-1)

5-2.21 List the functions of dressing and bandaging.(C-1)

5-2.22 Describe the purpose of a bandage.(C-1)

5-2.23 Describe the steps in applying a pressure dressing.(C-1)

5-2.24 Establish the relationship between airway management and the patient with chest injury, burns, and blunt and penetrating injuries.(C-1)

5-2.25 Describe the effects of improperly applied dressings, splints, and tourniquets.(C-1)

5-2.26 Describe the emergency medical care of a patient with an impaled object.(C-1)

5-2.27 Describe the emergency medical care of a patient with an amputation.

5-2.28 Describe the emergency care for a chemical burn.(C-1)

5-2.29 Describe the emergency care for an electrical burn.(C-1)

Affective Objectives

No affective objectives identified.

Psychomotor Objectives

At the completion of this lesson, the EMT-Basic student will be able to:

5-2.29 Demonstrate the steps in the emergency medical care of closed soft tissue injuries.(P-1,2)

5-2.30 Demonstrate the steps in the emergency medical care of open soft tissue injuries.(P-1,2)

5-2.31 Demonstrate the steps in the emergency medical care of a patient with an open chest wound.(P-1,2)

5-2.32 Demonstrate the steps in the emergency medical care of a patient with open abdominal wounds.(P-1,2)

5-2.33 Demonstrate the steps in the emergency medical care of a patient with an impaled object.(P-1,2)

5-2.34 Demonstrate the steps in the emergency medical care of a patient with an amputation.(P-1,2)

5-2.35 Demonstrate the steps in the emergency medical care of an amputated part.(P-1,2)

5-2.36 Demonstrate the steps in the emergency medical care of a patient with superficial burns.(P-1,2)

5-2.37 Demonstrate the steps in the emergency medical care of a patient with partial thickness burns.(P-1,2)

5-2.38 Demonstrate the steps in the emergency medical care of a patient with full thickness burns.(P-1,2)

5-2.39 Demonstrate the steps in the emergency medical care of a patient with a chemical burn.(P-1,2)

5-2.40 Demonstrate completing a prehospital care report for patients with soft tissue injuries.(P-2)

LESSON 5-3 MUSCULOSKELETAL CARE
Cognitive Objectives

At the completion of this lesson, the EMT-Basic student will be able to:

5-3.1 Describe the function of the muscular system.(C-1)

5-3.2 Describe the function of the skeletal system.(C-1)

5-3.3 List the major bones or bone groupings of the spinal column; the thorax, the upper extremities, and the lower extremities.(C-1)

5-3.4 Differentiate between an open and a closed painful, swollen, deformed extremity.(C-1)

5-3.5 State the reasons for splinting.(C-1)

5-3.6   List the general rules of splinting.(C-1)

5-3.7   List the complications of splinting.(C-1)

5-3.8   List the emergency medical care for a patient with a painful, swollen, deformed extremity.(C-1)

Affective Objectives

At the completion of this lesson, the EMT-Basic student will be able to:

5-3.9   Explain the rationale for splinting at the scene versus load and go.(A-3)

5-3.10 Explain the rationale for immobilization of the painful, swollen, deformed extremity.(A-3)

Psychomotor Objectives

At the completion of this lesson, the EMT-Basic student will be able to:

5-3.11 Demonstrate the emergency medical care of a patient with a painful, swollen, deformed extremity.(P-1,2)

5-3.12 Demonstrate completing a prehospital care report for patients with musculoskeletal injuries.(P-2)

LESSON 5-4 INJURIES TO THE HEAD AND SPINE

Cognitive Objectives

At the completion of this lesson, the EMT-Basic student will be able to:

5-4.1   State the components of the nervous system.(C-1)

5-4.2   List the functions of the central nervous system.(C-1)

5-4.3   Define the structure of the skeletal system as it relates to the nervous system.(C-1)

5-4.4   Relate mechanism of injury to potential injuries of the head and spine.(C-3)

5-4.5   Describe the implications of not properly caring for potential spine injuries.(C-1)

5-4.6   State the signs and symptoms of a potential spine injury.(C-1)

5-4.7   Describe the method of determining if a responsive patient may have a spine injury.(C-1)

5-4.8   Relate the airway emergency medical care techniques for the patient with a suspected spine injury.(C-3)

5-4.9   Describe how to stabilize the cervical spine.(C-1)

5-4.10 Discuss indications for sizing and using a cervical spine immobilization device.(C-1)

5-4.11 Establish the relationship between airway management and the patient with head and spine injuries.(C-1)

5-4.12 Describe a method for sizing a cervical spine immobilization device.(C-1)

5-4.13 Describe how to logroll a patient with a suspected spine injury.(C-1)

5-4.14 Describe how to secure a patient to a long spine board.(C-1)

5-4.15 List instances when a short spine board should be used.(C-1)

5-4.16 Describe how to immobilize a patient using a short spine board.(C-1)

5-4.17 Describe the indications for the use of rapid extrication.(C-1)

5-4.18 List steps in performing rapid extrication.(C-1)

5-4.19 State the circumstances when a helmet should be left on the patient.(C-1)

5-4.20 Discuss the circumstances when a helmet should be removed from the patient.(C-1)

5-4.21 Identify different types of helmets.(C-1)

5-4.22 Describe the unique characteristics of sports helmets.(C-1)

5-4.23 Explain the preferred methods to remove a helmet.(C-1)

5-4.24 Discuss alternative methods for removal of a helmet.(C-1)

5-4.25 Describe how the patient's head is stabilized to remove the helmet.(C-1)

5-4.26 Differentiate how the head is stabilized with a helmet compared with stabilizing without a helmet.(C-3)

Affective Objectives

At the completion of this lesson, the EMT-Basic student will be able to:

5-4.27 Explain the rationale for immobilization of the entire spine when a cervical spine injury is suspected.(A-3)

5-4.28 Explain the rationale for utilizing immobilization methods apart from the straps on the cots.(A-3)

5-4.29 Explain the rationale for utilizing a short spine immobilization device when moving a patient from the sitting to the supine position.(A-3)

5-4.30 Explain the rationale for utilizing rapid extrication approaches only when they indeed will make the difference between life and death.(A-3)

5-4.31 Defend the reasons for leaving a helmet in place for transport of a patient.(A-3)

5-4.32 Defend the reasons for removal of a helmet prior to transport of a patient.(A-3)

Psychomotor Objectives

At the completion of this lesson, the EMT-Basic student will be able to:

5-4.33 Demonstrate opening the airway in a patient with suspected spinal cord injury. (P-1,2)

5-4.34 Demonstrate evaluating a responsive patient with a suspected spinal cord injury.(P-1,2)

5-4.35 Demonstrate stabilization of the cervical spine.(P-1,2)

5-4.36 Demonstrate the four person logroll for a patient with a suspected spinal cord injury.(P-1,2)

5-4.37 Demonstrate how to logroll a patient with a suspected spinal cord injury using two people.(P-1,2)

5-4.38 Demonstrate securing a patient to a long spine board.(P-1,2)

5-4.39 Demonstrate using the short board immobilization technique.(P-1,2)

5-4.40 Demonstrate procedure for rapid extrication.(P-1,2)

5-4.41 Demonstrate preferred methods for stabilization of a helmet.(P-1,2)

5-4.42 Demonstrate helmet removal techniques.(P-1,2)

5-4.43 Demonstrate alternative methods for stabilization of a helmet.(P-1,2)

5-4.44 Demonstrate completing a prehospital care report for patients with head and spinal injuries.(P-2)

MODULE 6 *INFANTS AND CHILDREN*

LESSON 6-1 INFANTS AND CHILDREN
Cognitive Objectives

6-1.1 Identify the developmental considerations for the following age groups:(C-1)
- Infants
- Toddlers
- Preschool
- School-age
- Adolescent

6-1.2 Describe differences in anatomy and physiology of the infant, child, and adult patient.(C-1)

6-1.3 Differentiate the response of the ill or injured infant or child (age specific) from that of an adult.(C-3)

6-1.4 Indicate various causes of respiratory emergencies.(C-1)

6-1.5 Differentiate between respiratory distress and respiratory failure.(C-3)

6-1.6 List the steps in the management of foreign body airway obstruction.(C-1)

6-1.7 Summarize emergency medical care strategies for respiratory distress and respiratory failure.(C-1)

6-1.8 Identify the signs and symptoms of shock (hypoperfusion) in the infant and child patient.(C-1)

6-1.9 Describe the methods of determining end organ perfusion in the infant and child patient.(C-1)

6-1.10 State the usual cause of cardiac arrest in infants and children versus that in adults.(C-1)

6-1.11 List the common causes of seizures in the infant and child patient.(C-1)

6-1.12 Describe the management of seizures in the infant and child patient.(C-1)

6-1.13 Differentiate between the injury patterns in adults, infants, and children.(C-3)

6-1.14 Discuss the field management of the infant and child trauma patient.(C-1)

6-1.15 Summarize the indicators of possible child abuse and neglect.(C-1)

6-1.16 Describe the medical legal responsibilities in suspected child abuse.(C-1)

6-1.17 Recognize the need for EMT-Basic debriefing following a difficult infant or child transport.(C-1)

Affective Objectives

6-1.18 Explain the rationale for having knowledge and skills appropriate for dealing with the infant and child patient.(A-3)

6-1.19 Attend to the feelings of the family when dealing with an ill or injured infant or child.(A-1)

6-1.20 Understand the provider's own response (emotional) to caring for infants or children.(A-1)

Psychomotor Objectives

6-1.21 Demonstrate the techniques of foreign body airway obstruction removal in the infant.(P-1,2)

6-1.22 Demonstrate the techniques of foreign body airway obstruction removal in the child.(P-1,2)

6-1.23 Demonstrate the assessment of the infant and child.(P-1,2)

6-1.24 Demonstrate bag-valve-mask artificial ventilations for the infant.(P-1,2)

6-1.25 Demonstrate bag-valve-mask artificial ventilations for the child.(P-1,2)

6-1.26 Demonstrate oxygen delivery for the infant and child.(P-1,2)

MODULE 7   OPERATIONS

LESSON 7-1 AMBULANCE OPERATIONS
Cognitive Objectives
At the completion of this lesson, the EMT-Basic student will be able to:

7 1.1 Discuss the medical and nonmedical equipment needed to respond to a call.(C-1)

7 1.2 List the phases of an ambulance call. (C-1)

7 1.3 Describe the general provisions of state laws relating to the operation of the ambulance and privileges in any or all of the following categories:(C-1)
- Speed
- Warning lights
- Sirens
- Right of way
- Parking
- Turning

7 1.4 List contributing factors to unsafe driving conditions.(C-1)

7 1.5 Describe the considerations that should by given to:
- Request for escorts
- Following an escort vehicle
- Intersections (C-1)

7-1.6 Discuss "Due Regard For Safety of All Others" while operating an emergency vehicle.(C-1)

7-1.7 State what information is essential in order to respond to a call.(C-1)

7-1.8 Discuss various situations that may affect response to a call.(C-1)

7-1.9 Differentiate between the various methods of moving a patient to the unit based upon injury or illness.(C-3)

7-1.10 Apply the components of the essential patient information in a written report.(C-2)

7-1.11 Summarize the importance of preparing the unit for the next response.(C-1)

7-1.12 Identify what is essential for completion of a call.(C-1)

7-1.13 Distinguish among the terms cleaning, disinfection, high level disinfection, and sterilization.(C-3)

7-1.14 Describe how to clean or disinfect items following patient care.(C-1)

Affective Objectives
At the completion of this lesson, the EMT-Basic student will be able to:

7-1.15 Explain the rationale for appropriate report of patient information.(A-3)

7-1.16 Explain the rationale for having the unit prepared to respond.(A-3)

Psychomotor Objectives
No psychomotor objectives identified.

LESSON 7-2 GAINING ACCESS

Cognitive Objectives

At the completion of this lesson, the EMT-Basic student will be able to:

7-2.1 Describe the purpose of extrication.(C-1)

7-2.2 Discuss the role of the EMT-Basic in extrication.(C-1)

7-2.3 Identify what equipment for personal safety is required for the EMT-Basic.(C-1)

7-2.4 Define the fundamental components of extrication.(C-1)

7-2.5 State the steps that should be taken to protect the patient during extrication.(C-1)

7-2.6 Evaluate various methods of gaining access to the patient.(C-3)

7-2.7 Distinguish between simple and complex access.(C-3)

Affective Objectives

No affective objectives identified.

Psychomotor Objectives

No psychomotor objectives identified.

LESSON 7-3 OVERVIEW

Cognitive Objectives

At the completion of this lesson, the EMT-Basic student will be able to:

7-3.1 Explain the EMT-Basic's role during a call involving hazardous materials.(C-1)

7-3.2 Describe what the EMT-Basic should do if there is reason to believe that there is a hazard at the scene.(C-1)

7-3.3 Describe the actions that an EMT-Basic should take to ensure bystander safety.(C-1)

7-3.4 State the role the EMT-Basic should perform until appropriately trained personnel arrive at the scene of a hazardous materials situation.(C-1)

7-3.5 Break down the steps to approaching a hazardous situation.(C-1)

7-3.6 Discuss the various environmental hazards that affect EMS.(C-1)

7-3.7 Describe the criteria for a multiple casualty situation.(C-1)

7-3.8 Evaluate the role of the EMT-Basic in the multiple casualty situation.(C-3)

7-3.9 Summarize the components of basic triage.(C-1)

7-3.10 Define the role of the EMT-Basic in a disaster operation.(C-1)

7-3.11 Describe basic concepts of incident management.(C-1)

7-3.12 Explain the methods for preventing contamination of self, equipment, and facilities.(C-1)

7-3.13 Review the local mass casualty incident plan.(C-1)

Affective Objectives

No affective objectives identified.

Psychomotor Objectives

At the completion of this lesson, the EMT-Basic student will be able to:

7-3.16 Given a scenario of a mass casualty incident, perform triage.(P-2)

MODULE 8 ADVANCED AIRWAY

LESSON 8-1 ADVANCED AIRWAY

Cognitive Objectives

At the completion of this lesson the EMT-Basic student will be able to:

8-1.1 Identify and describe the airway anatomy in the infant, child, and adult.(C-1)

8-1.2 Differentiate between the airway anatomy in the infant, child, and adult.(C-1)

8-1.3 Explain the pathophysiology of airway compromise.(C-1)

8-1.4 Describe the proper use of airway adjuncts.(C-1)

8-1.5 Review the use of oxygen therapy in airway management.(C-1)

8-1.6 Describe the indications, contraindications, and technique for insertion of nasal gastric tubes.

8-1.7 Describe how to perform the Sellick maneuver (cricoid pressure).(C-1)

8-1.8 Describe the indications for advanced airway management.(C-1)

8-1.9 List the equipment required for orotracheal intubation.(C-1)

8-1.10 Describe the proper use of the curved blade for orotracheal intubation.(C-1)

8-1.11 Describe the proper use of the straight blade for orotracheal intubation.(C-1)

8-1.12 State the reasons for and proper use of the stylet in orotracheal intubation.(C-1)

8-1.13 Describe the methods of choosing the appropriate size endotracheal tube in an adult patient.(C-1)

8-1.14 State the formula for sizing an infant or child endotracheal tube.(C-1)

8-1.15 List complications associated with advanced airway management.(C-1)

8-1.16 Define the various alternative methods for sizing the infant and child endotracheal tube.(C-1)

8-1.17 Describe the skill of orotracheal intubation in the adult patient.(C-1)

8-1.18 Describe the skill of orotracheal intubation in the infant and child patient.(C-1)

8-1.19 Describe the skill of confirming endotracheal tube placement in the adult, infant, and child patient.(C-1)

8-1.20 State the consequence of, and the need to recognize, unintentional esophageal intubation.(C-1)

8-1.21 Describe the skill of securing the endotracheal tube in the adult, infant, and child patient.(C-1)

Affective Objectives

At the end of this lesson the EMT-Basic student will be able to:

8-1.22 Recognize and respect the feelings of the patient and family during advanced airway procedures.(A-1)

8-1.23 Explain the value of performing advanced airway procedures.(A-2)

8-1.24 Defend the need for the EMT-Basic to perform advanced airway procedures.(A-3)

8-1.25 Explain the rationale for the use of a stylet.(A-2)

8-1.26 Explain the rationale for having a suction unit immediately available during intubation attempts.(A-2)

8-1.27 Explain the rationale for confirming breath sounds.(A-2)

8-1.28 Explain the rationale for securing the endotracheal tube.(A-3)

Psychomotor Objectives

At the end of this lesson the EMT-Basic student will be able to:

8-1.29 Demonstrate how to perform the Sellick maneuver (cricoid pressure).(P-1,2)

8-1.30 Demonstrate the skill of orotracheal intubation in the adult patient.(P-1,2)

8-1.31 Demonstrate the skill of orotracheal intubation in the infant and child patient.(P-1,2)

8-1.32 Demonstrate the skill of confirming endotracheal tube placement in the adult patient.(P-1,2)

8-1.33 Demonstrate the skill of confirming endotracheal tube placement in the infant and child patient.(P-1,2)

8-1.34 Demonstrate the skill of securing the endotracheal tube in the adult patient.(P-1,2)

8-1.35 Demonstrate the skill of securing the endotracheal tube in the infant and child patient.(P-1,2)

Index